Genetic Diversity in Plants

BASIC LIFE SCIENCES
Alexander Hollaender, General Editor
Associated Universities, Inc.
Washington, D.C.

A Continuation Order Plan is available for this series. A continuation order
will bring delivery of each new volume immediately upon publication. Volumes
are billed only upon actual shipment. For further information please contact
the publisher.

This book is to be returned on or before
the last date stamped below.

PLYMOUTH POLYTECHNIC LIBRARY

Telephone
Ply. 21312
Ext. 219

Telex
45423

A book may be renewed by telephone or by personal visit
if it is not required by another reader.
CHARGES WILL BE MADE FOR OVERDUE BOOKS

Genetic Diversity in Plants

Edited by

Amir Muhammed

University of Agriculture
Lyallpur, Pakistan

and

Rustem Aksel and

R. C. von Borstel

The University of Alberta
Edmonton, Alberta, Canada

PLENUM PRESS • NEW YORK AND LONDON

Library of Congress Cataloging in Publication Data

· International Symposium on Genetic Control of Diversity in Plants, Lahore, 1976.
  Genetic diversity in plants.

  (Basic life sciences; v. 8)
  Includes bibliographies and index.
  1. Plant-breeding – Congresses. 2. Plant genetics – Congresses. I. Muhammed,
  Amir, 1930-   joint author. II. Aksel, Rustem, joint author. III. von Borstel,
  R. C., joint author. IV. Title.
  SB123.I72 1976   631.5'3   77-9475
  ISBN 0-306-36508-1

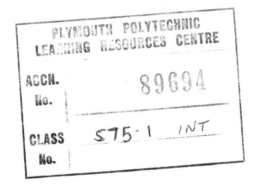
Proceedings of an International Symposium on Genetic Control of
Diversity in Plants held at Lahore, Pakistan, March 1–7, 1976

© 1977 Plenum Press, New York
A Division of Plenum Publishing Corporation
227 West 17th Street, New York, N.Y. 10011

Printed in the United States of America

Foreword

For the last eighteen years we have been deeply involved in a cooperative effort with our Latin American colleagues in genetics, biochemistry, physiology, and molecular biology. We have been in close contact with scientists in a number of centers and have helped to organize symposia, workshops, and so forth, in an effort to accelerate their development and make their substantial work known. These symposia in Latin America have been quite successful. The fifteenth will take place in Brasilia in 1977.

At the request of colleagues, we are in the process of developing a similar series in Asia. The first very successful symposium was held in Calcutta in 1973. We were most pleased when Dr. Amir Muhammed, Vice Chancellor of the University of Agriculture, Lyallpur suggested that we hold a symposium on a topic of great importance to Pakistan, Genetic Control of Diversity in Plants, under the auspices of the University of Agriculture.

It is our hope that this symposium will be followed by additional ones in Pakistan as well as in other countries in the Far East. Leadership is quickly developing in the hands of outstanding scientists in these countries, and we appreciate the opportunity to cooperate with them.

We are especially grateful to the National Science Foundation for making PL-480 funds available which made this symposium possible.

Alexander Hollaender
Associated Universities

Preface

Most of the chapters in this volume are based on papers that were read at the International Symposium on Genetic Control of Diversity in Plants held at Lahore, Pakistan, March 1–7, 1976. Several were submitted by persons who had been invited to attend but could not. The main objective of the symposium was to draw the attention of agronomists and plant breeders to the genetic variability which occurs naturally or which can be induced in cultivated and noncultivated plants.

At this symposium the environment and plant varieties of the host country are naturally emphasized. This serves to illustrate an overriding characteristic of the field of study. Plant genetics does have universal principles, but the principles must be applied under local conditions. Thus, like geology and meteorology, plant genetics is both universal and parochial. Plant genetics is one of the important sciences in a nation that must import its food. It is of interest that there is a correlation between the amount of food produced per acre by a nation and the degree of commitment of that nation to the disciplines of plant genetics and plant breeding. Obviously, this may be more closely related to the development of extension services, means of distribution, and good credit systems for the farmers, rather than to the support of plant genetics and plant breeding. However, it is more likely that the one could not survive without the other. The dramatic success of dwarf Mexican wheat in increasing world food production is an example of what plant genetics and plant breeding can do suddenly by the introduction of varieties with potential for high grain yield. Of course, the introduction of such varieties forces other factors to change, but not always for the good. For example, alteration of these factors causes the disuse and eventual loss of local varieties, thereby depleting the gene pool. Unless active countermeasures are brought to bear, this still could be a detrimental effect of the Green Revolution.

Sudden universally applicable breakthroughs are rare. Cereal and forage production will increase slowly but surely in most places, because local plant breeders will breed into imported strains the necessary factors of resistance to local diseases and pests, of adaptation to local soils, of resistance to lodging, and of adjustment to the months of maximum rainfall. The local breeder cannot depend on the conditions in Mexico to improve the cereal yield where he lives. The local strains are, therefore, a precious heritage which will provide the variability necessary to breed into universal strains in order to guarantee increased local yield. In recent years attention has been focused on new and exciting areas of genetic research such as plant cell cultures, restriction enzymes, and nitrogen fixation ability in Gramineae, where spectacular advances were reported. These novel approaches hold tremendous promise of a revolution in the realm of creativity and experimental evolution.

The symposium on which this volume is based served very well to bring together some of the plant genetics, plant physiology, and storage-protein specialists from Pakistan and a number of other countries. The guest participants visited the plant-breeding institutions of the host country, where Pakistani breeders work enthusiastically and successfully in producing better and more efficient cultivars for the agriculture of the country.

The organizers of the symposium were Amir Muhammed, Chairman; and Alexander Hollaender, R. C. von Borstel, R. A. Nilan, R. D. Brock, S. H. Mujtaba Naqvi, A. Shakoor, M. Akbar, and K. A. Siddiqui. They had considerable help in the initial stages from C. O. Person and D. E. Foard.

A number of individuals were helpful in reviewing the manuscripts. Particularly, we should like to thank O. H. Frankel, W. R. Scowcroft, A. Rehman, G. W. R. Walker, C. Y. Sullivan, and G. Kimber. We are indebted to Margaret Brennan and Dorothy Woslyng, who readied the manuscripts for publication.

Amir Muhammed
Rustem Aksel
R. C. von Borstel

Contents

I. Introduction

II. Natural and Induced Genetic Variability

III. Genetic Variability and Resistance to Disease

IV. Genetics of Quantitative Characters

V. Prospects of Breeding for Physiological Characters

VI. Seed Storage Proteins

VII.   Genetic Manipulation in Cell Cultures

I

Introduction

1

Perspective

Amir Muhammed

University of Agriculture
Lyallpur, Pakistan

Science has played a predominant role in the socioeconomic uplift of human society. It has conferred on humanity powers rarely imagined to exercise a kind of control over the environment that has in many ways made humans master of their own destiny. Practically the entire agricultural and industrial development in the world today owes itself to the concept of science in harness, and the tempo of this transformation is being maintained and even accelerated through rapid advances occurring in scientific knowledge and technological innovations. Whereas the developed countries have attained increasingly greater heights in scientific and technological achievements, the less developed countries such as Pakistan, plagued as they long have been with ignorance and inertia compounded by alien rule and exploitation, lagged far behind, although in recent years economic progress in such countries has picked up momentum owing to political awakening, more enlightened attitudes, and increased resource availability. Because the overall economy of the majority of the developing countries is critically linked with agriculture, the modernization of the agriculture sector has been given a top priority in our development programs. As a result, the agriculture of Pakistan is gradually changing from a way of living to a way of making a living. To accelerate this transition from the domain of arts and crafts to the world of science and technology, the People's Government in Pakistan is making all-out efforts to provide the necessary infrastructure with special emphasis on developing the requisite institutions, economic incentives, a backlog of technology, and so forth. These efforts have no doubt paid off, and handsome gains have been made in agricultural productivity through the use of the current improved crop varieties and management practices. But that is not enough to eliminate completely from our land the hideous specter of hunger and misery.

Far more work is required in this area to support a rapidly growing population. This is a great challenge; indeed it is a challenge to our research scientists and to their creative genius to pursue research with a purpose as well as a sense of urgency. Only then will this mission of alleviating human sufferings and of retrieving human dignity from abysmal despair have been carried through.

I believe that the symposium on which this volume is based witnessed a great exhibition of knowledge, a spectacular march of new ideas, and stimulating exchanges at a personal level which should go a long way to generate new enthusiasm among scientists, faculty members, and graduate students, and inspire them to more imaginative and dedicated work. Such symposia provide a forum, not only for comprehensive discussions on the subject matter, but also for creating durable personal relationships among the scientists and academicians of various countries, to be assiduously maintained and strengthened by common interests of science, as well as for the general benefit of humanity. Dr. Hollaender deserves sincere compliments from his colleagues, young scientists, and students alike for his initiative and foresight in organizing a series of such symposia in several Latin American countries. He is also actively associated with the present symposium volume; I am personally indebted to him for the inspiration, guidance, and support he gave us in making it a reality.

The subject matter of genetic diversity discussed in this volume is at once fundamental and applied in nature; it is of crucial importance to the welfare and future of humanity. Diversity is an important attribute of living organisms that has for centuries fascinated the human mind and captured the imagination in an effort to unveil the secrets of its origin and continuity. To begin with, this curiosity produced a profusion of ideas—many naive and even weird,—yet capable of inspiring more logical and systematic thinking. It ultimately led to the historic enunciations by Gregor Mendel in the latter part of the nineteenth century that diversity in plants is genetically controlled and ruled by definitive laws in its transmission through the generations. From this premise began to take shape an imposing superstructure of a new science—the science of heredity and variation, that is, genetics. With the new truths and realities unfolding gradually about the nature of genetic variation came about a clearer comprehension of many biological phenomena uppermost in contemporary thought. Perhaps the most intriguing and fascinating question was the one concerning organic evolution. Darwin had violently shaken the foundations of centuries-old popular beliefs as to the immutability of living species by propounding his revolutionary concept that coincident in time and space new species have evolved from the old through natural selection. Giving due allowance to the orthodox, there is hardly any doubt that variation provides a multiplicity of life, and nature selects the fittest to reproduce and multiply. Thus came not only a better understanding of the mechanics of organic evolution but also an increased awareness of the prospective use of variation in experimental evolution, that is, plant breeding.

Scientists working with all domesticated forms of life needed the types that could stand an ever-expanding disease complex and physiological stresses as well as be able to respond more profitably to various management practices. Genetic diversity provided scientists with the elements from which they were able to raise the desired genetic edifices. Hybrid and high-lysine maize, hybrid sorghum, short, fertilizer-responsive varieties of wheat and rice, and high-quality cottons, which have had tremendous impact on agricultural productivity and thus belied Malthusian predictions, are but a few of the magnificent examples of the scientist's ingenuity skillfully at work with genetic diversity. In Pakistan too, the introduction of short-statured, stiff-stemmed, and rust-resistant varieties of wheat and rice capable of responding to high fertilizer application levels, has resulted in remarkable yield increases that have amounted to as much as more than 50%. This upsurge in acre yields has brought us near self-sufficiency in food grains. However, because a major part of the small grain acreage in this country grows under stress conditions produced by various constraints, such as drought, salinity and waterlogging, disease and pest incidence, and other factors, there is an urgent need to breed better-adapted varieties that have a potential to carry us over the hump. A similar effort is needed in the case of cash crops, although research on cotton and sugarcane has already brought about modest but significant improvement in their yield and quality.

The modest achievements made in the field of agriculture should by no means induce our scientists to drift into a state of complacency. In view of the ever-growing complexities of life, there is hardly any occasion for them to rest on their laurels. Much of the world's population is still groaning under the weight of want and pestilence; these less fortunate people are looking up to scientists for their salvation. Surely, this is a great challenge, and genetic diversity undoubtedly remains one of our major hopes. The prosperity and continued existence of humanity is fatefully linked to our ability to create and manipulate variability in order to evolve more productive crop plants. To this end, some of the most efficient approaches used by plant scientists include routine variety crosses, wider crosses among species and genera, induction of polyploidy, chromosome substitution and engineering, and induced mutations. Furthermore, sophisticated methods and models have been developed for quantitative evaluation of variability to help design efficient breeding strategies. More recently a better insight has been obtained into the molecular structure of the gene and gene–character relationships. Such investigations, I am sure, will have far-reaching implications, and the day may not be far off when we shall have plants and even babies made to order.

I would like to take this opportunity to offer our sincerest thanks to the National Science Foundation of the United States, the University Grants Commission of Pakistan, and the Pakistan Science Foundation for their generosity in providing the financial assistance that made it possible to organize the symposium. I would also like to express a deep sense of gratitude to the members of the organizing committee for their great initiative and effort in holding the symposium. I shall be amiss if I don't acknowledge here the hard work done so conscientiously by my Pakistani colleagues to help make necessary arrangements for the symposium. Sincere thanks are also due to many philanthropist organizations for having so considerately extended their hospitality to the distinguished delegates to make the occasion more enjoyable.

It was a matter of great honor to have Nawab Sadiq Hussain Qureshi, chief minister of the Punjab, with us at the symposium as the chief guest. As a progressive farmer, a minister of agriculture, and now as chief minister of the province, Nawab Sadiq Hussain Qureshi has made commendable contributions to the growth and development of agriculture. His presence here today, in spite of his many preoccupations, bears ample testimony to his abiding concern and interest in this field, which is extremely reassuring to all of us.

2

Inaugural Address

Sadiq Hussain Qureshi

Chief Minister
Punjab, Pakistan

The subject of this volume is of great significance to the development of new plant types of superior merit, and thus has tremendous potentialities to reinvigorate and modernize agriculture and the way of life in the less developed countries of the world. People have been conscious of persistent diversity in biological populations and through the ages have exploited it to evolve more productive types of plants and animals. These crop plants and animals are probably still the best under conditions of minimum care, but this kind of starvation culture has no place in today's world, which is faced with a terrific population-growth pressure and a precarious imbalance between supply and demand. The days of a static agriculture are gone, and our farmer is no longer content with the pursuit of agriculture as a merely subsistence-oriented family occupation.

Agriculture has now developed into an industry increasingly dependent on science and technology. This evolution in concept and practice must be promoted and sustained. For its part, the People's Government in Pakistan, under the dynamic and inspiring leadership of Prime Minister Zulfiquar Ali Bhutto, is fully aware of its responsibilities to provide the necessary wherewithal for a progressive and forward-looking agriculture. Top priority is assigned to the development of the agriculture sector, as it is intricately linked with the whole spectrum of economic development. But then agriculture is not a simple process. It is a complex trade that encompasses many disciplines and variables and requires planning with idealistic realism and implementation with resourceful perseverance. Substantial progress has already been made in boosting agricultural productivity in this country by adopting improved production practices. Such practices include the use of high-yielding crop varieties, chemical fertilizers, effective plant protection measures, and better land use and management. Economic incentives by way of commodity procurement prices and credit facilities for various inputs are also liberally provided. The Punjab Agricultural College and Research Institute at Lyallpur, a famous seat of learning in Asia, was upgraded to a full-fledged University of Agriculture, which in its formative years received generous aid and cooperation from Washington State University in developing curricula and training of the faculty. Since its inception, the University of Agriculture at Lyallpur has played its part well to integrate the functions of resident teaching, research, and extension in order to develop healthy relationships between the researchers and farmers, as well as to ensure a steady supply of competent workforce for effective leadership. Moreover, agricultural research institutes have also been reorganized and expanded to provide better facilities and a congenial atmosphere for meaningful research. The extension wings of the Agriculture Department have also been considerably strengthened, keeping in view the requirements of the farmers.

Although all these measures have made valid contributions to the progress and revitalization of agriculture in Pakistan, conditions leave much to be desired and a great deal to be accomplished. Compared with the developed nations and even some of the developing countries, the crop yields of Pakistan are low—a stark reminder of the magnitude of the task ahead and of the challenge both to overcome the lingering food shortages in the country and to produce an exportable surplus. In addition to aiming at quantitative advances in food production, emphasis should also be placed on the qualitative improvement of the grain to help avert a growing protein crisis in the developing countries. The protein-deficient diet that has become the common destiny of the millions in these countries could be corrected more conveniently and expeditiously through plant sources. In this connection our plant scientists should make a concerted effort to develop not only edible legumes, such as soybean, gram, and other pulses, but high-protein cereals, particularly high-lysine maize and sorghum, as well.

Another area of research that has enormous potential but has remained rather neglected and unexploited is that of organized farming under rainfed conditions. To date, the research in this country has, for all intents and purposes, been oriented to the needs of irrigated farmlands with the result that this huge tract of unirrigated land, which constitutes about one-third of the country's total cropped acreage, has failed to make its full impact on agricultural production. In this regard, you, the plant scientists, can make a major contribution by developing crops and varieties adapted to such conditions.

This was just a little food for thought. I am sure that these papers will raise many other interesting points and questions; from such deliberations new ideas and inspiring proposals will emerge to accelerate the pursuit of excellence in the art and science of this vital area.

3

The World Food Crisis: Population, Food, and Environmental Issues as They Affect Pakistan

Joseph C. Wheeler

United States Agency for International Development
Islamabad, Pakistan

ABSTRACT

It is inevitable that Pakistan will double its population—there is even a possibility of a quadrupling. Because of an unusual resource base, Pakistan has an opportunity to more than double its agricultural production in the next generation and to go into business as a provider of food to the international market on a substantially larger scale. The first imperative in achieving this goal is for the people and government of Pakistan to want to achieve it. Once the will is there, policies and practices are available to make it happen. By implication, the fruits of such a policy will be only temporary unless humanity succeeds in finding the keys that will shift sociological attitudes toward family size. Although nobody has those keys to offer Pakistan today, together humanity must continue to search for them or suffer the penalties that overcrowding will inevitably exact on us. There is a need for more efficient food production to make possible nonfood consumption and the relationship of this to controlling population. Increasingly, food and population mathematics have become matters of worldwide concern. More than ever we human beings recognize each other as kindred and recognize each other's problems as belonging to us all. These next 25 years offer extraordinary challenges to the human race; Pakistan's scientists, working closely with colleagues around the world, are in an excellent position to help find the answers.

INTRODUCTION

Most readers are scientists concerned with the development of plant varieties in order to increase their value to earth's human population. I am a development administrator concerned with organizing people and funds to put to work the product of your scientific output. Our roles are complementary. I very much respect the achievements of plant scientists. They have made crucial contributions to the solution of the ever-changing food problem and promise to make many more. Indeed, they had better make more contributions, because the problems ahead are enormous.

It is the purpose of this chapter to suggest the dimensions of the problems ahead. In so doing I discuss first, the population peril; second, the food situation; third, the interrelationships among population, food, other forms of consumption, and the environment; and fourth, some policy perspectives.

THE POPULATION PERIL

World population in 1975 passed the 4 billion mark; it is expected to increase to somewhere between 6 and 7 billion by the year 2000.

South Asia contained about one-fifth of the world's population in 1975— more than 800 million people. The rate of population increase for South Asia is higher than the world rate. Hence, while the whole of earth's population increases by 50–75%, we can expect the population of South Asia to about double in the next 25 years to a level of more than 1.6 billion. Pakistan (including Azad Kashmir and the northern areas) probably passed the 75 million mark in 1975. This could be off by several million, as we lack a detailed analysis of the 1972 census which would indicate how much of an error occurred in the count. That census put the population of Pakistan at about 64.9 million, excluding roughly 1.5 million in Azad Kashmir and the northern areas, or a total "economic population" of 66.5 million. Using a 3% growth rate, the population of Pakistan increases by 2 million each year.

By the year 2000 the population of Pakistan will reach about 150 million, plus or minus 20 million, depending on trends in rates of fertility.

Because of the population pyramid in which more than one-half of the population of Pakistan is under 16 years of age, the eventual doubling of Pakistan's population is an inevitability unless there is a human catastrophe on a scale practically unknown in earlier periods. This doubling could take place as early as the year 2000, or it could be put off for at least an additional generation. The mathematics of this doubling can be understood by the realization that there are now about 19 million women under 16 years of age. Except for 2 million or so who will die prematurely, primarily because of poor health and nutrition as well as too-frequent childbirth, these 19 million young women will pass through at least an important portion of their reproductive period during the next 25 years; the older among them will already be having grandchildren by the year 2000. Meanwhile, most of the 10 million women already in their fertile period have not yet completed their families. Therefore, even if entirely unforeseen success in family planning were to cause changes of attitude and practice such that the average family size were quickly reduced to half its present level, the population of Pakistan would eventually double to more than 150 million people.

The issue before us—before the generation already born—is whether or not the population of Pakistan will quadruple to 300 million. Let us consider what doubling or quadrupling of population densities means in more detail. First, we must avoid the temptation to assume that every acre of Pakistan is habitable. There simply is no prospect of substantial numbers of people living in the high mountains and the arid deserts. Whereas a few million will be supported in these areas, the fact is that both the grazing areas of Baluchistan and the mountain terraces of the low hills to the north are already in severe ecological crisis. Hence, almost the entire doubled or quadrupled population of Pakistan will live in the rich irrigated areas to the south of Lahore.

Let us look at the potentially extraordinarily productive irrigated area between Lahore and Multan. It is surprising to many Pakistanis that Lyallpur District is even more populous than are Karachi and Lahore Districts. In fact, Multan is the second most populous district in Pakistan. Yet Lyallpur is a town that hardly existed at the beginning of this century.

It is common these days to talk about Bangladesh as an extraordinarily overpopulated country. Some districts in Bangladesh contain more than 2000 persons per square mile. This represents more than three persons per acre. Yet we know that more than half of Bangladesh is flooded each year, and much of its total area is utilized by rivers, roads, and villages so that a density of 2000 per square mile represents five to seven persons per arable acre.

There are some districts in Bangladesh that have a density more like that of the Punjab irrigated areas, that is, in the neighborhood of 1000 per square mile. Lyallpur District already contains more than 1100 people per square mile. This means that many parts of the irrigated Punjab are reaching toward 1.5 persons per acre or three persons per arable acre. It also means that by the year 2000 the irrigated, more populous parts of the Punjab (and I am speaking of the agricultural portions) will almost certainly have densities as great as now exist in the most densely populated districts of Bangladesh. The farmer who came to Lyallpur District 50 years ago and got an allocation of 25 acres was probably supporting his own family of eight, plus several families of farm labor. Let us guess that at that time he supported 20 people on the 25 acres. With a doubling every 25 years, if younger generations stayed on the farm, that 25 acres would be supporting 80 people today, and by the year 2000, 160 people. In fact, that

25 acres is supporting less than this because of off-farm employment and migration to the cities, but the implications of this doubling every generation are enormous in terms of sheer space both on land and in the cities.

The problem with the population issue is that nobody really knows what to do about it. We are wringing our hands. The government of Pakistan is energetically moving to make contraceptives available throughout the country and has taken a number of other steps as well. But in the end it will be necessary for Pakistan to undergo a fundamental sociological shift in attitudes if the increase in population is to be kept to only a doubling, and nobody really knows enough about how societies operate to be able to push the right buttons and be sure this sociological shift in attitudes will actually occur—and in time. There is a growing sense of desperation in the developing world as leaders come to appreciate the inexorable forces of nature and their implications on numbers and on standards of life for future generations.

One further point. Numbers in these magnitudes represent a problem that goes well beyond the problem of feeding people. People want more than food—they want education, health, security, and privacy—and all of these wants are jeopardized by such enormous population densities. I shall return to this point subsequently.

THE FOOD SITUATION

Having discussed the demand side of the equation, let us turn to the supply side. I have mentioned that the population of South Asia may double in as little as 25 years. A doubled population means a need for at least twice as much grain. A very rough estimate puts annual grain consumption in the less developed world at about 400 lb per capita, perhaps a little less in South Asia. That means that the 800 million people in the subcontinent today—directly or indirectly—consume something like 150 to 160 million tons of grain. If my assumptions are correct, Pakistan, with 75 million people, is consuming about 15 million tons of grain. Official statistics suggest that Pakistan is eating more than 9 million tons of wheat, 2 million tons of rice, and lesser quantities of maize, barley, and other coarse grains. Additional grain is fed to poultry and animals. With the inevitable uncertainties about statistics, a figure of 15 million tons for Pakistan grain consumption in 1975 seems to be a reasonable round number.

For the future, then, South Asia, will have to double grain production over the next 25 years in order to feed the inevitably increased population. Pakistan will need to produce another 15 million tons of grain. Wheat production should probably increase from the 1975 7.5-million-ton level to close to 20 million tons by the year 2000. This more than doubling takes into account the likelihood that wheat as a percentage of total grain consumption will probably continue to increase somewhat during this period and that with increased incomes, per capita consumption will also increase. However, even if the same proportions hold it will be necessary to double wheat production over the next 25 years.

Actually, doubling grain production in Pakistan over a 25-year period should be a relatively easy thing to achieve. Pakistan enjoys an unusually good agricultural resource base, and we know from the per-acre production statistics that Pakistan is grossly underproducing today. The important thing is to see Pakistan in the perspective of total world requirements.

Today the United States and Canada have a virtual monopoly on internationally traded wheat. Outside North America only Australia is a regular important participant in intercontinental wheat trade. The United States, blessed by relatively good rainfall conditions and other positive climatic features, has increased its production over the past years by a remarkable amount. A major difference between Pakistan and the United States is that the United States is already producing closer to its practical maximum than is the case in Pakistan. Doubled wheat production in the United States is considered to be quite possible. However, because of the diminishing returns to be expected from additional allocations of fertilizer, it will be a more difficult task than it will for Pakistan. One wonders if it is not increasingly dangerous for any country to remain dependent on imports from North America.

Would it not be safer and wiser to add more countries to the list of wheat exporters? If so, with Pakistan's agricultural potential, even with its rapid population growth rate, there is a real possibility that Pakistan will join the United States, Canada, and Australia in becoming one of the major wheat exporters. Pakistan has already accomplished this in a significant way for rice and now needs to ask itself whether or not it should become a regular international trader in wheat.

FOOD, POPULATION, AND THE ENVIRONMENT

Having briefly discussed the world population and the world food trends let me add a dimension to these by discussing standards of living and the environment. Recent concern with the shortages of wheat to feed a fast-growing world population have led many people to suggest that the principal goal of the plant scientist and the development administrator should be to produce more food to feed a starving world. I would argue that this is much too modest a goal.

In looking at the food situation in Pakistan I have suggested that Pakistan will have no particular problem in producing enough food to feed its population for at least the next two generations, even if population policy ends in failure and the population of Pakistan quadruples. Although in the long run the sheer problem of numbers would constitute a feeding problem, this is not the primary issue for the next 50 years. Rather, the Pakistan food issue revolves around the relationship between size of population and quality of life and the environment.

Let's face it. Too many people can be downright unpleasant. Two thousand people per square mile is no way to live. It is precisely this fact that gives the United States a population problem—not the notion that we can't feed more people. The fact is that we are feeding more people. No, our population problem grows out of the feeling we have that life is happier when there are fewer of us.

The other problem with more people is their use of the limited resources of this planet. If we have less people, we can achieve a balance between numbers and the environment that will permit each of us to consume more of those limited resources. Consuming more resources per capita is what economic development is all about. The problem in the so-called developed countries is that even with our generally much lower densities of population we are putting pressure on the environment with our huge per capita consumption. We are now becoming more sensitive to this and have begun measuring smog levels, noise levels, temperature changes, ozone layers, fish counts, mercury content, and many other factors. Gradually we are modifying our way of life in the United States in order to strike the balance among numbers of people, consumption levels, and pressure on the environment. Scientists are devoting their talents increasingly to finding ways to permit higher consumption levels with less negative impact on the environment.

Coming back to the less developed world, we now know that population densities are such that countries like Pakistan cannot achieve the consumption levels of the developed country without destroying their environment. Indeed, the pressure on Pakistan's environment is enormous. Forests have largely disappeared, grazing lands are overpopulated, and Lahore is suffering from increasing smog levels. Yet the fact remains that higher levels of per capita consumption of both food and nonfood items is the primary and very important goal of economic development.

From what has been discussed, you might wonder whether it is the author's opinion that scientists are working on the right subject. Instead of working on more productive strains of plant varieties one might suggest that plant scientists work on something else. Not at all.

What the author sees is a symbiotic relationship among several factors—population, food, nonfood consumption, and the environment. One way to make possible higher consumption levels of all those things which make life more pleasant is to produce food more efficiently. If one person produces food for 20, as is the case in the United States, than there is room in the process for more teachers, more health workers, and more producers of nonfood consumption items. Efficiency in food production is needed not simply to feed more people, but to make possible the other components of a higher standard of living.

Another aspect of the plant scientist's work that bears on the simultaneous equation I have described interrelating population numbers, food, nonfood consumption, and environment, is the direct impact plant scientists can have on the last, the environment. If we can extend the miniaturized fertilizer factory concept from the soybean to the grasses, we can avoid the nonrenewable resource use of petroleum products by those huge fertilizer plants we are now constructing. Likewise, if we can control insects by changing plant varieties rather than by means of ecology-disturbing pesticides, we can save "environmental room" for other forms of consumption. Thus, the plant scientist can be enormously helpful in our quest for the highest possible standard of living for humanity wherever it is located, however many its numbers.

From the narrower economic point of view of Pakistan, if Pakistan can produce a surplus of food and sell it, this will permit the importation of more raw materials and capital equipment to produce the items that will give Pakistan's people a higher standard of living.

Now let us add one more dimension. Thus far, this discussion has concentrated on interrelationships among population, food, nonfood consumption, and the environment. There is always the question of which comes first. The answer is that we don't really know and we can't wait to find out. However, we are developing some theories, one of which seems very reasonable—people with higher standards of living will have fewer children. If by the wave of a wand or the simple expenditure of funds we could suddenly give all Pakistanis adequate food, eight years of education, a standard of health that permitted them to live 70 years, and otherwise to consume things that constitute their concept of the "good life," we now agree that they would have fewer children and that the problem of population growth would be solved. Unfortunately, there are no such magic wands, and money alone cannot achieve this sort of change. But if the concept is right, then it has important policy implications for any government interested in achieving a better balance among population, food production, nonfood consumption, and the environment.

POLICY PERSPECTIVES

Having put on the table for your consideration a number of thoughts about the population problem, the food problem, the need for nonfood consumption, and the need for concern about the environment, as well as having suggested the symbiotic relationships among all these factors, what would be some of the policy precepts that would lead to our goal of a happier life by the shortest possible route?

1. We must accelerate our direct assault on the population problem. We should use our many powers of persuasion to convince people to want less children. Obviously, anybody who already wants to limit family size should be given the means to do so.

2. We should increase the consumption levels of the broad mass of people, not only because this is desirable in itself, but also to create the set of conditions whereby they will be more receptive to persuasion on the population issue. This

means that rather than concentrate increased resources in providing a higher standard of living for the already better-off portions of society, we should spread the resources over the whole population. Examples of consumption items that should be provided to the whole population are education, basic health services, and village services, such as roads, electricity, and safe drinking water.

3. We should produce more food and in so doing we should encourage every farmer, particularly the smallest farmers, to participate in the process. This is not the place to go into detail, but the agricultural policies that will ensure production of more food include price policies, fertilizer policies, water-use policies (with particular emphasis on the farm end of the irrigation system), and agricultural research. In all four of these areas of agricultural policy Pakistan is making constructive progress. Perhaps the point of view of plant scientists places particular importance on renewed determination to accelerate the pace and improve the quality of agricultural research. The United States is pleased to be associated with this new effort, which combines increased funding and more carefully developed national crop strategies with direct help to individual research stations and scientists. Fundamental to a successful agricultural research strategy is its interrelationships with the academic and scientific community and with the tillers of the soil. We are just beginning to implement this new research effort, but we have high hopes that the role of the scientist will be enhanced and that his contribution will continue to play the important role it has in the past. It will be out of the successes of the plant scientist that we will feed the doubled levels of population that will exist to feed in the twenty-first century. It will be your discoveries that will help us to find a better balance between man and his environment—making possible a faster rate of growth in nonfood consumption and thereby making possible an earlier and more constructive solution to the ever more critical population problem.

II

Natural and Induced Genetic Variability

4

Natural Variation and Its Conservation

O. H. Frankel

CSIRO Division of Plant Industry
Canberra, A.C.T. 2601, Australia

ABSTRACT

1. The diversity of species used by preagricultural peoples contracted as a result of domestication, but intraspecific diversity greatly expanded with world-wide migrations of crops, to be drastically contracted as a consequence of modern plant breeding.

2. Wild progenitors and other relatives of crops have much to contribute to plant breeding, but this is inhibited by inadequate collections and quite insufficient information. Although many of these crops are still relatively safe in their natural habitats, they should be extensively collected and studied.

3. The natural gene pools of many of the wild species directly used by humans, and particularly many tropical forest species (including tree fruits as well as forestry species) will be lost through replacement of indigenous forests by farmland and by planting with selected forest species. Extensive nature reserves are essential for gene-pool conservation, which would also help to preserve species that may become useful in the future.

4. In general, wild species are best preserved within the community of which they form a part. *Ex situ* preservation presents many difficulties, but it may be inevitable in some cases. Seed conservation is a practical alternative and should be more widely explored.

5. Because of the enormous genetic diversity between and within the local land races of crops evolved over long periods in diverse areas with traditional farming systems, they constitute a most valuable source of genetic materials for plant improvement. Such crops are threatened by the rapid advances of much

higher-yielding advanced cultivars, and efforts for their preservation are of the highest priority. The situation in Pakistan and neighboring countries is discussed.

6. Advanced cultivars (produced by modern plant-breeding methods) have been the principal genetic resources used in developed countries, but there are good reasons for enlarging gene pools used by plant breeders, one being the danger of "genetic vulnerability" that results from homogeneity. "Primitive" gene pools are of special importance for plant improvement in the countries in which they are situated.

7. Methods for the exploration and collection of genetic materials have been clarified. The urgent need now is to safeguard representative samples of what is left in the field, as well as the material now in collections, much of which is inadequately maintained.

8. Methods and procedures for the long-term conservation of seeds have been worked out, and the organization for international collaboration of seed-storage laboratories is in an advanced stage of preparation.

9. The conservation of genetic resources is solely directed toward utilization by present and future generations; hence, the evaluation and documentation of collected material is of the greatest importance. Evaluation must be directed toward the practical objectives of breeding projects, and information made available to all users.

10. Current developments are briefly recorded.

INTRODUCTION

The "natural diversity" of the plants we live on evolved in the course of the last 10,000 years. The ancestors of many of our crops were among the much larger number of species used by hunter–gatherers for unknown millenia. Thus there is an evolutionary continuum from prehistoric predomesticates to current cultivars (Fig. 1). Many early domesticates were abandoned. Some remained endemic, presumably in their area of domestication. But many more spread in their own hemisphere, and, in the last four or five centuries, around the globe, diversified as they adapted to different environments and cultures. Thus, genetic diversity underwent dynamic change at specific and intraspecific levels—initially it contracted at the species level, then expanded enormously at intraspecies levels to contract drastically at both levels in the last 100 years. This phase is still in progress, with evolutionary consequences that are causing growing concern. The author's intention is first to categorize the existing genetic diversity in its evolutionary context as well as examine which categories should be safeguarded and why, and second to show how this can be done both effectively and economically.

As this volume is based on a symposium held at the rim of the Near East center, probably the oldest nucleus of domestication, and also on the rim of the

Southeast Asian region, which gave rise to some of the world's most significant tropical species; seeing further that descendants of these early domesticates persist, though precariously, in this and in other countries of these regions, as do the wild ancestors of many of our principal crop species; and above all, because many participants in this symposium live and work in or near these cradles of plant domestication, I shall wherever possible refer to plants and circumstances of these historic regions.

WILD SPECIES

All domesticated species derive, directly or indirectly, from wild species, and many of these have been identified, although the progenitors of some crops including maize and hexaploid wheat, are still subjects of research and argument. Many of the progenitors were among the species that had been gathered by preagricultural peoples at productivity levels that may not have been greatly inferior to those under primitive cultivation (Harlan, 1967) (Fig. 1, WS). Other species, which so far as we know had not been gathered for food, also became progenitors of domesticates, in some instances by natural hybridization [Fig. 1 (5)]. Although never domesticated, many species have been used by peoples throughout the ages; they include nearly all species used in forestry and in unimproved pasture and range lands, and some fruits and drug plants (Fig. 1, WS, LR). Finally, it is likely that some species that are neither domesticated nor even used at present may come into prominence in the future, e.g., for pharmaceutical or other industrial purposes (Fig. 1: WS, DS). From the viewpoint of their past and potential utilization, there are three main categories of wild species— progenitors and other relatives of domesticates, species that are used but not domesticated, and species that may become domesticates at some future stage. These relationships are indicated in the schematic representation in Fig. 1.

Progenitors and Other Relatives of Domesticated Species

In recent years a great deal of information on the evolutionary relations of domesticates and their wild and weedy relatives has been generated from a spectrum of different sources, including archaeology, anthropology and ethnology, taxonomy, plant geography, climatology, ecology, and, of course, cytogenetics and experimental evolution. There are still many gaps in our knowledge of the ancestry of our crops, as already indicated; nor is the location, time, and mode of domestication of most crops known—it may never be known. However, a convincing attempt at integrating the various sources has been made recently by Harlan (1975a) who himself has contributed a great deal to the range of disciplines listed earlier, as well as to the interpretation of the evidence. This improved understanding of the evolution of crops should heighten the apprecia-

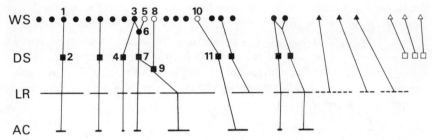

Figure 1. Schematic description of relationships between wild and domesticated species and of changes in the genetic diversity of domesticated species (indicated by length of horizontal lines). Wild species now used (▲) and potential domesticates (△□) shown at right of diagram. *Wild species* (WS): (●) Used by gatherers; (○) not used by gatherers; (▲) used, but not domesticated; (△) wild progenitors of potential domesticates. *Domesticated species* (DS): (■) Domesticated species; (□) potential domesticate. *Land races* (LR): Extensive genetic diversity. *Advanced cultivars* (AC): Genetic diversity reduced. *Examples:* (1) *Hordeum spontaneum;* (2) *H. vulgare;* (3) *Triticum boeoticum;* (4) *T. monococcum;* (5) *Aegilops* sp.?; (6) *T. dicoccoides;* (7) *T. dicoccum;* (8) *Aegilops squarrosa;* (9) *T. aestivum;* (10–11) *Trifolium subterraneum.*

tion of the wild progenitors and other related species as valuable sources for the improvement, and even the radical restructuring, of crop species.

In the main, the use of wild relatives of crop species has so far been restricted to breeding for resistance to diseases and pests. In recent years some new avenues have opened up which promise to extend significantly the boundaries of plant breeders' gene pools. Some of them are the subject of other chapters in this volume; I shall therefore be brief. One area derives from the detailed knowledge of the genetic architecture which has resulted from work such as that of Kihara, Sears, Riley, and others on the wheat genomes. This has already led to sophisticated transfers, from chromosome or half-chromosome substitutions to gene transfers. Another prospect is the technique of cell hybridization which, however, at least for the time being, is likely to be restricted to closely related species, such as the cell hybridization of *Nicotiana glauca* and *N. langsdorffii* effected by Carlson et al. (1972).

Zohary et al. (1969) drew attention to "the wild diploid progenitors of wheat [which] constitute large gene pools largely unexplored and untapped by plant breeders." The three diploids differ in ecological adaptation and in many other respects; incorporation by crossing (followed by backcrossing) should be easier and more readily exploitable than the more popular distant crosses. These workers urge that such species be extensively collected and studied.

The general observation is that most of the wild relatives of domesticates have been little collected (except by students of their evolution), and those few collections that are made for specific studies are often dissipated at their conclusion. For many of the principal crops—let alone minor ones—the number of wild accessions in existing major collections is pitifully small. Whereas wild biota are not as exposed to rapid extinction as are the land races discussed in the next section, representative collections should be established for observation and use by plant breeders. After all, one cannot use what one neither knows nor can obtain.

Availability and conservation of representative gene pools is one need, intensive study is another. We know next to nothing of the population structure of wild relatives of domesticates; hence, we have no information with which to guide collection and utilization. The nearest available evidence comes from population studies on introduced weed species, *Avena fatua* and *A. barbata,* in California, where considerable differences among regions were shown to exist in the degree of polymorphism of both morphological characteristics and isozymes (Jain, 1969; Marshall and Allard, 1970). There is also a need for information on physiological characteristics of wild relatives, and some recent studies have yielded interesting results. In comparing wild and domesticated wheats at the three ploidy levels, Evans and Dunstone (1970) found that evolution has involved a parallel increase in leaf and grain size, but coupled with a reduction in the rate of photosynthesis per unit leaf area. The wild species showed a fall in leaf photosynthesis during grain development, whereas in the domesticates it rose during that phase.

We should now turn to a consideration of the centers which are to be given special attention in this chapter—the Near Eastern region, which stretches from the eastern Mediterranean to Afghanistan, and Southeast Asia; but a comprehensive treatment is well beyond the scope of this discussion. Suffice it to remind you that in the Near East are found the progenitors and the wild (and weed) relatives of wheat, of barley, rye, chickpea, peas, broad beans, beets, rape, olive, safflower, flax, and an array of vegetables and fruits; in Southeast Asia are found those of a large range of tropical crops—cereals (rice and millet), pulses (pigeon pea and mung bean), and roots and tubers (yam, taro), to mention only a few of the most important ones, and, of course, oil, starch and sugar crops, and a large number of vegetables and drug plants.

Here I want to draw attention to the fruit species that tend to receive a low priority in the pecking order of genetic conservation, partly because many of them cannot be preserved as seeds and the conservation of trees is difficult and expensive and partly because some people rate them as luxury rather than food crops. One would scarcely place the dates and olives, the plums, apricots, or nuts of the Near East in the former category, no more than would anyone who has seen the array of nourishing fruits in the market of a country town in Java. As Zohary and Spiegel-Roy (1975) have shown, olive, grape, date, and fig were the first fruit species to be cultivated in the Near East, from the early fourth millenium B.C. onward. They are highly heterozygous; hence, domestication was associated with the shift to vegetative reproduction—quite easy in the four fruits—of superior individuals. The authors believe that these clones persisted for hundreds or even thousands of years. But the wild gene pools provided evolutionary opportunities for expansion into new environments. It is clear that such opportunities continue for new recombinations as long as the wild and feral gene pools persist.

Some of the tree fruits in Southeast Asia have less clearly defined boundaries between cultivated and wild types. But the establishment of selected cultivars tends to reduce the interest in and concern for the wild and semiwild types, which for the most part are forest trees and as such are exposed to erosion or virtual eradication in the many areas where large-scale destruction of primeval forests is now extensive. This process is having a drastic effect on the genetic reservoirs of tree crops in other tropical areas, e.g., of coffee in the rain forests of Ethiopia.

Wild Species of Direct Economic Concern

The observations made in the preceding paragraph lead to the consideration of those wild species that have not been domesticated yet are extensively used by humans. Foremost among these are the forestry species, which have their genetic reservoirs in primeval, or at any rate natural, forests. Although continuously shrinking—in some parts of the world with increasing rapidity—for most species there is still scope for the salvage of a broad range of genetic diversity, although perhaps not very much longer where pressure is most acute. In 1967, Richardson (1970) was able to say that the main threat to forest genetic resources came not from a rapid increase in the tempo of utilization, but from population pressure on cultivable land. This pressure has greatly intensified, especially in the tropics, and has been further increased by new timber-using technologies, which are replacing selective tree removal by clear felling. Today, foresters are increasingly concerned with the renewal of timber resources by planting fast-growing species. Quoting an ECAFE report of 1974, Whitmore (1975) predicts that "both Malaysia and the Philippines will have no remaining accessible virgin forests within a decade." Indeed, "silviculture in natural forests has virtually ceased." Whitmore lists the Southeast Asian and Melanesian species currently planted for industrial purposes, and others planted as whole timber species (for veneer, paneling, furniture, and so forth, with the former predominating. He also names many others worthy of immediate silvicultural trial. Guzman (1975) compiled a comprehensive list of forest species in the Philippines that can be utilized for the production of food, including fruits, oil, beverages, vegetables, and spices. Indeed, tropical forests are the main reservoir of as yet untapped resources of economic plants.

From the foregoing it is clear that indigenous forests have a dual function as genetic resources. First, with regard to the species planted either in monoculture, or, less frequently, into existing stands, the role of indigenous forests parallels that of land races and advanced cultivars with respect to domesticates. They are resources of genetic diversity for the adaptation of species to new environments (Guldager, 1975) as well as for selection and breeding. Second, indigenous forests are, as stated in the preceding paragraph, a reservoir for potentially useful species (*vide infra*).

The threat to these invaluable and irreplaceable genetic resources is world-wide, but it is especially acute in the tropics of Asia, America, and Africa. Many species have disappeared (see Guzman, 1975, for the Philippines), and many more are acutely threatened. The need for conservation is obvious and increasingly acknowledged.

Many wild species are used in pasture and range lands as well as for raw materials for chemical industries. In recent years some of these have become domesticated, generally in countries other than their own, as for example Mediterranean, African, and South American pasture grasses and legumes in Australia. Large collections of such species have been established, but material continues to be collected in the countries of origin to obtain types adapted to new ecological conditions or for specific purposes. On the whole, such species are not under acute threat except in specific areas in which rough grazing land is turned over to agriculture or forestry.

Wild Species of Potential Value to Man

Reference was made in the preceding section to wild species of prospective value. Such species are difficult to define. They stretch from plants that are now gathered as major vegetable food or as condiments in many parts of the world, in the forests of southern Asia or the wasteland and scrub in Mediterranean countries, to potential raw materials for chemical and pharmacological industries. Indications that species are worthy of attention come either from past usage, from taxonomic or other associations with species now used, or from new requirements by industry. The history of crop production fails to suggest that new major crops are likely to be discovered (as against new plants deliberately engineered by man). But there is reason to assume that species may be taken into cultivation for specific ecological niches or for requirements that arise in nutritional, medical, chemical, or other industrial research. Such leads should be taken up as they arise, but it hardly seems appropriate to collect and preserve a range of wild species on the basis of vague prospects. It would seem more purposeful to regard the preservation of potentially useful species as partial justification for the conservation of ecosystems.

Conservation of Wild Species

The conservation of wild plants is most effective in their natural environment, i.e., within the community in which they are adapted. A community in balance with a stable environment—the stability being subject to the general vagaries of natural environments—is the ideal model of long-term conservation. Such a community can be a primeval forest, a savanna landscape exposed to grazing and periodic fires, a Mediterranean scrub community, or weed populations of fields or roadsides. It can be exposed to environmental change resulting in physical or biological selection pressures, yet remain a significant genetic resource. But the genetic resource is wholly or partly invalidated if the community is destroyed or reduced below the level of self-reproduction, or if its genetic variance is drastically reduced. In such circumstances a genetic resource can be preserved in other ways—in living collections *ex situ,* as seeds, as pollen, or possibly in some form of tissue culture.

In situ conservation is the continuing maintenance of a population within the community of which it forms a part, in the environment to which it is adapted. For example, a wild form of *Aegilops squarrosa* is likely to be destroyed by cultivation, whereas a weed form could thrive. Many of the wild relatives of annual crop species are reasonably safe in their habitats, but this must not be taken for granted. Weeds of cultivated fields or species in roadside communities (e.g., wild peas in Turkey) can be very rapidly destroyed by the introduction of modern weedicides. Since, as has been urged before, representative collections should be established for study and use, these would constitute an insurance against erosion or loss. The position is probably similar for range and pasture plants and other short-lived wild plants used directly by man.

For long-lived woody biota the position is different. Many belong to forest or scrub communities and lack the faculties of recovery possessed by most short-lived organisms. Their survival *in situ* depends on the degree of integrity of the community as a whole. With the pressures on land and natural resources, *in situ* conservation becomes increasingly dependent on deliberate measures to protect specific sites or areas. The degree of protection required varies with the end purpose of the reserve as well as the "time scale of concern" (Frankel, 1975*a*), i.e., the notional period for which the projected protection is designed. For nature reserves which are to function as habitats for continuing evolution and to serve distant generations, this time scale should be open-ended, and the areas large and representative. A blueprint for such long-term reserves was provided for the establishment of biosphere reserves under Project 8 of Unesco's program *Man and the Biosphere* (Unesco, 1973, 1974). Such reserves are eminently suitable for the long-term conservation of forest-based genetic resources (*vide supra*), especially for tropical forests where the enormous diversity of species may hold resources only the future may appreciate and need. However, where the main protection targets are more limited and specific, e.g., the preservation of a population of a forest species, the standards of protection could sensibly be lowered, because the time scale of concern for a currently used resource, although not precisely definable, is of a different order of magnitude from the evolutionary time scale subsumed in nature conservation per se

(Frankel, 1976). This is recognized by foresters in the layout of provenance and other forest reserves (FAO, 1975*b*).

Ex situ conservation is practiced by botanical gardens the world over, many of which give prominence to species of economic significance. It must be recognized that the varied functions and responsibilities of botanical gardens as well as their limited resources restrict the amount of material they are able to maintain. The widest experience of large-scale conservation of wild species comes from conservation stands of forestry species, especially in the tropics, both in the countries of origin and in countries of adoption. The appropriate population size and structure must be considered in relation to reproductive and mating systems of species under *ex situ* conservation (Guldager, 1975).

Seed storage as a form of genetic conservation is discussed subsequently in the section on conservation. Here attention is drawn to the specific difficulties attaching to the seed storage of wild species. Many, especially those with dry, small seeds can be stored under conditions that are standard for many crop species, viz. $-10°$ to $-20°C$ at less than 10% moisture content, but many others require individual treatment which must be ascertained (Thompson, 1974). Seeds of many tree fruit and forestry species are short-lived and can endure only very limited drying and cold storage treatment. Storage of pollen presents similar difficulties, and storage life is generally shorter than that of seeds (Harrington, 1970; Wang, 1975).

PRIMITIVE CULTIVARS (LAND RACES)

Archaeological evidence shows that many of the newly domesticated species spread fairly rapidly throughout the known world. Wherever they went they were modified by the cultural methods adopted by different civilizations. Thus there emerged distinctive races adapted to the many variants and interactions of natural and cultural environments to which crop species were gradually exposed. We have come to call them land races, or, rather unhappily "primitive cultivars" (many of their cultivators were far from primitive) as distinct from the "advanced cultivars," which are the highly selected varieties produced by scientific breeding methods over the last 100 years.

Primitive cultivars have been given prominence recently as "genetic resources," a term which emerged at an international conference organized by FAO and IBP in 1967. There are several reasons for this. First, their value as reservoirs of genetic diversity (in contrast with the advanced cultivars) has been widely recognized, especially for the improvement of crops in the region in which they are located. Second, their continued existence is increasingly threatened by the introduction of high-producing varieties as part of accelerated agricultural development. Third, the scientific background, methodology, and technology of genetic conservation have been clarified and developed (Frankel and Bennett, 1970*a*; Frankel and Hawkes, 1975). Finally, scientific, political, and popular concern have been generated (Bennett, 1965; Frankel, 1967; Frankel and Bennett, 1970*a*; UN, 1972; Harlan, 1972, 1975*b*; and various references in journals and the press). The following is an assessment of the evolutionary and population—biological features of primitive cultivars:

1. Primitive cultivars evolved over long periods, exposed to natural selection under a diversity of natural and cultural environments; presumably they were subjected to some deliberate selection by cultivators, but prior to the introduction of individual selection in the latter part of last century.

2. In the main they evolved under production systems with low levels of cultivation, fertilization, and plant protection.

3. It follows from (1) that their heterogeneity has two dimensions—*between* sites and populations and *within* sites and populations, the former generated chiefly by heterogeneity *in space,* the latter in addition by heterogeneity *in time,* i.e., short-term variation between seasons, and longer-term variations in response to climatic, biological, and social changes.

4. Migration must have played a part in diversifying gene pools through addition and recombination. Wild and weed relatives, as we know, have continued to introgress with cultivated populations (Harlan, 1951; Zohary and Feldman, 1962).

5. It follows from (2) and (3) that a primitive variety is typically a population with a subtly balanced population structure (including genetic polymorphisms for resistance characteristics), capable of producing in any but disaster seasons at a level which safeguards the survival of the cultivator. This can be seen as a symbiotic relationship between crops and humans, which results from interactions between biological and cultural evolution.

6. In consequence, primitive cultivars accumulated resistance genes to limiting factors in the physical and biological environment—drought, cold, diseases, pests, and so forth—which provides the main reason for the current interest.

7. It does not, however, follow that land races were solely or even principally selected for survival of crop and cultivator. Although this was necessarily so in stress environments, the fact that the first advanced cultivars, selected from land races in Western, Northern, and Central Europe, gave remarkably high yields shows that under favorable conditions land races contained high-producing components.

8. An exception to the typical population structure of land races are the vegetatively reproduced crops, many of which were domesticated as clones. However, many of these crops retained a broad range of genetic diversity in wild or feral populations, as discussed earlier.

9. It must be recognized that land races have generally outlived their economic usefulness in present-day agriculture. Wherever improved varieties

appropriate to the physical, economic, and social environment are available, land races should, and progressively are, being replaced.

Ever since Vavilov (1926) discovered and systematically studied extensive collections of land races from many parts of the world, their enormous genetic diversity has come to be recognized as a resource for plant breeders. For a number of reasons the extent of the genetic diversity as well as its usefulness are as yet not fully appreciated and exploited. First, apart from the great collections assembled by Vavilov, his colleagues, and present-day successors, not a great number of existing collections have a good representation of primitive material; hence, study and evaluation have been limited. Second, evaluation has been restricted to a relatively narrow range of characters, related mainly to re-sistances. Future selection targets will at once be broader and more specific thanks to a greater knowledge of the chemical and physical properties of plant products.

So far one has looked at primitive materials primarily as donors of single, observable genes, such as resistance genes, or as genes controlling the content of a chemical product. Too little attention has been given "the enormous diversity of gene complexes determining adaptation and productivity, assembled and incorporated over centuries of cultivation in differing environments" (Frankel and Bennett, 1970b), coadapted gene complexes of fundamental importance in the adaptation of populations to their environments (Dobzhansky, 1970). Some of these have indubitably been incorporated in the many cultivars selected from land races, but there must be many more, and especially some which confer adaptations to extreme conditions, such as salt tolerance, which is of great significance in southern Asia and elsewhere. Moreover, as emphasized by Vavilov (1926), the combination of parents adapted to widely different environments may provide opportunities for major advances—presumably through the com-bination of different adaptive complexes. This is a precept that has been practiced by some of the most successful plant breeders—William Farrer in Australia nearly a century ago and Norman Borlaug in our time. But it must be admitted that genetic information on such complexes is scant, apart from reports on genes with adaptive connotations being associated in supergenes (see Bennett, 1970a). We generally know all too little about the population structure of primitive cultivars, perhaps even less than what we know of their wild and weedy relatives. As Marshall and Brown (1975) emphasize, this limits efficiency in exploration, conservation, and utilization.

If, as I have endeavored to show, primitive cultivars are valuable genetic resources, and because for the most part they are rapidly disappearing, steps are needed to conserve an appropriate representation for use and study. The first question is where they are to be found. Obviously, first thoughts will turn to the "centers of origin" of domesticated crops. But it had long been recognized—even by Vavilov himself—that there are centers of diversity which are not centers of origin. Some such "secondary centers," such as Ethiopia for barley, contain greater diversity than the center of origin (Harlan, 1975*a*) and, as has already been emphasized, they add greatly to the genetic diversity of crop species. Moreover, as a number of authors (quoted by Harlan, 1971) have pointed out, not all crops originated in Vavilov's centers, nor in any "center" at all. Recently Harlan (1971, 1975*a*) proposed a distinction between "centers" and "noncenters" of origin. The centers gave rise to a group of crops which together provided the basis of an agricultural and cultural system; whereas "noncenters"—a rather unfelicitous term—are *regions* of domestication, large areas in which species were domesticated independently, i.e., wherever they happened to be, with considerable spread in space and time of domestication and diversity in the cultures of the original cultivators. Vavilov recognizes a Near Eastern center, and an African noncenter stretching across the continent in a broad belt; the Yang-shao center in China and a vast and prolific noncenter comprising South East Asia and Oceania; a Meso-American center and a South American noncenter. Harlan acknowledges that apart from some areas in which Vavilov had insufficient information, his presentation generally does not differ drastically from Vavilov's. In fact, if Vavilov's and Harlan's maps are combined one obtains a fair idea of the ancient regions of genetic diversity, including primary and secondary centers, and noncenters. To these must be added those regions in which diversity evolved in more recent times, especially as a result of post-Columbian migrations between the hemispheres. Many Western Hemisphere crops, such as maize, formed distinctive secondary centers in Europe, Africa, and Asia, as did, for example, peas in Brazil. These are under threat of extinction as much as the land races in the ancient regions of diversity. The types of maize that had differentiated in Europe would have been wiped out by hybrid maize had it not been for the efforts by maize geneticists who established germ plasm collections in Italy, Bulgaria, and elsewhere before it was too late.

It is, of course, all too clear that the areas of genetic diversity identified by Vavilov and others have in many parts undergone a process of what we have come to call genetic erosion. This process has been greatly accelerated in areas in which the drive for intensification of agricultural production—the so-called green revolution—has been most effective. But even in countries where traditional cultivars seemed reasonably secure a few years ago the advance of introductions acutely threatens the traditional stocks, some of which, like Ethiopian barleys resistant to the barley yellow dwarf virus, are quite unique.

For some of the worst affected areas we are now entirely dependent on older collections, and more will have to be said about these. If a fair proportion of what is left is to be salvaged before it is too late, one must know where it is. For a number of years the FAO Panel of Experts urged that such a survey be rapidly undertaken (FAO, 1969, 1970) to indicate where there was a good chance of locating material in the field, and in particular, where it was acutely threatened. This survey was carried out through visits of experts to some areas, but for the most part through inquiries from plant explorers and from experts on the spot.

The outcome was the *FAO/IBP Survey of Crop Genetic Resources in their Centres of Origin* (Frankel, 1973). For some regions the reports provide a useful guide for availability and urgency. In other regions they were disappointing mainly because the remnants were few, scattered, and ephemeral. This was the case with many crops, particularly with the cereals in the Near Eastern center, which as we had seen earlier had been perhaps the richest of the ancient genetic treasuries. Even in Afghanistan a map drawn by Erna Bennett of FAO in 1973 shows substantial incursions of introduced wheat varieties; by now they have spread a good deal further. In Pakistan, there was relatively little wheat left to be salvaged, mainly in the southwest and in isolated mountain areas of the northwest and east of the country. Since the publication of this report, J. R. Witcombe, University College, Bangor, and A. R. Rao, University of Agriculture, Lyallpur, carried out a successful collecting expedition in North Pakistan and secured representative collections of wheat, barley, and maize, as well as samples of a number of other crops, from more than 100 villages at altitudes between 1100 and 3300 m. They reported that modern varieties were beginning to enter even this isolated mountain region, and that before long the traditional germ plasm was likely to be threatened.

Land races of grain legumes—peas, broad beans, lens, vetches, lupins, and chickpea—are fairly abundant in Near Eastern countries. A map of the distribution of wild, primitive, and modern chickpeas, prepared at FAO from information supplied by L. J. G. van der Maesen, shows land races still widespread but in danger of replacement in the Mediterranean and Near Eastern countries (Frankel, 1973).

The ancient fruits and nuts of Near Eastern countries constitute rich but all too little appreciated and now fast vanishing genetic resources. Replacement by newly introduced varieties is widespread, and in some important areas old trees in home gardens may be the main or only residues of a rich heritage. The FAO/IBP report contains information provided by workers in Near Eastern countries; maps provided by Inayat Ali Razi of the Government Fruit Research Station, Mirpurkhas, Sind, indicate the distribution in Pakistan of indigenous stocks of apples, pears, plums, grapes, peaches, apricots, and almonds. As in other Near Eastern countries, the main horticultural areas in Pakistan are now planted in introduced fruit varieties.

The situation appears to be similar in Iran, but the distribution of indigenous stocks could not be ascertained at the time of the survey. However, Turkey still has considerable possibilities for salvage of important germ plasm of a range of fruits and nuts (Zagaja, 1970; Sykes, 1972). Pistachio (*Pistacia vera*) is a nut that has considerable market potential and economic prospects as an irrigation crop. Pistachio savannas and scattered trees, which may be degraded savannas, are widespread throughout the desert fringes of Asia (Maggs, 1972, 1973). Maggs states that the gene pool, although widespread, is being depleted by land clearance, kill-out grazing, and the use of wild pistachio as rootstocks. He urges that research stations interested in this crop establish representative collections; he suggests the types and numbers of representatives of each to be assembled in a reference collection.

It will be appreciated that in view of the scarcity of remaining resources, and in many instances the urgency of the situation, there is a need for careful planning, preparation, and execution in the collecting of primitive cultivars (see Bennett, 1970b). Moreover, even in circumstances of extreme scarcity—whether it be a handful of crops or orchards—there will be problems of sampling, as it is hardly ever possible to collect and retain even one entire population. As a rule there are limits to the number of samples that can be collected, evaluated, and conserved. This issue has been examined by Marshall and Brown (1975) who conclude that sampling techniques should focus on locally common alleles, and that the aim should be to include "at least one copy of each variant occurring in the target population with a frequency greater than 0.05." Generally, the optimum strategy will be to collect 50–100 individuals per site, to sample as many sites as possible, and to include a representative range of environments within the target area.

Conservation methods appropriate to primitive cultivars are discussed in the section on conservation (*vide infra*).

ADVANCED CULTIVARS

There is a curious contradiction in the relative prominence given advanced cultivars, the products of scientific plant breeding and the mainstay of modern agriculture. Whereas they have been and continue to be the principally used genetic resources of plant breeders, they have received little attention in the discussions and publications on genetic resources during the last 10 or 15 years. There were several reasons for this that were recognized early in the discussions of genetic conservation (e.g., IBP, 1966). Advanced cultivars were well represented in many existing collections, whereas primitive cultivars were for the most part poorly represented in relatively few collections. Many advanced cultivars were closely related, differing only in minor respects, whereas primitive cultivars, as we have seen, possessed a broad genetic diversity. Advanced cultivars could, as a rule, be obtained from their breeders or from national collections; primitive cultivars were not readily available, either from collections or from the areas in which they were still grown, even if these were known. Above all, primitive varieties were rapidly vanishing. Hence, the collection and preservation of primitive material received, and should continue to receive, foremost consideration.

Yet the advanced cultivars must not be neglected. One may assume—albeit with some doubt—that the currently used cultivars incorporate most of the coadapted complexes at the genic or the character level assembled in their predecessors in the earlier stages of plant selection. This may be partially justified, but it is not unlikely that the early varieties selected prior to the widespread use of fertilizers, intensive cultivation, or irrigation possessed adaptive characteristics which later became redundant, yet which may be needed again for less favored environments and low-input agricultural systems. Similarly, resistance to currently infrequent biotypes may again be required should they build up in the future. The most convincing reason for retaining representative collections of obsolete cultivars is that they are, or should be, documented for many characteristics associated with performance. The question arises which to preserve, in view of their enormous number. Judicious culling is inevitable, but along what principles?

These remarks apply also to "genetic stocks" of various kinds—natural or induced mutants, breeding lines with specific characteristics, and, of course, to the large array of cytologically and/or genetically characterized stocks that have become tools of trade in current cytogenetic, evolutionary, and breeding research. The maintenance and distribution of the latter—an essential service to current research—has become a burden on individual institutions and calls for cooperative action. These, and perhaps other genetic stocks, should be looked after by appropriate institutions and, in some instances, by cooperatives of scientists. Initiatives might come from international organizations, such as the International Genetics Federation, Eucarpia, SABRAO, and so forth.

CONSERVATION

Exploration and conservation are the kingpins of the current problems of genetic resources. Exploration is to salvage threatened resources in the field, conservation to preserve new as well as existing collections. Even if no further material were to be added, the effective conservation of material now in possession of institutions the world over is an important issue that requires serious attention. If in exploration the need is for urgent action in the field, on as broad a front as possible, the need in conservation is for effective organization. Exploration emphasizes crops and areas, conservation, facilities and their operation and coordination.

Conservation *in situ,* clearly the most effective form for wild biota, as discussed earlier, as a rule is not practicable for domesticates. Nor is the use of bulk populations, as has been suggested, appropriate, because conservation should aim to preserve the integrity of allele frequencies and adaptive character and gene assemblies which have evolved in response to environmental and deliberate selection (Frankel, 1970).

Conservation is safest and cheapest if life processes are reduced to the minimum level. This is the case in seeds preserved under conditions appropriate to each species. Live plants are subject to genetic change and to losses through parasites, climatic extremes, or human error, but in some plants seeds are either not produced or cannot be stored for extended periods. The great majority of seed-reproduced economic species can be safely stored over long periods—

decades, and probably centuries—without undue genetic change or loss of viability (Roberts, 1975). The advantages of long-term storage as opposed to frequent reproduction are the avoidance of genetic erosion and loss referred to in the previous paragraph, and the economy of maintenance. The FAO Panel of Experts has specified storage conditions for long-term storage of "conventional" seeds, i.e., those which can be stored at low temperatures and low moisture content, at two levels—"preferred" and "acceptable." The preferred standard specifies storage at $-18°C$ or less in air-tight containers at a seed moisture content of $5 \pm 1\%$, the acceptable standard is storage at $5°C$ or less, in air-tight containers at a seed moisture content of 5–7%, or if stored in unsealed containers, in an atmosphere of not more than 20% relative humidity (FAO, 1975a). A number of storage laboratories, including some of the largest, are in the "acceptable" class, but some of these, and new storages now projected, are concerned to reach the "preferred" standard. The panel has also specified operating procedures, including entry procedures, accession size, routine germination tests, regeneration, documentation, and duplication in other laboratories as a safety measure. None of these would be found burdensome by a well-run storage laboratory.

The organizational pattern required for operating the system is to consist of "base collections" which have the facilities outlined above and the function of providing safe long-term seed conservation. Associated with these collections are "active collections" whose functions include the multiplication and distribution of seed, regeneration of samples when required as a consequence of loss of viability or near-exhaustion of seed stocks, evaluation, documentation, and medium-term seed storage. The latter is required for the storage of the center's own collection and of seed stocks for distribution to other users. Such storages can be smaller and of somewhat lower standard compared with base collections. The great majority of existing collections are "active collections," actively engaged in some or all activities in genetic resources work, from exploration to evaluation and utilization. According to a survey conducted by FAO's Crop Ecology and Genetic Resources Service, a substantial number of seed storage laboratories are adequately equipped and prepared to participate in a cooperative seed conservation network. The biggest gaps, however, are in the developing countries. There are vast areas without any storages of base collection standard, including South and Southeast Asia, Central America, and large parts of Africa. Clearly, it is neither possible nor necessary to have substantial base collections in every country. But regional quarantine restrictions, let alone technical needs and convenience, make regional distribution of base collections an absolute necessity.

The preservation of the so-called "recalcitrant seeds," i.e., those which cannot be stored at low moisture contents, presents individual problems for species or groups of species. Some of these have been solved, but research is required to improve and extend existing information. An interesting discovery that some seeds can be successfully preserved in a fully imbibed state is being further explored (Villiers, 1975). Research on recalcitrant seeds is of special relevance in tropical species, especially in the many fruit species of Southeast Asia.

Living collections of species that cannot be preserved as seeds are difficult and expensive to maintain but are inevitable where valuable germ plasm would otherwise be lost. As has already been emphasized, this represents a real and present danger for the tree fruits of both the Near East and Southeast Asia. There is particular interest, therefore, in research into the preservation of parts of plants, as meristem, tissue, or cell culture, and their subsequent regeneration (Frankel and Hawkes, 1975, chaps 25–27). There are now good prospects that the genetic instability of tissue culture may be overcome by storage at very low temperatures (−196°C) [for references, see Frankel (1976)]. The real bottleneck is now the regeneration of plants from cell or tissue culture which so far has been accomplished only in a limited number of species (discussed in Chapter 37, this volume).

UTILIZATION, EVALUATION, DOCUMENTATION, AND ORGANIZATION

Although only the briefest outline can find place in this chapter, for a more comprehensive treatment reference should be made to the relevant chapters in Frankel and Bennett (1970a) and Frankel and Hawkes (1975). Genetic conservation would have little meaning without the prospect of utilization in plant breeding or other branches of research. Utilization in plant breeding depends on the evaluation of relevant characteristics as an essential preliminary and on the availability of the resulting information through a documentation and information system as well as stocks from a well-organized network of collections.

Evaluation may involve no more than a site description of the place of origin and a few morphological or phenological characteristics, or it may extend to multidisciplinary studies including physiological, genetic, biochemical, plant pathological, or other examinations. All such studies have, and indeed should have, the common motivation of being related to utilization, whether in some area of research, plant introduction, plant breeding. Many of these examinations are carried out in laboratories, i.e., are no longer environment-specific. Laboratory methods are applied not only on chemical, biochemical, or technological characteristics, but in entomology, plant pathology, genetics, physiology, and other areas. Such work requires expertise and equipment of a high order; furthermore, it is expensive. Agreement on labor sharing and cooperation, on methods, and on the sharing of information would benefit all nations, all of which could give a new dimension to the usefulness of genetic resources.

A systematic descriptive documentation of collections is the key to their utilization. It is no overstatement that the relatively limited use which has been made of large existing collections is mainly attributable to the deficiencies of existing documentation which may restrict the usefulness of a collection even within the institution that owns it, and much more so to other potential users. The difficulty arises from the vast amount of information and from the lack of mutual standards and procedures to facilitate the communication of information among collections as well as between collections and users. Developments that have taken place during the past two years have shown how to overcome most of the problems of documentation and information. Based on research carried out by information specialists over a number of years, a project was established jointly by FAO, the Consultative Group on International Agricultural Research (CGIAR), and the University of Colorado, under the title Genetic Resources Communication, Information and Documentation System (GR/CIDS). The system is based on the application of the EXIR (TAXIR) computer system especially developed for genetic resources requirements. The system is undergoing practical tests and, it is hoped, will be found widely acceptable.

Information is one cornerstone of utilization, availability of plant materials to bona fide users another. Elaborating on institutional arrangements that have passed the test of time, the FAO Panel of Experts has proposed a hierarchy of collections that would jointly be responsible for the conservation, multiplication, regeneration (when needed), distribution, and documentation of the collections in their charge (FAO, 1970, 1975a). The components—base collections for long-term conservation and active collections which produce seed for distribution and regeneration as required—have already been described. Base and active collections must cooperate in maintaining adequate stocks for distribution and in continuing storage and documentation. Plant breeders' collections, although often not of active collection standard, are expected to make valuable contributions to evaluation through the GR/CIDS, as just discussed.

The best of blueprints and organization charts are ineffective without firm conviction and continuing drive, without the appropriate technical background, professional competence, and public support, and finally, without administrative and financial backing. To a large degree all this has been forthcoming during the last 10 years largely through the efforts of a small group of people associated with FAO and IBP, the devoted but all too small FAO staff, and collaborators in many countries. J. R. Harlan, a member of the FAO panel since its inception, recently gave an outline of the main events of this period (Harlan, 1975b). What was almost completely lacking was financial support for plant exploration and an adequate administrative base for stimulating and guiding international and national activities in all other relevant fields. But most of what was needed to establish an active program had been done, and as Riley (1976) remarks, in the new phase which has now begun "it will be necessary for those concerned to draw to a large extent on the philosophies and methodologies developed during earlier work." The final success of this period was the establishment of the International Board for Plant Genetic Resources (IBPGR) by the Consultative Group on International Agricultural Research (CGIAR).

The new board has been in action for two years; it is not surprising that this time was largely spent in examinations and preparations. Though closely associated with FAO, the board is developing policies of its own, and because hardly any of its members have shared the experience of the previous phase it is not surprising that action, especially in the crucial field of exploration, has not been extensive. However, very considerable progress has been made in advancing the GR/CIDS project, which had been initiated by FAO and has been developed with substantial support from IBPGR/CGIAR. IBPGR has published its Annual Report for 1974 and Programme and Budget Proposals for 1976 (IBPGR Secretariat 1975a,b). The program for 1976 is wide ranging, with substantial financial support in key areas, as is evident from the main headings:

GR/CIDS	$360,000
Support for germ plasm activities	
International centers	$115,000
Regional Programs	$218,000
Exploration of priority crops and facilities in base collections	$250,000
Crop committees, workshops	$ 60,000
Quarantine problems	$ 10,000
Support for training programs	$ 35,000
Board meetings and missions	$130,000
Secretarial expenses (the secretariat is provided by FAO)	$ 60,000
Contingencies	$100,000

At this stage only general comments are possible. I shall make three.

First, the program specifies priority regions and signifies the designation of priority crops to be announced shortly. It would appear that both, with few exceptions and changes of emphasis, follow the priorities designated by the panel in its recommendations. These were intended as guidelines rather than as administrative rules. It is to be hoped that the board will take a similarly liberal attitude and avoid rigid observance. Exploration depends on the availability of competent and willing explorers; considering the short supply of such people, exploration policies should therefore be mercurial within reasonable limits following up initiatives and opportunities. Moreover, urgency or even emergency arises quickly, or it is suddenly discovered to exist, in species or areas not considered priorities even a few months earlier.

Second, it seems unlikely that the exploration activities of 1976, considering the state of planning and preparation, will be able to absorb a greater part of the allocated $250,000. There is a strong case for supplying storage facilities as a matter of urgency to base and to active collections in the developing countries, especially in Southeast and South Asia where there are none at present.

Third, cooperative networks, leading up to a figurative global network, have been advocated and negotiated for years, with no tangible result as yet. The Near East network, of which Pakistan is a member, is under discussion by the board; it is possible that agreement has been reached. The lesson that has emerged is that a network will work only if it has functions that have clear advantages to the participants and if they themselves are in a position to make a major contribution rather than depend on the internationally funded Big Brother—whether a regional center or an international institute. Such a cooperative network appears to be emerging in Southeast Asia with the participation of IBPGR.

Perhaps I may be permitted a philosophical comment. As I have said earlier, the advent of an international body with the ability to procure and distribute funds is a very great step forward. Furthermore, together with FAO it has the capacity to stimulate coordination and rationalization. But it must be borne in mind that the bulk of genetic resource activities remains the responsibility of institutions all over the world, which will continue to have the largest collections, with all their immanent shortcomings, and most of the scientific competence and leadership. It would be a mistake should the board attempt to assume the role of a world government of genetic resources rather than strive to stimulate and support the activities of institutions, individuals, and the emerging cooperative moves which the board can do much to encourage.

CONCLUSIONS: IS IT WORTHWHILE?

In his review of *Crop Genetic Resources for Today and Tomorrow* (Frankel and Hawkes, 1975), Riley (1976) suggests that a devil's advocate might have been appropriate as a contributor. Here are some of the arguments he might have advanced.

Natural diversity, as we have seen, is a useful source of individual alleles that confer adaptive advantages, such as resistance to pests or diseases, or some physiological characteristics, such as insensitivity to the length of day. However, as Brock (1971) states, "we can induce any mutation that has occurred naturally, and probably many which have either never occurred spontaneously, or have been lost from the natural populations." Because Dr. Brock discusses induced mutation in Chapter 12 of this volume I confine myself to this basic proposition.

Second, it can be argued that primitive cultivars have not been used extensively by plant breeders as sources of either coadapted gene complexes or the coadapted characters that Darwin (1859) recognized as the basis of ecological adaptation; it is possible that they have largely confined themselves to advanced cultivars, assuming, as already discussed, that they incorporate most of the adaptive advantages of their primitive predecessors combined with greater productivity.

Third, the assembly, multiplication, and conservation, as well as the evaluation and use of primitive cultivars are replete with technical and organizational difficulties. Success depends on consensus at national and international levels, so far rarely achieved except under the impact of worldwide emergency.

Fourth, it would be "very expensive" (Harlan, 1975a).

It may be that the first point can be conceded, although our knowledge of the physiology and genetics of disease resistance, both natural and induced, seems scarcely sufficient to declare redundancy of natural resistance sources. At any rate, this is not the case with resistance conferred by related wild species.

What little we know of coadaptation suggests that natural selection and no doubt artificially induced (or influenced) selection have been operative in the evolution and fine adjustment of crop races. While as yet we fail to use, and indeed to recognize, these stores of adaptations, the sciences, which assist and instruct the plant breeder, are likely to do so in years to come. New approaches, such as the analysis of the effects of individual chromosomes, demonstrate previously unsuspected relationships, such as the association in wheat between vernalization requirement and cold resistance, and also between genes for resistance to eyespot and to freezing (Law and Worland, 1973), both relationships at least partly attributable to linkage. The areas that stand most to lose, should their genetic resources be lost, are presumably those in which they evolved and where their adaptations may be most needed.

I believe that what has been said in earlier sections of this chapter and elsewhere (e.g., Frankel, 1976) indicates that the biological basis has, to a large degree, been clarified, that many of the technical problems are solved, and that answers to organizational issues are in sight. Documentation can provide the operational link for all participants to a degree that could make coordination of effort possible and profitable at all levels and in all countries. What is needed is maximum cooperation, which results from flexibility, and minimal bureaucratic restraints. Above all, there is the need to enlist the willing collaboration of the worldwide scientific community, which results not from financial support alone!

The cost of genetic conservation is hard to estimate. The major expense would not come from exploration—which does not have many years to go—but rather from the establishment and operation of conservation facilities and from the operative expenses of conservation on the one hand, the many facets of utilization on the other. None of these is of the order of capital and operating expenses of a small number of modern aircraft, if we take the world as a whole. In raising the cost−benefit issue, the real question is: Is it worthwhile?

If, after what has been said, the question remains open, perhaps the only remaining answer is to consider genetic conservation as an evolutionary insurance. The needs and the scientific advances of future generations are unforeseen and unforeseeable. Who foresaw the need for cytoplasmic diversity before the disastrous corn leaf blight epidemic? The very understandable emphasis, especially it seems on the part of IBPGR, on satisfying the needs of present-day plant breeders tends to obscure the responsibility toward the needs of future genera-

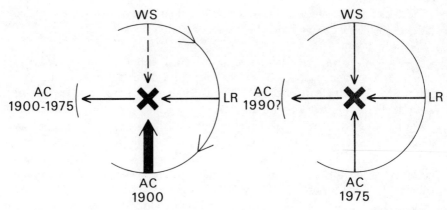

Figure 2. Genetic resources of yesterday (left) and for tomorrow (right). (WS) Wild species; (LR) land races; (AC) advanced cultivars.

tions, which are as real as those of the present, considering that they will have no means of recovering what we now let go by default. It is this responsibility which may help divert our thinking from cost–benefit reasoning to evolutionary resolve.

The future of plant adaptation to human needs, as shown in subsequent chapters, is bright indeed, with likely advances in several fields. In the field of genetic resources one can foresee a shift from the predominant use of advanced cultivars (Fig. 2, *left*) to the use of primitive cultivars, and, perhaps to an equal extent of the almost untapped resources of the wild relatives of our crops (Fig. 2, *right*).

REFERENCES

Bennett, E. (1965). Plant introduction and genetic conservation: Genecological aspects of an important world problem. *Scott. Plant Breed. Sta. Rec.* 27–113.

Bennett, E. (1970*a*). Adaptation in wild and cultivated plant populations. In *Genetic Resources in Plants–Their Exploration and Conservation* (Frankel, O.H. and Bennett, E., eds.), pp. 115–129. Blackwell, Oxford.

Bennett, E. (1970*b*). Tactics of plant exploration. In *Genetic Resources in Plants–Their Exploration and Conservation* (Frankel, O.H. and Bennett, E., eds.), 157–179. Blackwell, Oxford.

Brock, R.D. (1971). The role of induced mutations in plant improvement. *Radiat. Bot.* *11*:181–196.

Carlson, P.S., Smith, H.H., and Dearing, R.D. (1972). Parasexual interspecific plant hybridization. *Proc. Natl. Acad. Sci. USA* 69:2292–2294.

Darwin, C. (1859). *The Origin of Species.* Murray, London.

Dobzhansky, Th. (1970). *Genetics of the Evolutionary Process.* Columbia Univ. Press, New York.

Evans, L.T. and Dunstone, R.L. (1970). Some physiological aspects of evolution in wheat. *Aust. J. Biol. Sci. 23*:725–741.

FAO (1969). *Third Session of the FAO Panel of Experts on Plant Exploration and Conservation, FAO, Rome.*

FAO (1970). *Fourth Session of the FAO Panel of Experts on Plant Exploration and Conservation, FAO, Rome.*

FAO (1975a). *Sixth Session of the FAO Panel of Experts on Plant Exploration and Conservation, FAO, Rome.*

FAO (1975b). *The Methodology of Conservation of Forest Genetic Resources.* FAO, Rome.

Frankel, O.H. (1967). Guarding the plant breeder's treasury. *New Scientist 35*:538–540.

Frankel, O.H. (1970). Genetic conservation in perspective. In *Genetic Resources in Plants– Their Exploration and Conservation* (Frankel, O.H. and Bennett, E., eds.), pp. 469–489. Blackwell, Oxford.

Frankel, O.H. (1973). *Survey of Crop Genetic Resources in Their Centres of Diversity.* FAO/IBP Rome.

Frankel, O.H. (1975). Genetic conservation: Our evolutionary responsibilities. *Genetics 78*:53–65.

Frankel, O.H. (1976). Conservation of crop genetic resources and of their wild relatives–an overview. In *Conservation and Agriculture* (Hawkes, J.G., ed.), Duckworth, London.

Frankel, O.H. and Bennett, E., eds. (1970a). *Genetic Resources in Plants– Their Exploration and Conservation.* (IBP Handbook No. 11.) Blackwell, Oxford.

Frankel, O.H. and Bennett, E. (1970b) Genetic resources. In *Genetic Resources in Plants– Their Exploration and Conservation* (Frankel, O.H. and Bennett, E., eds.), pp. 7–17. Blackwell, Oxford.

Frankel, O.H. and Hawkes, J.G. eds. (1975). *Crop Genetic Resources for Today and Tomorrow.* Cambridge Univ. Press, Cambridge.

Guldager, P. (1975). *Ex situ* conservation in stands in the tropics. In *The Methodology of Conservation of Forest Genetic Sources,* pp. 85–92. FAO, Rome.

Guzman, E. (1975). Conservation of vanishing wood species in the Philippines. In *South East Asian plant genetic resources.* LIPI, Bogor.

Harlan, J.R. (1951). Anatomy of gene centers. *Am. Naturalist 85*:97–103.

Harlan, J.R. (1967). A wild wheat harvest in Turkey. *Archaeology 20*:197–201.

Harlan, J.R. (1971). Agricultural origins: Centers and noncenters. *Science 174*:468–474.

Harlan, J.R. (1972). Genetics of disaster. *J. Environ. Quality 1*:212–215.

Harlan, J.R. (1975a). *Crops and Man.* American Society of Agronomy, Madison, Wisc.

Harlan, J.R. (1975b). Our vanishing genetic resources. *Science 188*:618–621.

Harrington, J.F. (1970). Seed and pollen storage for conservation of plant gene resources. In *Genetic Resources in Plants– Their Exploration and Conservation* (Frankel, O.H. and Bennett, E., eds.), pp. 501–521. Blackwell, Oxford.

IBP (1966). Plant gene pools. *IBP News 5*:48–51.

IBPGR (1975a). *Annual Report 1974.* IBPGR Secretariat, Rome.

IBPGR (1975b).*Programme and Budget Proposals for 1976.*IBPGR Secretariat, Rome.

Jain, S.K. (1969). Comparative ecogenetics of two *Avena* species occurring in Central California. *Evolut. Biol. 3*:73–118.

Law, C.N. and Worland, A.J. (1973). Chromosome substitutions and their use in the analysis and prediction of wheat varietal performance. *Proc. 4th Int. Wheat Genetics Symposium.* Missouri Agr. Exp. Sta. Columbia, Mo.

Maggs, D.H. (1972). Pistachios in Iran and California. *Plant Introd. Rev. 9(1)*:12–15.

Maggs, D.H. (1973). Genetic resources in pistachio. *Plant Genet. Res. Newsl. 29*:7–15.

Marshall, D.R. and Allard, R.W. (1970). Isozyme polymorphisms in natural populations of *Avena fatua* and *A. barbata. Heredity 25*:373–382.

Marshall, D.R. and Brown, A.H.D. (1975). Optimum sampling strategies in genetic conservation. In *Crop Genetic Resources for Today and Tomorrow* (Frankel, O.H. and Hawkes, J.G., eds.), pp. 53–80. Cambridge University Press, Cambridge.

Richardson, S.D. (1970). Gene pools in forestry. In *Genetic Resources in Plants—Their Exploration and Conservation* (Frankel, O.H. and Bennett, E., eds.), pp. 353–365. Blackwell, Oxford.

Riley, R. (1976). Review of Frankel, O.H. and Hawkes, J.G. (eds.). *Nature 259*:347–348.

Roberts, E.H. (1975). Problems of long-term storage of seed and pollen for genetic resources conservation. In *Crop Genetic Resources for Today and Tomorrow* (Frankel, O.H. and Hawkes, J.G., eds.), pp. 269–296. Cambridge University Press, Cambridge.

Sears, E.R. (1956). The transfer of leaf-rust resistance from *Aegilops umbellulata* to wheat. *Brookhaven Symp. Biol. 9*:1–22.

Sykes, J.T. (1972). Tree fruit resources in Turkey. *Plant Gen. Res. Newsl. 27*:17–21.

Thompson, P.A. (1974). The use of seed-banks for conservation of populations of species and ecotypes. *Biol. Conserv. 6*:15–19.

United Nations (1972). *Report of the United Nations Conference on the Human Environment, Stockholm, 5–16 June 1972.* General Assembly A/Conf. 48/14.

Unesco (1973). Programme on Man and the Biosphere (MAB). Expert Panel on Project 8: Conservation of natural areas and of the genetic material they contain. *MAB rep. ser. No.12.*

Unesco (1974). MAB Task Force on Criteria and guidelines for the choice and establishment of biosphere reserves. *MAB rep. ser. No.22.*

Vavilov, N.I. (1926). *Studies on the Origin of Cultivated Plants.* Institute of Applied Botany and Plant Breeding, Leningrad.

Villiers, T.A. (1975). Genetic maintenance of seeds in imbibed storage. In *Crop Genetic Resources for Today and Tomorrow* (Frankel, O.H. and Hawkes, J.G., eds.), pp. 297–315. Cambridge University Press, Cambridge.

Wang, B.S.P. (1975). Tree seed and pollen storage for genetic conservation: Possibilities and limitations. In *The Methodology of Conservation of Forest Genetic Resources* pp. 93–103. FAO, Rome.

Whitmore, T.C. (1975). S.E. Asian forests as unexploited source of fast growing timber. In *South East Asian Plant Genetic Resources.* LIPI, Bogor.

Zagaja, S.W. (1970). Temperate zone tree fruits. In *Genetic Resources in Plants—Their Exploration and Conservation* (Frankel, O.H. and Bennett, E., eds.), pp. 327–333. Blackwell, Oxford.

Zohary, D. and Feldman, M. (1962). Hybridization between amplidiploids and the evolution of polyploids in the wheat (*Aegilops—Triticum*) group. *Evolution 16*:44–61.

Zohary, D. and Spiegel-Roy, P. (1975). Beginnings of fruit growing in the Old World. *Science 187*:319–327.

Zohary, D., Harlan, J.R., and Vardi, J. (1969). The wild diploid progenitors of wheat and their breeding value. *Euphytica 18*:58–65.

5

On Germ Plasm Conservation with Special Reference to the Genus *Medicago*

R. C. von Borstel and K. Lesins

Department of Genetics
University of Alberta
Edmonton, Alberta, Canada T6G 2E9

ABSTRACT

As Frankel has indicated, there is ample justification for maintaining international germ plasm centers for preservation of land races and species of a genus; this would appear self-evident on the grounds that extinction involves a permanent loss of gene pools that have required from several centuries to millions of years to evolve. Monoculture is causing extinction of some *Medicago* species, yet all species of the genus *Medicago* are of economic importance. Examples are drawn from recent crosses involving wild species of this genus, and we note the rapidly increasing appreciation of the value of annual *Medicago* species. Their potential future use in the South Temperate Zone countries is discussed.

INTRODUCTION

Frankel (1976) asks the rhetorical question of whether it is worthwhile to assemble, multiply, and conserve the primitive cultivars or samples of wild populations of species from which advanced cultivars have been developed or which may have the potential of being cultivated. Several corollary arguments can be added to Frankel's general argument that the discarding of a land race and the extinction of a species constitute a permanent loss. How important such collections could be would depend, of course, on the purposes for which they were initially established, especially on the subsequent policy of their management. Although never explicitly stated, it seems that there have been a number of cases in which painstakingly assembled collections of genetic stocks have been lost or the gene pool they initially contained has been greatly impoverished because of ignorance or a shortsighted management policy. An analysis of the geographic patterns of variation in some cultivated plants made by Harlan (1975), wherein he refers to the pioneering works of Vavilov, concludes as follows:

> The world of N. I. Vavilov is vanishing and the sources of genetic variability are drying up. The patterns of variation we have been discussing here may no longer be discernible in a few decades and the living traces of the long coevolution of cultivated plants may well disappear forever.

There are two approaches to the task of preventing the erosion of the gene resources of the economically important plant species: (1) to maintain collections of live seeds, and (2) the suggestion of Dr. Clayton O. Person (personal communication) that large sanctuaries be established in the centers of origin and diversity where the plant species of interest grow naturally in the company of other species, including the parasitic ones (e.g., insects, fungi, bacteria, viruses), with which they have evolved. According to Person, there is no point in growing the plants in sanctuaries away from their parasites and, generally, away from the natural selective forces operating on them.

However, even tiny sanctuaries of a few square meters would be of great value in saving some species from extinction. For example, the rare species *Medicago heyniana* Greuter, an annual, is endemic only on the island of Karpathos in the Aegean archipelago. The goats roaming freely in the area snap off every edible shoot and pick up ripe pods that have fallen on the ground. A few small, well-fenced patches scattered over the rocky island would serve the purpose of preserving this species and would not be objectionable, as would a large sanctuary, to the users of common pastures. One is surprised at the richness of species and varieties found in somewhat protected small areas, such as old cemeteries, and tourist attractions, such as the ancient ruins. In Athens goats are not permitted to browse freely; hence we still find *Medicago arborea* at the Acropolis and on Lycabettus Hill. This shrub *Medicago* is now seen only very rarely in the Greek countryside.

The importance of the plant collections or natural sanctuaries, or both, becomes increasingly self-evident, from both the scientific and the economic–utilitarian points of view, to those directly involved, and to the public at large. After these general remarks, let us consider the case of domesticated alfalfa and annual *Medicago*.

ALFALFA (LUCERNE)

Alfalfa, as we know it in the North Temperate Zone, has originated from crosses of the two perennial species—the northern *Medicago falcata* and *M. sativa,* the latter having been brought to Greece during the Greco-Persian wars. It was taken into cultivation as horse fodder in ancient Persia following the revolutionary change in warfare when horse-drawn chariots were introduced (Lesins, 1976). Under cultivation the originally diploid *M. sativa* (*M. coerulea*) became tetraploid. It is not possible to decide whether the stronger tetraploid plants, which arose naturally, attracted the attention of growers who collected seeds from them, or whether the tetraploids under cared-for conditions simply crowded out the less vigorous diploids. The *Medicago sativa* × *M. falcata* hybrids from Greece, now known as *M. varia* or *M. media,* spread to Italy and from there traveled everywhere with the Roman armies and colonists. With the collapse of the Roman Empire, alfalfa cultivation disappeared for about 1000 years.

It was not until this century that *M. sativa* was again crossed with *M. falcata.* This was done by Hansen in 1914 at the Agricultural Experiment Station in Brookings, South Dakota. Improved alfalfa varieties have now been made by crosses within populations of Hansen's original cross, or by crossing *M. falcata* from Hansen's collection with cultivated alfalfa. Some of these crosses and their advantages are listed in Table I.

The Teton variety, shown in Table I, was selected from within populations that survive from Hansen's original cross. All the others were new crosses. A common thread runs through the strains for the characters introduced, and why not? Offspring still resemble parents, and similar selections yield similar advantages.

There is no doubt that a cost accounting of the increased profits and tax monies realized from the alfalfa production produced by the crosses shown in Table I, when compared to prior strains, would be enough justification for support of an international germ plasm center for the genus *Medicago.* But let us look further.

OTHER PERENNIALS

Other useful characters exist in the wild perennial species of *Medicago*—glandular hairs in some varieties of *M. falcata* confer resistance to the alfalfa weevil and to the potato leafhopper (R. D. Shade, unpublished); *M. cancellata,* which makes viable hybrids with *M. sativa,* has a high level of resistance against Stemphylium leafspot (Borges et al., 1976). Self-pollinating varieties with high forage yield and high tolerance against inbreeding depression have been developed from crosses of *M. falcata* and *M. sativa* (K. Lesins, unpublished). These perennial species of *Medicago* can be crossed with each other, especially after the

Table I. Varieties of Alfalfa Derived by Inclusion of Germ Plasm from Wild Species

Cross Wild sp. × cult.	Variety	Place	Characters introduced	Ref.
M. falcata × M. media	Rhizoma	British Columbia	Low-temperature tolerance High seed and forage yield Spreading growth	Nilan (1951)
M. falcata × M. media	Narragansett	Rhode Island	Winter hardiness Tolerance to foliar diseases High seed and forage yield	Graber (1953)
M. falcata × M. media	Vernal	Wisconsin	Wilt resistance Yellow-leaf blotch tolerance Winter hardiness High forage yield	Brink et al. (1955)
M. falcata × M. media	Rambler	Saskatchewan	Winter hardiness Creeping rootedness Drought resistance	Heinrichs and Bolton (1958)
M. falcata × M. sativa	Teton	South Dakota	Some wilt resistance Common leaf spot resistance Wide, spreading crown Winter hardiness Frost resistance	Adams and Semeniuk (1958)

chromosome doubling technique had been introduced into plant breeding. If collections of *Medicago* did not exist, their characteristics would not be available for improvement of alfalfa on demand.

ANNUAL *MEDICAGO* SPECIES

Many of the species of *Medicago* are annuals. Appreciation of their value is rapidly increasing. Not less than 10 cultivars belonging to four species (*M. truncatula, M. littoralis, M. rugosa,* and *M. tornata*) are already available for agriculture in Western Australia (McComb, 1974). A vigorous search for special annual *Medicago* species and varieties has been launched by the South Australia Department of Agriculture. Expeditions have been sent to countries around the Mediterranean to collect endemic annual *Medicago* species (M. J. Mathison, personal communication). Annuals used for grazing in rotation with cereal (wheat) crops considerably increase the returns from the land. Some annual species have been introduced and are components of rangeland stands in the southern states of the United States and in some South American countries. Pakistan is one of the South Temperate Zone countries in which several species of annual *Medicago* grow naturally (D. R. Cornelius, personal communication). It would be timely for Pakistan's agricultural authorities to turn to studies of the use of endemic as well as introduced annual *Medicago*. According to our observations, great variations in growth, vigor, maturing time, spininess, and other agriculturally significant characters can be found in the same species.

CONCLUSION

It would be a useful enterprise for agricultural economists to prepare cost—benefit analyses for introduced wild species in agriculture and to sum up useful characters from wild species, land races, or primitive strains against commonly used cultivars of economic plants as well. Such analyses would provide ample economic justification for maintaining representative germ plasm collections for each genus. A cost—benefit justification is often adamantly required by governmental agencies before they endorse support for any scientific endeavor. Unfortunately, keeping a species or land race alive for its own sake or for future generations is often, in the eyes of governmental agencies, not justification enough.

REFERENCES

Adams, M. W., and Semeniuk, G. (1958). Teton alfalfa, a new multipurpose variety for South Dakota. Agriculture Experiment Station, South Dakota State College, Brookings. Bull. 469.

Borges, O. L., Stanford, E. H., and Webster, R. (1976). Sources and inheritance of resistance to *Stemphylium* leafspot in alfalfa. *Crop Sci. 16*:458–461.

Brink, R. A., Jones, F. R., Smith, D., and Graber, L. F. (1955). Vernal alfalfa. Univ. Wisconsin Spec. Circ. 37.

Frankel, O. H. (1976) Natural variation and its conservation. In *Genetic Diversity in Plants* (Muhammed, Amir, Aksel, R., and von Borstel, R. C., eds.), pp. 21–43. Plenum Press, New York and London.

Graber, L. F. (1953). Registration of varieties and strains of alfalfa, II. *Agron. J. 45*: 330–331.

Harlan, J. R. (1975). Geographic patterns of variation in some cultivated plants. *J. Hered. 66*:182–191.

Heinrichs, D. H. and Bolton, J. L. (1958). Rambler alfalfa. Can. Dept. Agr. Publ. No. 1030.

Lesins, K. (1976). Alfalfa, lucerne, In *Evolution of Crop Plants* (N. W. Simmonds, ed.), pp. 165–168. Longman, London.

McComb, J. A. (1974). Annual *Medicago* species with particular reference to those occurring in Western Australia. *J. Roy. Soc. West Australia. 57(3)*:81–96.

Nilan, R. A. (1951). Rhizoma alfalfa: Chromosome studies of the parent stocks. *Sci Agr. 31*:123–126.

6

Distribution Patterns of Indigenous Wheat Varieties in Northern Pakistan

Altafur Rehman Rao

Department of Botany
University of Agriculture
Lyallpur, Pakistan

ABSTRACT

Phytogeographic distribution of genetic variability pertaining to eight characters recorded in 115 primitive wheat accessions of *Triticum aestivum vulgare* L. was studied by dividing the qualitative characters into two and the quantitative ones into five categories. The categories so devised were plotted on maps of the area of exploration. Clear-cut patterns of distribution emerged for the qualitative characters, i.e., disease reaction, awns, and the auricle color. However, the "single-character graphs" of quantitative characters showed a generally diffuse, but in some areas nonrandom, distribution for length of flag leaf, height of stem, and days to heading. Even less-pronounced geographic patterns emerged for length of ear and yield per plant. These investigations afford useful information for future expeditions.

INTRODUCTION

Northern Pakistan is on the rim of the vast area between the Caucasus and Western Iran where hexaploid wheat originated and evolved (see, e.g., Harlan and Zohary, 1966; Johnson, 1972). It is a mountainous region, having many peaks that exceed 15,000 ft, including Nangaparbat (26,660 ft), one of the world's highest mountains. The valleys are reached by high mountain passes and are largely isolated from each other as well as from the outside world. Crops were collected from altitudes of 4000 ft to over 10,000 ft. Most of the region is dry; wheat is grown under irrigation in the valley bottoms or on river terraces (Figs. 1 and 2).

In this isolated area the indigenous varieties have presumably remained relatively undisturbed by introductions, hence are of great interest. Affinities or differences among individual collections among groups of collections with similar environments, and among river valleys could be attributable to natural selection, deliberate selection, or social selection (i.e., introductions from other villages or valleys) or combinations of these. Close studies in the region itself and of plantings in a single environment could provide some answers. This study is a first attempt, using transplant populations planted at Lyallpur.

Unfortunately, detailed studies of this kind have scarcely been undertaken on land-race material in its original state. An exception is the study of primitive cereals conducted by the author in Eastern Nepal (Rao, 1974), in which clear distributional patterns of genetic variability were demonstrated. The present studies were undertaken to determine the nature of patterns of genetic variability in Northern Pakistan.

MATERIALS AND METHODS

One hundred and fifteen accessions of *Triticum aestivum* were collected by the Bangor–Lyallpur Universities Expedition in Northern Pakistan in 1974. The

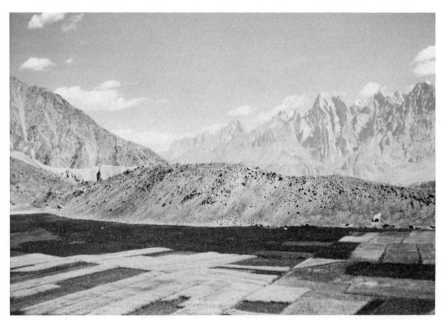

Fig. 1. A flat piece of land surrounded by denuded hills near Khaplu and Skardu.

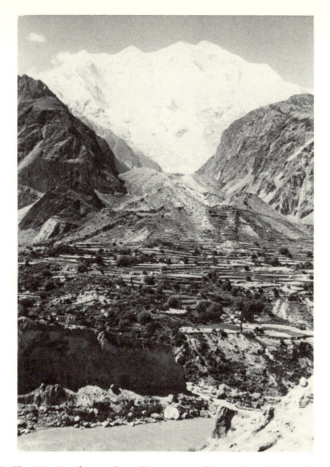

Fig. 2. The irrigational water from the snowy peak is used to cultivate the terraces.

collection sites are shown in Fig. 3. They were sown at Lyallpur in a field fertilized with 8.1 kg (18 lb) of P_2O_5 and 33.8 kg (75 lb) of nitrogen per acre. Seeds were planted in November at distances of 30.5 cm (12 in.) between and 15.2 cm (6 in.) within rows. Nearly 40 plants of each accession were raised. The following qualitative and quantitative characters were recorded on approximately 10 plants per accession:

Disease reaction	Days to heading
State of awns	Height of stem
Color of auricle	Length of ear
Length of flag leaf	Yield per plant

Eight single characters were plotted on the map of the exploration area (Figs. 4–11). The qualitative characters were divided into two and the quantitative characters into five classes (character states). An attempt was made to keep the classes in the quantitative characters about equal in size. The range of variability in characters observed is shown in Table I, and the symbols for the range of characters correspond to those plotted in Figs. 4–11.

RESULTS AND DISCUSSION

Qualitative Characters

It will be seen from Figs. 4–6 that the qualitative characters show well-marked geographic patterns of variability for the three characters plotted. With regard to disease reaction (Fig. 4), more than 80% of the accessions were severely attacked by leaf and stem rusts. Some resistant accessions came from collections from the lower villages of the Chitral and Skardu regions; others were scattered in the Kaghan and Nangaparbat valleys. Not a single rust-resistant accession was observed from the Yasin, Ishkuman, and Gilgit regions; yet at the site of the collection in 1974, these stocks rarely showed any sign of disease, possibly owing to differences in the environments or in the pathogen itself.

The map for awns (Fig. 5) also exhibited a pattern of geographic distribution. Peripheral areas show awnless accessions, and the awned wheats are confined to the central (Yasin, Ishkuman, and Gilgit) regions. However, there is a sporadic occurrence of awned accessions from the Kaghan and Nangaparbat valleys. Such a geographic distribution of awned and awnless wheats can result from either deliberate or natural selection pressures, or both. The former are thought to have had a more pronounced effect than the latter, thanks to sociological contacts between the valleys in the almost insurmountable mountain barriers. The scarcity of birds in the area is perhaps a factor responsible for restricting conscious selection for awns.

Approximately 80% of the accessions showed white auricle color. The remaining 20% exhibited anthocyanin pigmentation, which is confined to the eastern part of the exploration area (Fig. 6).

Quantitative Characters

As might have been expected, the quantitative characters did not show similarly clear-cut patterns of geographic distribution. For the length of the flag leaf (Fig. 7) there are some marked local patterns and an otherwise a random distribution. The longest flag leaf was found in the wheats of Eastern Indus and Skardu, the shortest in the Chitral, and upper Hunza and Nangaparbat valleys. Elsewhere all categories are well scattered. In the Nepalese materials the shortest flag leaf was confined to high altitudes, and the longest to low altitudes (Rao, 1974); this is not in accord with the present results which suggest a near-random altitudinal distribution.

The number of days to heading shows a more consistent distribution pattern (Fig. 8). The latest flowering collections are confined to the Yasin and Ishkuman regions, whereas those of the adjoining Hunza valley are midflowering. In the Chitral and Nangaparbat valleys early flowering is prevalent. Elsewhere there are no clear patterns.

The height of stem (Fig. 9) in the Hunza and Yasin valleys is tallest, whereas the lower portion of the map shows a predominance of short stems. The remaining entries showed a random geographic distribution of the remaining states of this character. These results fail to corroborate the Nepalese observations where high-altitude villages had high frequencies of tall-stemmed wheats and the low altitude villages the reverse.

Length of ear (Fig. 10) and yield per plant (Fig. 11) do not show a consistent pattern apart from similarities among a few adjacent collections. With the exception of the highest class, length of ear and yield per plant frequently coincide on the maps, which suggested that these characters might be correlated. However, this has not been verified statistically. In fact, the highest class of ear length and yield showed the reverse pattern. The Hunza and parts of Ishkuman valleys, situated at the highest elevations, have the longest ears but not the heaviest yields; the heaviest yielders are confined to the Chitral, Kaghan, and Nangaparbat regions.

Table I. Range of Variability in the Qualitative and Quantitative Characters[a]

	Qualitative characters				
Figure	State I ◑		State II ◎		
4. Disease reaction	Disease free		Diseased by rust		
5. State of awns	Awned		Awnless		
6. Color of auricle	Anthocyanin pigmentation		No anthocyanin pigmentation		

	Quantitative characters				
Figure	State I ◑	State II ◎	State III ●	State IV ○	State V ⊘
7. Length of flag leaf (cm)	18.7–25.8	25.9–28.3	28.4–29.7	29.9–31.1	31.2–42.2
8. Days to heading	102.1–126.6	126.7–131.6	131.8–134.8	134.9–138.6	138.7–147.2
9. Height of stem (cm)	64.0–103.3	103.4–109.5	109.7–114.0	114.1–118.5	118.6–131.5
10. Length of ear (cm)	7.0–11.4	11.5–12.4	12.5–13.2	13.3–14.0	14.1–16.5
11. Yield per plant (g)	0.7–2.5	2.6–5.9	6.0–8.7	8.8–12.4	12.5–26.6

[a]Symbols correspond to those shown in Figs. 4–11.

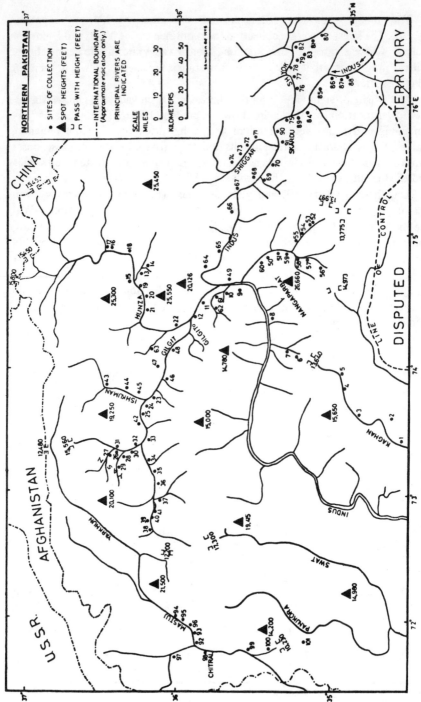

Fig. 3. Map and names of villages (collection sites) and their altitudes.

Names of Villages at the Collection Sites Shown in Figure 3, and Their Altitudes

	Village	Altitude m	Altitude ft		Village	Altitude m	Altitude ft		Village	Altitude m	Altitude ft
1	Balakot	1100	3600	35	Tangai	2440	8000	69	Katzarah	2190	7200
2	Urni	2560	8400	36	Pingal	2560	8400	70	Pakora	2160	7100
3	Plunder	2240	7350	37	Chhashi	2770	9100	71	Shigar	2230	7300
4	Battakundi	2830	9300	38	Barsat	3230	10,600	72	Hushupa	2290	7500
5	Dunga Banse	2900	9500	39	Teru	3140	10,300	73	Sildi	2320	7600
6	Babusar	2960	9700	40	Serbal	2930	9600	74	Huno	2350	7700
7	Thaknala	1920	6300	41	Phandar	2930	9600	75	Gol	2320	7600
8	Gunarfarm	1280	4200	42	Sumal	2100	6900	76	Gwali	2440	8000
9	Thelichi	1490	4900	43	Imit	2380	7800	77	Kurphak	2500	8200
10	Jaglot	1490	4900	44	Chatorkhand	2100	6900	78	Bara	2530	8300
11	Parri Bungla	1490	4900	45	Hasis	1980	6500	79	Khapalu	2500	8200
12	Minawar	1580	5200	46	Singal	1770	5800	80	Kustang	2680	8800
13	Nagir	2590	8500	47	Sherqila	1720	5650	81	Dou	2590	8500
14	Hoppar	2770	9100	48	Shirot	1740	5700	82	Surmo	2590	8500
15	Baltit	2290	7500	49	Bunji	1460	4800	83	Hanjore	2990	9800
16	Alnabad	2470	8100	50	Harchu	2130	7000	84	Parkutta	2260	7400
17	Shishkot	2530	8300	51	Idgah	2380	7800	85	Tolti	2380	7800
18	Kamadas	2290	7500	52	Palagnot	3260	10,700	86	Chuksido	2410	7900
19	Tashot	2230	7300	53	Khirim	3080	10,100	87	Bagicha	2530	8300
20	Gulmat	2040	6700	54	Gudai	3020	9900	88	Garekhdo	2590	8500
21	Sikandarabad	1980	6500	55	Kushnat	2960	9700	89	Sermi	2560	7400
22	Jutal	1675	5500	56	Junji	2990	9800	90	Thorgubala	2230	7300
23	Gakush	1890	6200	57	Rattu	2620	8600	91	Skardu	2290	7500
24	Haim	1980	6500	58	Rampur	2560	8400	92	Rag	1550	5100
25	Yangal	2060	6750	59	Gurikot	2440	8000	93	Pine Mor Shagf	1680	5500
26	Yasin	2470	8100	60	Mushkin	1680	5500	94	Buni	2130	7000
27	Ishkaibar	2590	8500	61	Chakarkot	1710	5600	95	Zaid	1830	6000
28	Taus	2470	8100	62	Jagot	1830	6000	96	Baranas	1830	6000
29	Baltiring	2740	9000	63	Naltar	3050	10,000	97	Shogor	1770	5800
30	Atkash	2440	8000	64	Sasi	1430	4700	98	Chitral	1460	4800
31	Sandhi	2470	8100	65	Shengus	1980	6500	99	Drosh	1280	4200
32	Hilter	2440	8000	66	Twa	2040	6700	100	Ashirat	1740	5700
33	Gupis	2210	7250	67	Byicha	2040	6700	101	Dir	1310	4300
34	Dahimal	2290	7500	68	Tsari	2190	7200				

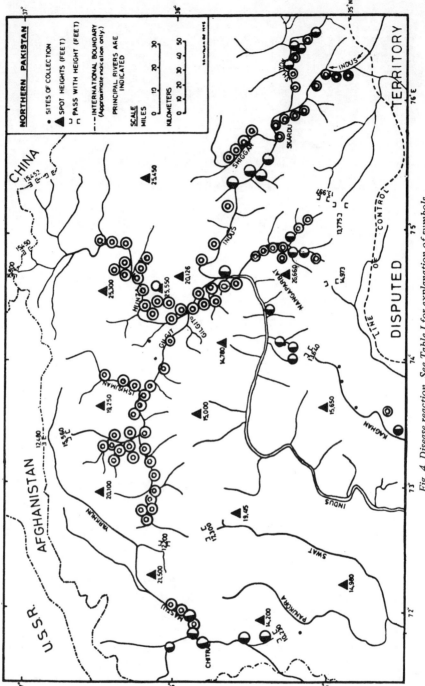

Fig. 4. Disease reaction. See Table I for explanation of symbols.

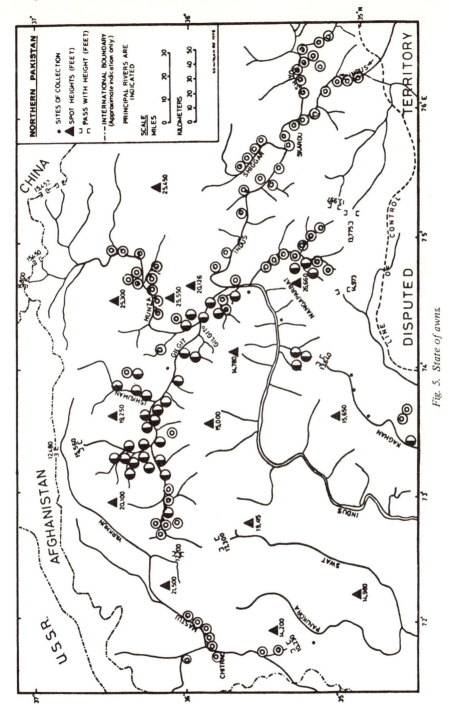

Fig. 5. State of awns

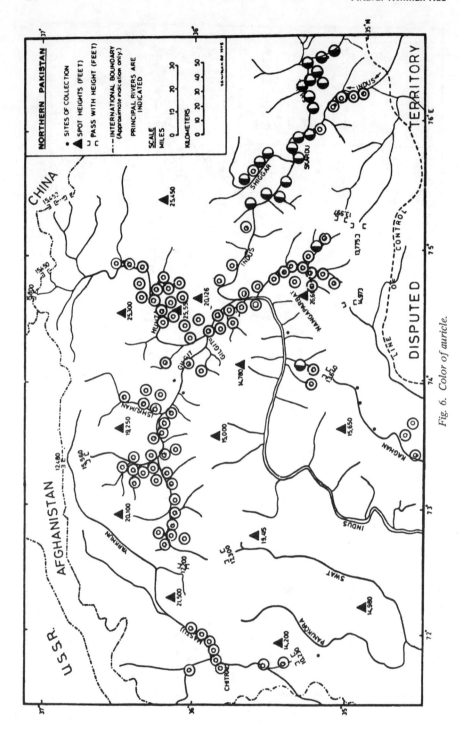

Fig. 6. Color of auricle.

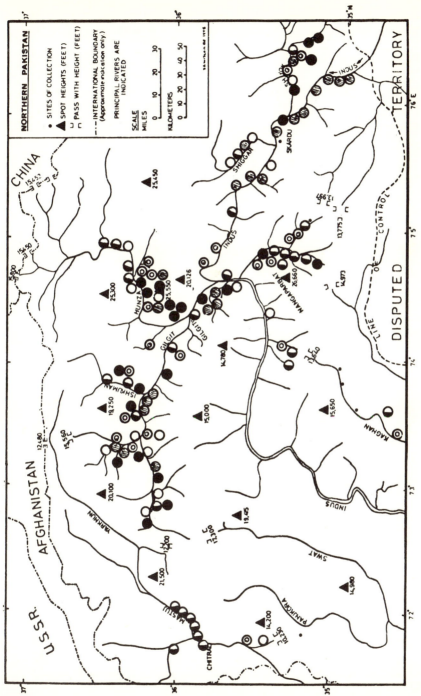

Fig. 7. Length of flag leaf.

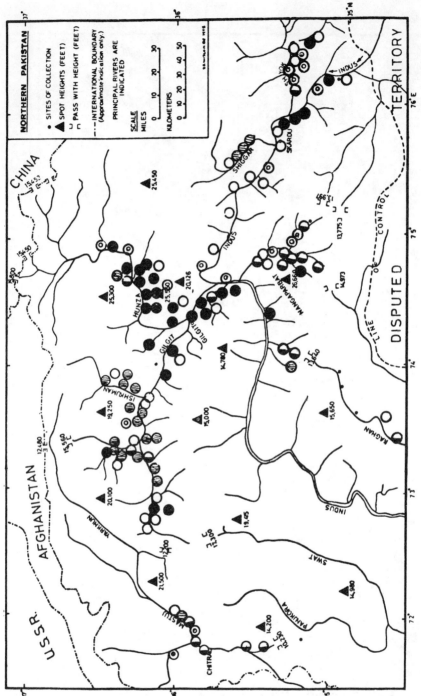

Fig. 8. Days to heading.

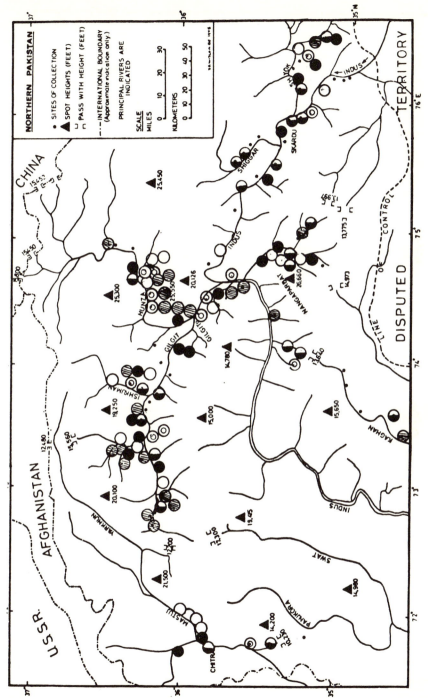

Fig. 9. Height of stem.

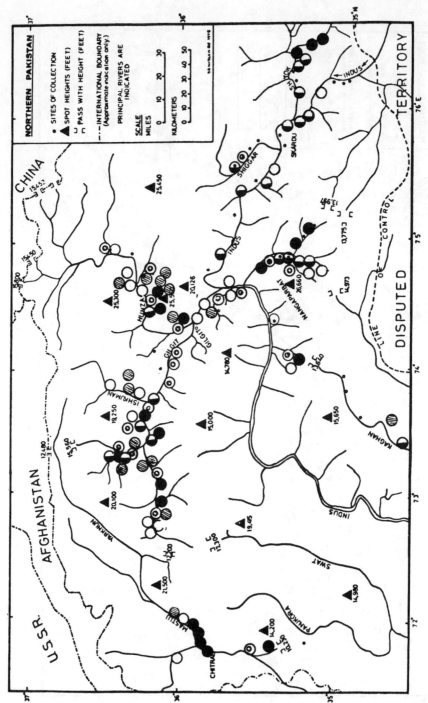

Fig. 10. Length of ear.

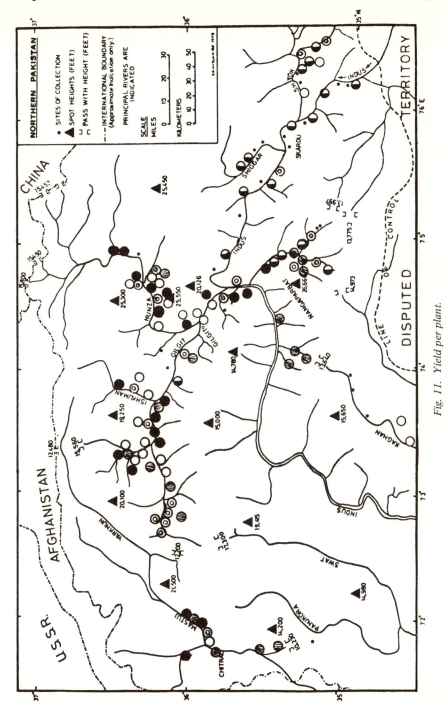

Fig. 11. Yield per plant.

The patterns of yield are not in agreement with those of Nepal where high-altitude areas are the poorest yielders, and conversely the low altitude areas are the highest yielding.

Apparently, the emergence of diffuse patterns indicated by quantitative characters, such as yield, height of stem, and length of ear, are at least partly the result of conscious selection. But the pressure of natural selection cannot be ignored—it stabilized the populations for the qualitative characters studied, much more so than for the quantitative characters, no doubt because of the heterogeneity of the environments.

It should be noted that haphazard introduction of wheat "varieties" from Iran, Afghanistan, Russia, and China was another factor that greatly increased the variability.

Among the people of this area, the understanding of a variety is rather vague. They could name many varieties of their region, but they were unable to identify any one of them in their field. The color of grain, the yield, and the "keeping" quality of "chapati" are the only criteria for varietal identification and introduction.

Of many stories narrated by the inhabitants, one appeared very interesting. In the Gupis valley, a wheat variety was named as Shiroti after the name of the village Shirot. The variety was fairly common in the Gupis valley; when its origin was traced we were told by the residents of this village that a couple of decades ago a swan was hunted whose gut was full of freshly eaten grains of wheat. The grains from the gut were thrown into a nearby field which, on maturity, proved to be a heavy yielding variety, and this is how the Shiroti variety of wheat was "evolved."

ACKNOWLEDGMENTS

The author is highly indebted to Misses Furrakh Saeed and Shamim Rukhsana for furnishing the data and helping him in many other ways. The author wishes to thank Dr. John R. Witcombe for the altitude data used in Figure 3.

REFERENCES

Harlan, J. R. and Zohary, D. (1966). Distribution of wild wheats and barley. *Science* *153*:1074–1080.

Johnson, B. L. (1972) Seed protein profiles and the origin of the hexaploid wheats. *Am. J. Bot. 59*(9):952–960.

Rao, A. R. (1974). The genecology of cereal varieties from Eastern Nepal. Ph.D. thesis, Univ. of Wales (U.K.).

7

Useful Genetic Sources of Economic Importance and Their Utilization in Wheat-Breeding Programs in Pakistan

S.A. Qureshi

Punjab Agricultural Research Institute
Lyallpur, Pakistan

ABSTRACT

Wheat breeders the world over have been utilizing genetic sources to tailor the varieties to meet ever-changing requirements. In the late 1940s Dr. Borlaug at CIMMYT recognized that further increase in yield would be possible only if lodging in the existing wheat varieties could be avoided, for which he began to look for a suitable source for dwarfness. The Japanese had developed semidwarf Norin strains through a series of crosses involving a local line, Daruma; American soft red winter variety, Fultz; and American hard red winter variety, Turkey Red. One of the Norin strains, Norin-10, was used in the breeding programs, first in Italy and then in the United States where Dr. Orville Vogel developed two to three semidwarf varieties. In 1953 Dr. Vogel supplied some F_2 seeds of Norin-10 Brevor to the CIMMYT program in Mexico, where this source was employed extensively in the breeding program; a large number of varieties were developed, some of which worth mentioning are Pitic, Penjamo, Lerma, Sonora, Inia, Tobari, and Siete Cerros.

INTRODUCTION

CIMMYT expanded its international wheat-breeding program in 1961–1962 both to provide plant materials to many developing countries, including India and Pakistan, and to train workers. The purpose of the materials provided was to breed semidwarf, fertilizer-responsive varieties that would combine disease resistance and acceptable quality. Wheat varieties, such as Mexipak, Sandal, PARI, and Lyallpur-73, are examples of selections from exotic materials, and varieties like Chenab-70, Pak-70, Khushal, Barani-70, SA-42, and Potohar have been developed from the local programs.

Present-day agriculture has at its disposal excellent purpose-specific varieties of field crops, orchard trees, and vegetables as well as a very advanced technology for producing high yields. As compared to their wild ancestors, today's varieties have a much higher-yielding ability, a broader range of adaptability to environmental conditions, and qualities that meet the requirements of the users of the produce.

Some 5 to 6 years ago a major genotype of wheat with a certain range of variability in its field characteristics in various environments became widely adopted in this part of the world. Because of its adaptability and high response to fertilizers, it has replaced all the old varieties of wheat in a very short time and has contributed toward the increase of wheat production in many countries.

This genotype is known as Mexipak in Pakistan, Kalyan-Sona in India, and Siete Cerros in Mexico. Derived from a cross between Penjamo and Gabo (cross II-8156), it is now becoming the progenitor of many new varieties. It carries a good combination of genetic characters, such as high responsiveness to fertilizers because of its semidwarf nature, resistance to diseases, a fairly short period to maturity, and a quality suitable for various systems of milling and baking. All these characteristics are derived from a good number of sources through a series of crosses independently made in Japan, Italy, and Mexico.

THE BEGINNING OF THE INCORPORATION OF DWARFNESS IN OTHERWISE ADAPTED VARIETIES

In fact, all the desired characteristics existed in nature in the form of wild ancestors commonly found in primary and secondary centers of origin. From these centers the wild ancestors have spread by means of natural phenomena, such as glaciation and floods as well as through human activities; human direction of the selection pressure led to the establishment of cultivars that met specific requirements.

Natural causes of variability, such as mutations and recombinations, further led to the creation of types that were better adapted to a wide range of climatic conditions. The plants that exist today represent only a small fraction of the total diversity that came into existence since plant forms first appeared. Many kinds of plants became extinct during the various geological epochs (Elliott, 1958).

The strains that possess a wide range of variability in economic characters were later utilized by man to tailor the varieties to suit his particular requirements. This approach became increasingly more fascinating as the knowledge of the mechanism of heredity became better understood and the means of communications better developed.

Japanese work to isolate sources for dwarfness and short maturity periods has given momentum to many wheat-breeding programs in major wheat-growing countries of the world. Japanese farmers were even handling the dwarf varieties in the nineteenth century, most of which were seldom taller than 2 ft. They claimed that their commercial varieties will never lodge even on the richest soils.

This was the type of characteristic that was eagerly sought by such workers as Dr. Orville Vogel at Washington State University and Dr. Norman Borlaug in Mexico, as their breeding efforts had run into a yield plateau caused by lodging under high levels of fertilization. In the words of Dr. Borlaug, cited after Dalrymple (1974)

> We had recognized the barriers on yield imposed by lodging as early as 1948, but we had been frustrated in our search for a useable form of dwarfness to overcome this problem until the discovery of the so-called Norin dwarfs. In 1953 we received a few seeds of several F_2 selections from the cross Norin-10 X Brevor from Dr. Orville Vogel. Our first attempts to incorporate the Norin-10 X Brevor dwarfness into Mexican wheat in 1954 were unsuccessful. A second attempt in 1955 was successful after which it immediately became evident that a new type of wheat was forthcoming with higher yield potential.

Norin-10, a dwarf variety originated in Japan, is thus the source of dwarfness for the major semidwarf commercial varieties all over the world.

Norin-10 itself is not an indigenous variety of Japan and has been obtained through a breeding program. In 1917 Japanese workers crossed a local dwarf variety Daruma with a strain of the American soft red winter wheat variety Fultz to produce a strain known as Fultz–Daruma. This strain was, in turn, crossed in 1924 with the American hard red winter variety Turkey Red. One of the strains derived from this cross later became known as Norin-10. It was released as a commercial variety in Japan in 1938. This variety was used in the breeding programs first in Italy and then in the United States and Mexico, and presently its derivatives are extensively used in Pakistan, India, and a few Middle East and African countries.

The F_2 selections made in Mexico from the original cross Norin-10 X Brevor received from Dr. Vogel provided the source for dwarfness for many dwarf and semidwarf varieties like Pitic–Penjamo-62, Sonora-64, Mayo-64, Inia-66, Tobai-66, Ciano-67, Norteno-67, and Siete Cerros. Most of these varieties became the commercial varieties in Mexico.

Other genetic traits of great economic importance that were incorporated into a large number of today's commercial varieties are earliness and tolerance to hot winds. The source of these traits was also found in Japanese wheat varieties. These varieties were used first in Italy to confer earliness and other useful traits to local varieties. Mentena is a classic example of Italian-bred wheats used as a source of earliness and resistance to stripe rust in many breeding programs. It played a key role in the Mexican wheat-breeding programs in the 1940s. Its traits were incorporated into Frontana and Kentana, which in turn became the progenitors of a large number of commercial varieties that now occupy almost two-thirds of the spring wheat acreage for the world (Borlaug, 1968).

A CHANGE IN BREEDING PROGRAM IN PAKISTAN

In the mid-1960s wheat breeders in Pakistan decided to change their philosophy; they subjected their segregating materials to high-fertility conditions and to screening for resistance to rusts under artificial infective conditions. This was the time when active cooperation was sought from the CIMMYT for technical assistance. The Ford Foundation, the Rockefeller Foundation, and the Food and Agricultural Organization of the United Nations provided the financial assistance. Until that time, major emphasis was on the development of high-quality wheats with semihard, plump white grains to be used in the preparation of white, palatable, and attractive Chapaties. The varieties with these grain characteristics were mostly the local tall selections, except for the Yalta and Dirk varieties from Australia, and Mentena from Italy. None of these were semidwarfs. The crosses made were local X local collections. Selections from them resulted in considerable improvement in grain characteristics, but the yields always remained very much the same. This situation could not meet the country's food requirements for a rapidly increasing population. The breeding philosophies therefore had to be changed by adopting the same course adopted by Dr. Borlaug a decade earlier under identical agricultural and social conditions (Qureshi et al., 1967).

HIGH-YIELDING VARIETIES OBTAINED IN PAKISTAN

In 1961 one set of crosses was received from CIMMYT. One entry among them, cross II-8156, was still segregating and had some promising peculiarities. From it two to three strains were obtained. One strain met the local requirements and was later named Mexipak. Within 3 years Mexipak became the major commercial variety and has now replaced all the old varieties. The genealogy of Mexipak is given in Fig. 1.

Under the accelerated program begun in 1965, segregating materials, advanced lines, and various international nursery entries began arriving in Pakistan

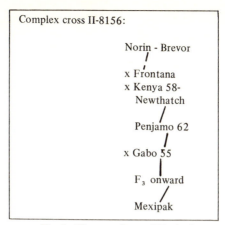

Fig. 1. The genealogy of Mexipak.

from CIMMYT. The breeding program was thus strengthened and diversified, and selections were directed to develop specific-purpose varieties.

The local program was then geared to select lines suitable for direct introduction as well as for local X exotic crosses to diversify the program. A number of varieties have been developed both by selections from the segregating materials received from CIMMYT and from hybrids that involve local varieties as one of the parents. Among the varieties developed from segregating materials obtained from CIMMYT are Sandal, PARI, LYP-73, as well as those obtained from crosses made in Pakistan, which involve the local varieties Chenab-70, Barani-70, SA-42, Potohar, Khushal, and Pak-70. The genealogies of Chenab-70, Barani-70, and SA-42 are given in Figure 2.

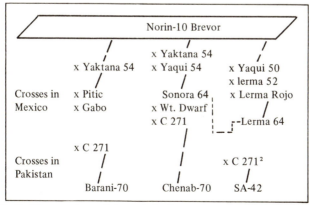

Fig. 2. The genealogy of the varieties Barani-70, Chenab-70, and SA-42.

In addition to the search for semidwarf fertilizer-responsive varieties, emphasis was placed on the incorporation of drought tolerance into varieties being developed. For this purpose, collections from Baluchistan have provided the ideal source. These collections have a long duration period and a high drought and winter tolerance, but are highly susceptible to most of the races of stem, leaf, and stripe rust. Therefore, the collections from Baluchistan fit well into our breeding program to develop wheat varieties for our rainfed areas where planting is made about 1 month earlier. This aspect of our program was also successful, as can be seen from the pedigree of the variety Potohar released for rainfed areas or in irrigated areas where irrigation water is a limiting factor (see Fig. 3).

FUTURE TRENDS

The imported production technology is highly efficient and economical. However, the production potential of the country has not yet been fully exploited. With the existing technology, the national average of yield could reach 1.25 tons per acre as compared with the 0.5 ton we are getting now. The amount of yield obtainable from the fertilizer-responsive varieties depends on the use of sufficient amounts of fertilizers, whereas the credits to purchase them are not yet properly provided. The technology in full has been adopted only by the well-to-do, educated farmers, i.e., by 7–8% of the farming population. As for the rest of the farmers, about 60% have adopted the varieties but cannot afford to use sufficient amounts of fertilizer, and even what is used is inadequate to create a proper balance of nitrogen and phosphorus. These farmers are convinced of the usefulness of fertilizers, but cannot afford to buy them. The country's resources to provide the necessary credits are limited. Therefore, whatever the constraints may be, we as wheat research scientists in Pakistan, have started to evolve another possible solution. This solution involves the development of varieties sufficiently efficient at lower levels of nitrogen and phosphorus. Some indications of differential varietal response to various levels of fertilizers offer the possibility of obtaining the necessary varieties. This will still involve credits, however, with much reduced pressure on the government.

The present commercial varieties with fairly high genetic potentials for yield are sensitive to abrupt rise in temperature in the month of March, a common phenomenon. Some unimproved indigenous strains have provided an excellent

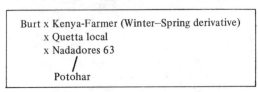

Fig. 3. The genealogy of Potohar.

source for gradual physiological maturity, which is being incorporated in the present disease-resistant, better-yielding varieties.

With the increased use of fertilizers and commercial importation of wheat seed from abroad, the weed problem is now becoming more serious. Cultural practices currently in use do not offer complete weed control. Herbicides may be very expensive and difficult to handle. One approach could be to establish wheat genotypes to suit extreme planting times: (1) long-duration types insensitive to high temperature for planting at the end of September or early October; and (2) extremely short-duration plants, particularly in the vegetative phase, which are suitable to plant up to mid-January yet which give slow physiologic maturity.

THE IMPORTANCE OF UNDERSTANDING THE USE OF FERTILIZERS

The development of varieties with a satisfactory efficiency at lower doses of fertilizers, adaptability to wide range of temperatures at different planting dates, disease resistance, and required quality are not enough in themselves to have a positive impact on wheat production unless proper cultivation methods are worked out.

It appears that it is not simply the quantity of fertilizers that matters, but rather the joint effect of nitrogen and phosphorus when used in a particular ratio at a specific stage of plant growth. This effect may vary in different types of soils, depending on their clay and salt content.

We believed the requirement of wheat plants for nitrogen and phosphorus to be in the ratio of 2:1, but recent experiments have demonstrated that better yields are obtained at a 1:1 ratio, or even when the proportion of phosphorus is somewhat higher. This is consistent with research findings elsewhere (Berkmen, 1952; Berkmen and Aksel, 1954).

Fertilizer–water interaction studies indicate that the water shortage to wheat crop can be compensated for by the adequate and balanced use of fertilizers. This is completely contrary to the common belief that the use of fertilizer requires additional water. However, the application of water must synchronize with the time for maximum contribution to root extension and sink development (Eckert, 1975).

We then believed that because phosphorus is slowly available to the plant it must be applied before or at planting time. There was a general impression in Pakistan that the cotton plant does not respond to phosphorus, but it was not reported anywhere in the world. One treatment of an experiment designed to study the effect of phosphorus on cotton at Multan, showed a positive response when the phosphorus was applied at the flowering stage (Mahboob, 1977). Recent experiments on wheat have shown that if nitrogen and phosphorus are given with the first irrigation the response is better than if the same dose is given at planting time. A recommendation cannot be made at the present time. Detailed studies are needed in order to find the exact stage of plant growth at which the phosphorus can be most efficiently used by the plant. The behavior of phosphorus in soils of different levels of salts, organic matter, and clay content also needs to be studied. However, there are strong indications that some of the phosphorus is lost or becomes ineffective during the period from planting up to the primary root stage.

Available genetic variability more efficient at lower levels of fertilizers as well as phosphorus-economizing techniques both provide prospects for developing a low-cost technology so badly needed in the developing countries.

REFERENCES

Berkmen, N. (1952). Fertilizer trials in Central Anatolia. (Turkish with summary in German and English.) Ministry of Agriculture, Ankara, Turkey.

Berkmen, N. and Aksel, R. (1954). Agrotechnical trials 1952–53 (Turkish with English summary). Annual Report of the Agricultural Research Institute of Ankara.

Borlaug, N. E. (1965). Accelerated Crop Improvement Report, West Pakistan, vol. 1, Ford Foundation, Pakistan.

Borlaug, N. E. (1968). Wheat breeding and its impact on world food supply. *Proc. 3rd Int. Wheat Genetic Symp., Canberra, 1968.* pp. 5. Australian Academy of Science, Canberra.

Dalrymple, D. G. (1974). Developmental and spread of high yielding varieties of wheat and rice in the less developed nations. Foreign Agr. Eco. Report, No. 95, July 1974. Economic Research Service, U.S. Department of Agriculture in cooperation with the U.S. Agency for International Development.

Eckert, J. B., Chaudhry, N. M., and Qureshi, S. A. (1976). Water and nutrient response of dwarf wheat under optimum management in Pakistan. Agronomic and economic implications. Presented at the Agronomy Society Meetings, Houston, and *Agron, J.,* submitted for publication.

Elliott, F. C. (1958). *Plant Breeding and Cytogenetics,* pp. 199. McGraw-Hill Book Co., New York.

Mahboob, A. (1977). Phosphorus responses on cotton. *J. Agr. Res.,* in press.

Qureshi, S. A. and Morales, I. N. (1967). Annual Technical Report, Accelerated wheat breeding program, July 1967. Agriculture Department, Government of West Pakistan. pp. 86. Lahore, Pakistan.

8

Natural and Induced Genetic Variability in Wheat

A. Shakoor, N. I. Hashmi, and M. Siddique Sadiq

Nuclear Institute for Agriculture and Biology
P.O. Box 128
Lyallpur, Pakistan

ABSTRACT

An account is given of the genetic variability in primitive wheats collected from the northwest Pakistan. Apart from genetic sources for disease resistance, drought tolerance, and other plant characters, new sources of possible height reduction in wheat were identified and described. The taller-growing primitive wheats have better emergence, perhaps largely because of their longer coleoptiles. A detailed account is given of comparative genetic studies of height-reducing genes, through both conventional genetic analysis techniques and induced mutation breeding procedures. Both approaches demonstrated the effect of height genes on grain size. At the present time there is a linear relationship between plant height and 1000-kernel weight. Possibilities of achieving a breakthrough in wheat yields through increased kernel size in short wheats are discussed.

INTRODUCTION

Man's interest in selecting certain types of plants was aroused when he developed a primitive agriculture to meet his needs. With the advancement of civilization the criteria for plant selection have changed. Vavilov was perhaps the first geneticist who made a systematic effort to collect genetic plant materials found in their centers of origin for the purpose of using them to improve different crop plants.

Up to 1920, wheat breeders in various parts of the world preferred tall and quick-growing wheats, but later we find an interest in decreasing the plant height; by 1950 most of the wheat cultivars ranged in height from 120 to 140 cm. Further reduction in plant height usually resulted in loss of grain yield. However, Japanese wheat breeders were able to develop high-yielding fertilizer-responsive semidwarf wheats in 1920 (Reitz and Salmon, 1968). Height-reducing and high-fertilizer-response genes from Norin-10 were first transferred into the American wheat Brevor (Briggle and Vogel, 1968). However, it was strongly felt that height reduction was always associated with loss in fertility and grain weight. Repeated backcrosses with Brevor resulted in the evolution of the Norin-10–Brevor-14 variety. A record yield of wheat was produced by the first semidwarf variety Gaines, developed at Pullman. Norin-10–Brevor-14 was the first variety to be used successfully all over the world in the evolution of most of the present-day semidwarf wheats.

The early semidwarf wheats had a poor emergence rate owing to their short coleoptile (Livers, 1958; Burleigh et al., 1965; Kaufman, 1968). The later efforts of the breeders resulted in breaking this undesirable association between height and coleoptile length (Chowdhry and Allan, 1963). The association between plant height and grain weight was also posing a difficulty to the breeders during early development of semidwarf wheats; in fact it is still in most cases one of the major obstacles to achieving higher, theoretically possible yields from still shorter wheats. Through their chromosome substitution work Law and Worland (1973) demonstrated that taller wheats had larger grain and there was a gradual decrease in grain weight with the reduction in height. Height reduction through induced mutations generally results also in reduced grain weight (Chaudhry, 1971; Konzak, 1973). Semidwarfing genes of Norin-10 isolated into a common genetic background indicated that the genotype carrying Rht_1 gene is taller than the one carrying Rht_2 gene (Allan and Vogel, 1968). The tall isogenic lines produced more yield and had a higher 1000-kernel weight than did relatively shorter ones (Allan, 1970).

MATERIALS AND METHODS

Northwestern Pakistan is quite rich in endemic wheat. Attempts have been made from time to time to collect and preserve this germ plasm. For the present study some of the primitive wheat lines maintained at the Agricultural Research Station in Quetta and the materials recently collected from the northern parts of Pakistan were grown at the Nuclear Institute for Agriculture and Biology in Lyallpur. The materials collected last year from Azad Kashmir have been studied only for their spike and grain characteristics. Crosses between some tall and dwarf varieties were studied at the Plant Breeding Institute of Cambridge, England. For the study of genetic variability caused by induced mutations the commonly grown cultivars of wheat—C-591, C-273, Mexipak-65, Chenab-70, and SA-42—were treated with various doses of gamma rays and ethyl methanesulfonate (EMS) and then subjected to selection. Various true-breeding mutant lines with differing heights obtained from these varieties were studied for various characters.

RESULTS AND DISCUSSION

Description of Some Promising Selections Made from Northwest Pakistan Collections

Preliminary observations made on primitive wheats collected from the north-western part of Pakistan are presented in sequence. Populations of *Triticum aestivum* and *T. durum* are cultivated in Kaghan, Gilgit, and Chitral areas. *Triticum turgidum,* probably introduced from Russia, was grown by a few farmers, as were two land races of *T. durum.* The race with a square, compact head was believed to be relatively drought resistant.

The variability for habit of growth, disease reaction, grain character, plant height, spike character, awning, and so forth, in these populations is extremely high. In a few places, the hooded character of spikes in *T. aestivum* was quite common. Some single plant isolations selected for semidwarfness may be of considerable interest. Preliminary data regarding this possibly new source of semidwarfness are presented in Table I.

NIAB-6B is an early maturing plant isolated at Kaghan near Babusar, at an altitude of about 1000 m (3000 ft). This strain has a characteristic rolling of leaves after the jointing stage, which tends to be more pronounced as the plants

Table I. Characteristics of Semidwarf Selections Made from the Northwestern Part of Pakistan

Accession No.	Habit of growth	Foliage color	Plant height (cm)	Awns	Flag leaf	Remarks
NIAB-6B	Spring	Light green	95.5	Awned	Narrow	Short duration
NIAB-42	Spring	Dark green	80.0	Awned	Broad and long	Short peduncle
NIAB-370	Intermediate	Dark green	65.5	Awned	Narrow	

enter the heading stage. The genetic basis of this characteristic is being investigated.

NIAB-42 is an isolation selected from bulk material obtained from Afghanistan from a farmer's field. It has dark green foliage with a relatively short peduncle.

NIAB-370 was collected last year from Azad Kashmir on the basis of its short straw. It was found in a farmer's field growing among the taller wheat plants. This line appears to be intermediate with regard to growth characteristics.

NIAB-155 had barbs on the leaf sheath and leaf margins. This character may not have immediate usefulness but may prove to be valuable in future breeding programs.

Induced Variability

Plants of various heights have been produced by mutagenic treatment of tall and semidwarf wheats (Table II). The height of the mutants obtained by treating the variety Chenab-70 (108 cm) varied between 65 and 114 cm. From Chenab-70 mutant lines were evolved with improved grain quality. Of these lines NIAB-432 and NIAB-503 are taller, and NIAB-504 and NIAB-506 are shorter, than the parent. Lines showing higher 1000-kernel weight (NIAB-244) and resistance to leaf rust (NIAB-546, NIAB-547, and NIAB-549) were selected form among the mutants induced in Mexipak-65. A uniculm mutant was obtained from the EMS-treated variety Bersee.

Coleoptile length is one of the important factors affecting the stand of a crop, particularly under conditions in which moisture is a limiting factor and the crop needs deep seeding. The primitive wheats grown by the farmer in the northern areas had longer coleoptiles ranging from 5.07 to 8.01 cm (Table II). Coleoptile length of improved tall cultivars varied from 5.68 to 7.96 cm, whereas the coleoptile length of new improved semidwarf wheats was < 5.00 cm. Plant height was positively correlated with coleoptile length ($r = 0.59$). This relationship between plant height and coleoptile length has been reported by various workers (Chowdhry and Allan, 1963; Favereau et al., 1968). Although some improvement in coleoptile length of Mexican wheats has been achieved, that length is still not sufficient, particularly for deep planting. It is interesting to note that the semidwarf isolate NIAB-6B, with a plant height of 95 cm, has a 7.03-cm-long coleoptile. NIAB-6B may prove a useful source for breeding varieties with short straw and sufficiently long coleoptiles.

Coleoptile length of improved tall cultivars and their induced mutants was found to be positively correlated with plant height ($r = 0.83$). A reduction in coleoptile length occurred in semidwarf mutants derived particularly from tall wheats C-591 and C-273.

However, mutant lines derived from semidwarf wheats with about the same plant height did not show much variation in coleoptile length, except in the case

Table II. Plant Height, Coleoptile Length, and 100-Kernel Weight of Different Primitive, Improved Varieties and Induced Mutant Lines

	Primitive, improved tall and semidwarf wheats			Induced mutants derived from tall and semidwarf wheats			
Var.	Plant height (cm)	Coleoptile (cm)	1000-kernel weight	Var./induced mutants	Plant height (cm)	Coleoptile (cm)	1000-kernel weight
1	118.5	8.01	28.0	C591	158.54	7.96	35.0
2	118.5	6.71	25.0	Mut 523	119.25	5.93	36.5
6B	85.0	7.03	32.0	C273	134.70	5.68	35.5
7	95.0	5.07	43.6	Mut 535	109.00	5.03	30.0
14	113.0	7.16	34.4	Mut 537	100.67	4.74	32.2
15A	132.5	7.08	33.0	Mut 502	104.79	5.05	44.1
18	110.5	7.02	29.0	Mut 508	99.92	3.99	43.5
28	131.0	7.07	29.0	Mexipak	106.65	4.83	31.40
31	125.0	7.88	29.0	Mut 521	108.95	3.58	32.4
32	118.0	7.14	31.0	Mut 17	99.73	4.65	33.55
36	114.5	6.99	34.4	Mut 244	97.69	4.60	35.13
43	100.5	6.80	41.0	Chenab 70	108.24	4.97	36.8
48B	117.0	6.95	27.2	Mut 503	114.77	4.83	41.50
83A	142.0	7.38	38.8	Mut 504	95.55	4.42	41.40
C273	134.70	5.68	35.5	Mut 506	98.26	4.36	39.0
C591	158.54	7.96	35.0	Mut 528	73.13	4.23	34.6
Ch.-70	108.24	4.97	36.8	Mut 432	108.98	4.35	36.50
PARI-73	71.0	4.52	33.4	Mut 399	65.06	3.66	29.63
Mexipak	106.65	4.84	31.8	Mut 527	97.15	4.58	43.0
SA-42	100.40	4.36	45.0	SA-42	100.40	4.36	45.0
				Mut 511	107.03	4.66	42.9
				Mut 509	97.83	4.49	46.0
				Mut 519	104.75	4.59	47.2

of NIAB-521 where reduction in coleoptile length occurred even though the height was almost equal to that of the parent. A drastic effect on coleoptile length occurred when the height of mutants was reduced below 80 cm.

Thousand-kernel weight is an important component of yield. In the primitive wheats, although there is a large amount of variation, 1000-kernel weight is lower than in improved types. A weak correlation ($r = 0.0121$) between plant height and 1000-kernel weight was found in the improved types. A positive correlation between plant height and 1000-kernel weight was reported by Johnson et al. (1966). In the case of induced mutants the correlation between these two characters was weak ($r = 0.0239$). Improvement in 1000-kernel weight with the increase in height was obtained in the induced mutants, such as NIAB-519 derived from SA-42, and NIAB-503 derived from Chenab-70. However, 1000-kernel weight was adversely affected when the height was reduced

Table III. Plant Height, 1000-Kernel Weight, and Yield from a Six-Variety Diallel

Varieties/crosses	Plant height (cm)	1000-kernel weight	Yield/plot (g)
Olsen	40.41	25.4	15.28
Mexipak	77.38	29.34	32.81
Rothwel Sprite	102.33	26.06	42.94
Maris Ensign	96.89	29.74	43.55
Kolibri	101.54	32.54	53.33
Fylgis	127.66	31.06	57.56
Olsen × MPK	60.89	27.70	37.40
Olsen × RS	76.38	31.10	39.80
Olsen × ME	73.16	29.96	54.48
Olsen × K	75.60	32.64	52.43
Olsen × F	83.09	30.74	62.00
MPK × RS	96.97	31.90	60.98
MPK × ME	92.58	32.04	62.52
MPK × K	92.90	35.60	62.08
MPK × F	105.12	31.44	74.28
RX × ME	97.21	29.80	54.23
RS × K	101.96	33.20	70.97
RS × F	112.53	29.94	56.83
ME × K	99.74	30.74	59.33
ME × F	112.67	28.70	61.28
K × F	116.47	36.50	72.90

below 80 cm. But mutants as tall as the parents in most of the cases did not differ from them.

In the study of a six-variety diallel representing three different levels of plant height, i.e., dwarf, semidwarf, and tall, a positive correlation ($r = 0.7219$) was found between plant height and 1000-kernel weight. The highest 1000-kernel weight was obtained from a cross between the tall wheat varieties, such as Kolibri and Fylgia. The cross between Olsen and Mexipak, short and semidwarf wheats, respectively, had low-grain weight. In only a few cases did these short wheats produce higher 1000-kernel weights, particularly in their crosses with tall parents.

Under British conditions Olsen dwarf and Mexipak were poor yielding; this was also true of the crosses between these two cultivars. Hybrids involving the tall parents exhibited a higher trend in yield with the increase in plant height. The highest yield was obtained in the cross involving Mexipak and Fylgia. A positive correlation ($r = 0.4332$) existed between plant height and grain yield. Most of the early workers also found a positive correlation between plant height and grain yield.

The present studies, as well as the previous ones, strongly indicate that a better emergence, higher 1000-kernel weight and yield are possible in tall wheats, but due to lodging the potential yield cannot be realized. Apart from other factors like a better root system, a stiff and short straw is, of course, one of the most important factors securing resistance to lodging. The semidwarfing genes of Norin-10, in fact, do not appear to be the sole factor for high yield potential of the present day Norin-10 derivative semidwarf wheats, but there appears to be a complex of genes which ultimately improve most of the other components of yield. With the present-day technology, this complex of genes can be utilized most profitably in semidwarf wheats showing tendency toward tallness but possessing resistance to lodging. However, another breakthrough in wheat-yield improvement can be expected if this complex of genes is successfully incorporated into short wheats showing better fertility and higher grain weight. This would require Vogel's patience, hard work, and ingenuity to make the short wheats more productive.

ACKNOWLEDGMENT

This work was supported in part by Pakistan Science Foundation Grant PU-AGR 16.

REFERENCES

Allan, R. E. (1970). Differentiating between two Norin 10–Brevor 14 semidwarf genes in a common genetic background. Seikhen ziho. (Report of the Nihara Institute for Biological Research.) 22:83–90.

Allan, R. E. and O. A. Vogel. (1968). A method for predicting semidwarf genotypes in *Triticum aestivum* L. *Agronomy Abst.* 2.

Briggle, L. W. and O. A. Vogel. (1968). Breeding short stature, disease resistant wheats in United States. *Euphytics,* Suppl. 1, pp. 107–130.

Burleigh, J. R., R. E. Allan, and O. A. Vogel. (1965). Varietal differences in seedling emergence of winter wheats as influenced by temperature and depth of plants. *Agron. J.* 57:195–198.

Chaudhry, A. S. (1971). Induced semidwarf mutants in *Triticum aestivum* L. *Pak. J. Agri. Sci.* 8:82–89.

Chowdhry, A. R. and R. E. Allan. (1963). Inheritance of coleoptile length and seedling height and their relation to plant height of four winter wheat crosses. *Crop Sci.* 3:53–58.

Favereau, G., P. Parodi, A. San Juan, and R. Avendano. (1968). Diferencias varieties en la emergencia de plantulas de trigo de primavera determindas por longitud de coleoptilo, temperatura y profundidad de slembra. *Agri. Tech. (Chile)* 28:103–110.

Johnson, V. A., K. J. Biever, A. Haunold, and J. W. Schmidt. (1966). Inheritance of plant height, yield of grain and other plant and seed characteristics in a cross of hard red winter wheat, *Triticum aestivum* L. *Crop Sci.* 6:336–338.

Kaufmann, M. L. (1968) Coleoptile length and emergence in varieties of barley, oats and wheat. *Can. J. Plant Sci.* 48:357–361.

Konzak, C. F. (1973). Using mutagens and mutations in wheat breeding and genetics research. *Proc. 4th Int. Wheat Genet. Symp. Missouri,* pp. 275–281.

Law, C. N. and A. J. Worland. (1973). Chromosome substitutions and their use in the analysis and prediction of wheat varietal performance. *Proc. 4th Int. Wheat Genet. Symp., Missouri,* pp. 41–49.

Livers, R. W. (1958). Coleoptile growth in relation to wheat seed emergence. *Agron. Abst.* 56.

Reitz, L. P. and S. C. Salmon. (1968). Origin, history and use of Norin 10 wheat. *Crop Sci.* 8:686–689.

9

The Exploitation of Natural Genetic Variability for the Improvement of Chickpea (*Cicer arietinum* L.)

A. K. Auckland and K. B. Singh

International Crops Research Institute
for the Semi-Arid Tropics (ICRISAT)
1-11-256 Begumpet
Hyderabad 500 016, A.P., India

ABSTRACT

The two main types of cultivated chickpeas of interest to plant breeders are the small-seeded desi types adapted to "winter" (Oct./Nov.) plantings in eastern Asia and the large-seeded kabuli types adapted to "summer" (Mar./Apr.) plantings in western Asia. These two types have most probably been separated for thousands of years. The total world area under chickpea cultivation is about 10.5 million hectares. India, Pakistan, and Ethiopia produce 74, 10, and 4% of the world's crop, respectively. The world's average productivity at approximately 710 kg/ha is very low. Breeding programs have to date made little impact on yield improvement, and most farmers continue to grow ancient land races on soils of low fertility and under rainfed conditions. ICRISAT began a breeding program in 1973 with the aim of producing elite lines and segregating populations to strengthen national and regional programs for the chickpea-growing countries of the world. Classic and recurrent selection breeding methodologies are being employed. In India, the breeding program of ICRISAT is carried out at Hyderabad (lat. 17°N) and at Hissar (lat. 29.5°N). In 1975 a "summer," off-season (for India) nursery was grown in Lebanon. The crop in Lebanon proved highly informative with regard to divergencies between kabuli and desi types. Adaptability of coadaptation appears to be most important in chickpeas. Transgressive segregation is greater in kabuli X desi crosses than between same-group crosses. The introgression of kabuli germ plasm into desi germ plasm is important for the improvement of the desi crop in eastern Asia and the introgression of desi germ plasm into kabuli germ plasm for the improvement of the kabuli crop in western Asia. A superior cultivar for eastern Asia is more likely to be produced from a (kabuli X desi) X desi backcross and for western Asia by a (kabuli X desi) X kabuli backcross. Whereas initial gains are more likely to come from intraspecific hybridization, current evidence suggests the potential importance of interspecific hybridization involving *Cicer arietinum* and *C. reticulatum.* Cytogenetic studies of hybrids between cultivars of *Cicer arietinum* and *C. reticulatum* indicate chromosome repatterning within *C. arietinum,* which may indicate cytogenetic differences between cultivar groups within the cultivated species.

INTRODUCTION

The cultivated chickpea (*Cicer arietinum* L.) is of ancient origin. Helbaek (1970) found specimens of chickpea at the Hacilar site in Turkey that dated back to about 5400 years B.C. Van der Maesen (1972) states that the first written evidence about chickpea is in Homer's *Iliad* (ca. 1000–800 B.C.).

Chickpea appears to have originated in western Asia. Recent work by Ladizinsky and Adler (1975) suggests a monophyletic origin of the cultivated species. Ladizinsky (1975) discovered *Cicer reticulatum* L. in Southeast Turkey, and this wild annual species appears from its seed protein profile as well as from interspecific crosses to be the progenitor of the cultivated species.

Van der Maesen (1972) compiled evidence about the spread of the cultivated species and presents an informal intraspecific classification in *Cicer arietinum* L. Of the four main classifications outlined by Van der Maesen in 1973, two, at this stage appear to be of practical value to plant breeders. These are as follows:

1. The large seeded, ramshead-shaped or rounded chickpeas (> 26 g per 100 seed) are of creamy color. The plants are medium to tall, no anthocyanin is present, and the flowers are white and the leaflets large (10–20 mm). This type is characteristic of the Mediterranean area and is generally known as the kabuli type in the Indian subcontinent.

2. The small seeded types are irregularly shaped and of various colors. The plants are small, sometimes prostrate and mostly with anthocyanin. The flowers are usually purplish pink and the leaflets are small (6–9 mm). This type is characteristic of eastern Asia, Ethiopia, and parts of Iran and Afghanistan. In India they are described as desi (indigenous) types.

Chickpeas can be grouped also according to either "winter" (Oct./Nov.) or "summer" (Mar./Apr.) plantings. The planting of the winter crop is largely of desi type, from Pakistan eastward; the desi type is also planted in Ethiopia, Sudan, Mexico, and Chile. The planting of the summer crop is largely of the kabuli type from Afghanistan westward into the Middle East, Southern Europe, and North Africa. There is an overlap of desi types adapted to summer plantings in Iran and Afghanistan.

The kabuli and desi types have most probably been separated for thousands of years. From the centers of origin in western Asia and the Mediterranean, the desi types spread eastward and the kabuli types westward. There are many land races to be found within these two types. Some kabuli types are grown in eastern Asia and were introduced about 1700 (Van der Maesen, 1972). The kabuli types have not yet become adapted and yield poorly in India. Chickpeas were introduced into the New World by the Spanish and Portuguese.

AREAS OF PRODUCTION, USES, AND YIELDS

The total world area grown to chickpea is estimated as 10.5 million ha. It is the most important pulse crop of India, Pakistan, and Ethiopia, producing 74, 10, and 4% of the worlds' crop, respectively. Other countries in which chickpeas are grown in decreasing order of crop production are Mexico, Burma, Spain, Morocco, Turkey, Iran, and Tanzania. In the Indian subcontinent and Ethiopia the bulk of the crop is of desi type. From Afghanistan westward the large seeded kabuli types are commonly grown. Mexico grows both desi (*garbanzo porquero*) and kabuli (*garbanzo blanco*) types. Most of the primary chickpea producers of desi types consume the crop locally and have a minimal export trade. There is an ever-increasing trade in the kabuli types, however. Mexico, for instance, exports *garbanzo blanco* to Spain, Portugal, Italy, Brazil, Cuba, Venezuela, and Puerto Rico. In the oil-rich but arid countries of Arabia there is an increasing consumer demand for the kabuli types, and countries such as Ethiopia and Sudan are attempting to supply these needs.

In India, Pakistan, and Bangladesh most of the chickpeas are used in the form of dhal, prepared by splitting the seeds in a mill and separating the husk, the split seeds then being cooked or boiled and eaten with rice and curry. Chickpea flour is also used in many forms of Indian confectionary. In Arab countries the kabuli types are prepared into a rather substantial hors d'oeuvre known as hommos. In Ethiopia chickpeas are eaten raw or roasted, made into biscuits, or more commonly boiled, ground, and mixed with spices to make Shero Wat. In Sudan it is boiled with salt and sesame oil to produce balilah, a popular and energy-giving food during the fasting period of Ramadhan, or it is mixed with onions, garlic, chillies, and baking powder and then fried in spoonfuls to make Ta'mmia for breakfast. Garbonzo beans are increasing in popularity for use in salads in the United States.

The world's average productivity at approximately 710 kg/ha is very low—breeding programs in various parts of the world have to date made little impact on yield improvement, and most farmers continue to grow ancient land races on soils of low fertility and under rainfed conditions. The highest per-hectare production is in Egypt (1660 kg/ha, under irrigation) and the lowest in Tanzania (190 kg/ha). In India average yields are about 700 kg/ha.

ICRISAT'S CHICKPEA BREEDING PROGRAM

The Technical Advisory Committee of the Consultative Group for Agricultural Research assigned to ICRISAT the international responsibility for the improvement of the chickpea crop. ICRISAT, based in Hyderabad, India, has a team of plant breeders, germ plasm botanists, entomologists, pathologists, physiologists, and biochemists working to achieve this goal.

Little fundamental research has been carried out on chickpeas. From the breeding point of view there have been studies on some simply inherited characters but few on quantitative gene inheritance or breeding methodologies. A germ plasm collection of more than 10,000 entries from various parts of the world and with a wide range of diversity for plant characteristics has now been assembled. In 1973 the variability between cultivars grown in Hyderabad ranged from 9 to 618 pods per plant, 6 to 68 g per 100 seed weight, 1 to 3 seeds per pod, 14- to 128-cm canopy width and plant height from 16 to 71 cm. Little was known, however, about genotype X environment interaction, the pedigrees of the cultivars, the breeding record of potential parents, or combining ability of parents. An ideotype for chickpea was difficult to quantify. However, it was known that chickpeas were entirely self-pollinated; a hybridization program was started in the 1973–1974 winter season at Hyderabad (Singh and Auckland, 1975).

Breeding Objectives and International Cooperation

The objectives of the breeding program are (1) high yield and good acceptance (palatability, seed color, seed size, etc.); (2) stability of yield; (3) resistance to pests and diseases—the chief insect pest is *Helicoverpa (Heliothis) armigera,* the main diseases are wilt (a complex of *Fusarium* sp., *Rhizoctonia, Opercullela, Sclerotium,* etc.) and blight (*Ascochyta rabei*); and (4) higher protein content and good amino acid profiles per unit per day.

We believe that, in the first instance, the greatest genetic gain can be made by deliberately delimiting our objectives to high yield and stability of yield, using the components of yield, such as pods per plant, number of seeds per pod, and seed size as selection criteria. Specific resistances to pests and diseases can be incorporated at a later stage when positive sources of resistance are identified, when the nature of their inheritance known and screening techniques have been perfected. Therefore, this chapter largely confines its discussion to yield improvement per se.

The objectives and scope for our international cooperation programs are (1) to make introductions of cultivars into other countries; (2) to supply segregating populations to strengthen national and regional programs; (3) to identify genotypes with wide-range adaptability for use in international breeding programs; and (4) to release cultivars with special characteristics, e.g., disease resistance, high protein, and so forth, to other countries.

Breeding Methodology

The breeding program is being approached from two standpoints.

The Classic Approach (Single, 3-Way, 4-Way, and Backcrossing)

Large-spaced F_2 populations are grown under conditions of good fertility. Phenotypic evaluation of yielding ability is made at this stage, and many crosses are eliminated. Single plants from good crosses retained after the F_2 undergo the pedigree method of breeding in ICRISAT's nurseries. A modified bulk method of selection may also be practiced within the good crosses or in other crosses considered useful for different environments; this bulk seed is available to cooperators in other countries as well.

Selected plants or segregating populations, or both, are advanced in off-season nurseries in the 10,000-ft Lahaul valley in northern India or in Lebanon; it is therefore possible to obtain two generations per year. It is not possible to grow a chickpea crop during the summer rains in peninsular India, because of root-rot diseases.

Recurrent Selection Approach

Hanson (1959) highlighted linkage as a tremendous conservative force inhibiting the frequency of genetic recombination. The classic approach to plant breeding offers limited means of maximizing recombination; various authors have recommended population improvement, using recurrent selection as a means of increasing the frequency of genetic recombination. Jensen (1970) suggested a "diallel selective mating system" for self-pollinated species, and later (Redden and Jensen, 1974) obtained success using this procedure for wheat and oats.

There is some evidence (Wallace, 1963) that too much genetic recombination in self-pollinated plants may cause a breakdown of coadapted gene combinations which may be essential for fitness. Continued crossing and recurrent selection methods may increase genetic recombination, but it may cause "genetic disintegration" of adaptive linkages which may have developed over the centuries in land races of chickpeas.

Nevertheless, it was felt that Jensen's diallel selective mating procedure may be of considerable value for the chickpea. It provides for the broad use of germ plasm, simultaneous input of parents, creation of persistent gene pools, breaking of linkage blocks, freeing of genetic variability, and the general fostering of genetic recombination. In the long term this method may be the means of achieving a breakthrough in yield for chickpeas. Male sterility has not yet been discovered in chickpeas, but fortunately in India we can employ 60–80 people per year to make large numbers of hand crosses.

Progress To Date

During the 1973–74 winter season in Hyderabad, 423 single crosses, utilizing nearly 100 parents, were made. The F_1 generation of these crosses was grown in summer advancement nurseries, and these produced enough seed for F_2 generation testing at Hyderabad in the 1974–1975 winter season from 324 crosses. Of these crosses 252 were of desi X desi parentage of Indian origin, and 72 were of kabuli X desi parentage. Transgressive segregation with respect to plant habit, seed size, pod number, and yield was greater in F_2 populations involving kabuli parents. The plants selected from these F_2 populations were advanced one generation in the summer of 1975 in Lebanon and are now (1975–1976 season) growing as F_4 progeny lines in Hyderabad. These lines, when harvested, will be an indication to us of progress made from the first cycle of breeding chickpeas at ICRISAT.

In the 1974–1975 season at Hyderabad we used 294 cultivars in the crossing program, making 1046 single crosses and 613 multiple crosses. More emphasis was placed on kabuli X desi crosses.

In the present 1975–1976 season we are concentrating on making crosses as a basis for initiating Jensen's diallel selective mating system. We are now in a better position to choose our parental material more judiciously. Three diallels have been initiated with 6, 11, and 22 parents, respectively. We will produce our future populations based on combining ability and genetic diversity. Some crossing programs have been initiated aimed at producing erect cultivars for mechanical harvesting, fertilizer-responsive cultivars, and disease-resistant cultivars.

Cultivar and Cross Performances in Lebanon, 1975

During the 1975 summer various F_2 populations of crosses were grown in Lebanon and this off-season (for India) nursery proved highly informative in relation to kabuli and desi divergencies and cross performances.

It was noted at an early stage in growth that the Indian desi cultivars were mostly susceptible to iron chlorosis, and that the kabuli X desi crosses were segregating for susceptibility and resistance. There is apparently little shortage of available iron in most East Asian soils growing chickpeas (and natural selection for resistance would not therefore have taken place among the desi types). In western Asia and North Africa there is apparently a shortage of available iron in many of these calcareous soils and iron-efficient cultivars are obviously needed for this area. The deficiency symptoms were corrected at an early stage by application of ferrous sulfate.

At plant maturity (selection time) it was apparent that F_2 segregating populations of crosses involving Indian desi X Indian desi parentage were showing little phenotypic variability and that it would be inexpedient to select individual plants from within them. The plants were of short stature and were low yielding. A modified bulk method of selection was therefore practiced on these crosses. Within F_2 populations of kabuli X desi crosses, and to a lesser extent within Indian desi X Iranian desi crosses, however, there were large phenotypic differences between plants; individual plant selection could therefore be carried out with impunity.

We hypothesized from these observations (made on 178 single crosses and 92 multiple crosses) that adaptability is important in chickpeas, and that the kabuli types are more adapted to western Asia and the desi types (with the exception of the Iranian desis) to eastern Asia. Conceptually, this would be the case if long-time separation of these major types had occurred. If this were true, it would be more likely, for instance, that a superior cultivar for eastern Asia would be produced by a (kabuli X desi) X desi backcross, and for western Asia by a (kabuli X desi) X kabuli backcross. This was exemplified in a spectacular fashion in Lebanon by two reciprocal backcrosses involving the cultivars F378 (an Indian desi) and Rabat (a Moroccan kabuli). The two populations, about 800 spaced plants for each, were grown contiguously.

The backcross of (F378 X Rabat) X Rabat was producing widely divergent segregants, and it was easy to select the best phenotypes. The backcross of (F378 X Rabat) X F378 showed no remarkable divergencies of plant type in the Lebanese environment. All plants within these two backcrosses were harvested and individual plant seed weight recorded. Results are shown in Table I.

From within each backcross we selected 15 high-yielding, 15 low-yielding, and 15 random-sample F_2 plants; these are now (as of Feb., 1976) growing as progeny rows in Hyderabad, India. It would appear, at this stage, that those plants obtained from the backcross to Rabat are not going to yield well in India—they are mostly late-maturing kabuli types, all of which look fairly similar. Those plants selected from the F378 backcross are mostly desi types, showing wide phenotypic divergences between progenies. The results should be available mid-March. These results will, of course, be preliminary, but they should be indications of the possibilities of future systematic breeding methodology studies to prove the hypothesis.

The present paucity of fundamental knowledge about the chickpea plant makes it difficult to ascertain the nature of adaptability or divergencies between

Table I. Production of Divergent Segregants by Backcrosses of
F378 and Rabat Strains of Chickpea[a]

Cross/parent	% Frequency: classes (g)				Mean seed wt (g/plant)
	0–40	40–80	80–120	120–140	
(F378 × Rabat) × Rabat	43.4	46.6	9.7	0.3	46.3
(F378 × Rabat) × F378	79.7	19.7	0.6	–	32.8
F378	90.0	10.0	–	–	22.4
Lebanese local[b]	85.0	15.0	–	–	25.5

[a]F_2 generation, Lebanon (1975).
[b]Rabat not grown. Lebanese local is a kabuli type.

cultivar types. In summarizing evidence of photoperiodism Van der Maesen (1972) said that differences between cultivars exist, but generally the chickpea is only moderately sensitive to photoperiodism. Ladizinsky and Adler (1975) studied 88 cultivars that "displayed tremendous variation in photoperiodical response." In Hyderabad, planting is done on a decreasing day length and in Lebanon on an increasing day length. Temperature, soil type, or strains of *Rhizobia* may be important. The physiology of adaptation in chickpeas deserves further study. It is interesting to note that the cultivar L 550 produced in India (Sandhu et al., 1975) from a desi × kabuli cross appears to be stable for moderate yield in a range of environments, such as Thailand, southern and northern India, and Lebanon.

Within the context of kabuli × desi crosses grown in Lebanon during 1975, the F_2 populations of the following types of cross were producing recombinants of possible future agronomic worth:

Single crosses	A × B
Backcrosses	(A × B) × B
3-way crosses	(A × B) × C

Four-way crosses made between individual F_2 plants from single crosses (i.e., after one generation of selfing) in Hyderabad in the 1974–1975 winter season were also producing recombinants of agronomic worth. However, F_2 segregants within 4-way crosses made between F_1 plants, i.e., F_1 (A × B) × F_1 (C × D) were producing segregants with undesirable agronomic characteristics, many of which looked distorted.

This may be taken as further evidence of the importance of adaptability or coadaptation in chickpeas. Random intercrossing between F_1's to produce 4-way crosses may be disturbing internal balances. We may be in danger of causing "genetic disintegration" of desirable linkages, rather than achieving the required useful "genetic recombination," if we carry out random intercrossing without pausing to allow for one, or maybe two, generations of selfing before continuing hybridization. Theoretically, it should be possible to recover useful recombinations from these $F_1 \times F_1$ 4-way crosses, if it were practically possible to grow out vast populations of segregants. It is pertinent to note that the CIMMYT wheat program obtained good recombinants from 4-way crosses produced between F_1 generations—perhaps with chickpeas, at this time, we are dealing with more ancient land races with more adaptive linkages than was the case for wheat.

These observations and the resultant hypothesis may, of course, profoundly affect our future breeding strategy for chickpeas on a global basis. Certainly, as far as breeding methodology is concerned we need to modify, by pausing to allow some selfing, before we continue to increase the heterozygosity of the gene pools we envisage creating by Jensen's diallel selective mating scheme.

FUTURE APPROACHES TO ICRISAT'S INTERNATIONAL CHICKPEA BREEDING PROGRAM

ICRISAT now has two main sites for chickpea breeding in India. The main breeding program takes place on the ICRISAT site at Hyderabad, (lat. 17°N). In 1975–1976 we initiated a cooperative program with Haryana Agricultural University in Hissar (Lat. 29.5°N), and we select from within late maturing populations there. Average maturity periods for cultivars grown in Hyderabad and Hissar are 110 and 165 days, respectively. This program should adequately cater to the needs of eastern Asia (mainly Pakistan, Nepal, India, Bangladesh, and Burma) in the winter production of high-yielding desi cultivars. It should also suffice the needs of most other chickpea-growing countries in the semiarid tropics growing chickpeas as a winter crop (although the Ethiopian high-altitude area of production may need special consideration).

However, it is unlikely that ICRISAT's breeding program in India can cater effectively to the many smaller, but important, countries growing kabuli chickpeas as a summer crop in western Asia and North Africa.

Two major programs are needed—the present one based in India and a future one in the Middle East. It is envisaged that when ICARDA (International Centre for Agricultural Research in Dry Areas) is established in the Middle East it will be possible to initiate this second program. The ICARDA and ICRISAT programs should be closely coordinated because of the scientific nature of the breeding strategy. It would appear that the introgression of desi germ plasm into kabuli germ plasm is necessary if quantum yield increases are to be achieved for kabuli types in western Asia. The reverse would be the case for the improvement of desi types in eastern Asia. This situation has arisen in other crops, e.g., the kafir × milo crosses for sorghum in the United States. However, the coadapted gene combinations of the desi and kabuli types appear to be a necessary basis for adaptation to eastern Asian and western Asian conditions, respectively; care must be taken to retain this adaptation in both cases.

During the 1975–1976 winter season we are cooperating with research workers in Pakistan, India, Bangladesh, Burma, Thailand, Philippines, Laos, Ethiopia, Sudan, Yemen Arab Republic, Mexico, and Chile in the testing of cultivars. The results of these trials will be of value in estimating genotype × environment interaction and in assessing specific national requirements. This cooperation will be extended in the 1976 summer season to various countries in western Asia.

INTERSPECIFIC HYBRIDIZATION

The natural genetic variability present within the cultivated *Cicer arietinum* L., has not yet been fully exploited, and for some time to come it is most probable that the improvement of chickpeas will depend on intraspecific hybridization.

However, the recent discovery by Ladizinsky (1975) of *Cicer reticulatum* L. and the fascinating cytogenetic study of Ladizinsky and Adler (1976) on interspecific hybridization between this new species, *Cicer echinospermum* Davis, and five cultivars of *Cicer arietinum* L. indicates future potentialities for the improvement of the cultivated chickpea.

These three species are all diploids with $2n = 16$. *Cicer echinospermum* and *C. reticulatum* produced a completely sterile hybrid and differed from each other by a major reciprocal translocation. *Cicer echinospermum* also differed from the cultivated species by the same reciprocal translocation, and their hybrid was highly sterile. *Cicer reticulatum* crossed readily with four red-flowered cultivars of *C. arietinum*—meiosis was normal and the hybrids were fertile. One white-flowered cultivar, when crossed with *C. reticulatum,* produced a quadrivalent, an anaphase I bridge and fragment at meiosis, which indicated that this cultivar and *C. reticulatum* differ by a translocation and a paracentric inversion—pollen fertility of the hybrid was low and not a single seed was formed. The difference in meiosis of the hybrids involving cultivars of *C. arietinum* and *C. reticulatum* indicates chromosome repatterning within *C. arietinum;* this leads one to suspect that there may be cytogenetic differences between cultivar groups within the cultivated species not hitherto suspected. We know that desi × desi crosses, for instance, are more successful than either desi × kabuli or kabuli × kabuli crosses, and that there may be a cytogenetic reason for this.

Paracentric inversions may also be of particular interest from an evolutionary point of view in chickpea. Sturtevant (1938) says that paracentric inversions offer one possibility of a change which will finally be sterile with its original parents. This may be of considerable evolutionary importance—if the change were to adapt it could account for the fact that paracentric inversions are the most common form of chromosome aberration found within the species of *Drosophila.*

The value of paracentric inversions in chickpeas deserves further study. We know that linkage is a conservative force ensuring the adaptation (fitness to a given environment) and continuance of a species. Naturally occurring paracentric inversions do not break down linkages to the extent that other chromosome exchanges do; therefore, they survive in greater numbers and may be of value in ensuring adaptability (flexibility or capacity for change in fitness). They may be a natural means of ensuring genetic recombination in an adaptive manner, rather than "genetic disintegration" caused by too-sudden changes.

It is pertinent to mention the improvement of yield obtained by the introgression of wild *Avena sterilis* germ plasm into the cultivated oat *Avena sativa* (Lawrence, 1974). Frey (1975) presented his ideas on the possibility of interspecific hybridization for other crops and states: "In reality, for a weedy or wild species to have value for improving a relative cultivated species, it should have evolved neither too close or too distant in relatedness."

There is much more to be learned about interspecific hybridization in chickpeas. In particular, studies of the special attributes of *Cicer reticulatum,* such as disease resistances, should be initiated.

APPENDIX

Since the presentation of this paper in Pakistan, additional results from the backcross selections (reported in Table I and in text discussion) are available. They are presented in Tables II and III. It can be seen that the backcross to F378 has produced a higher mean yield than the backcross to Rabat and that the possibilities of selecting higher-yielding plants are greater in the former cross in India. This is as predicted. It would appear, in both crosses, that there may be an inverse relationship between segregant yield in Lebanon and India. Selection for one environment in another would therefore be inappropriate; even advancement of early-generation material would be inadvisable.

**Table II. Production of Divergent Segregants by
Backcrosses of F378 and Rabat Strains of Chickpea**[a]

	% frequency (g classes)			Mean seed wt (g/plant)
Cross	0–40	40–80	80–120	
(F378 × Rabat) × Rabat	95.9	3.6		22.4
(F378 × Rabat) × F378	72.7	27.0	0.3	31.7

[a]F_3 generation, India (1976).

Table III. Selected Segregants from
Backcrosses of F378 and
Rabat Strains of Chickpea

| | Mean seed wt (g/plant) | | |
Cross	Lebanon (F_2)	India (F_3)	Correlation (F_2/F_3)
(F378 × Rabat) × Rabat			
High-yielding segregants	90.7	21.7	+ 0.25
Random segregants	46.4	22.2	+ 0.18
Low-yielding segregants	10.4	23.4	− 0.47[a]
Cross mean	49.8	22.4	− 0.10
(F378 × Rabat) × F378			
High-yielding segregants	73.3	30.6	+ 0.37
Random segregants	33.0	32.9	0.00
Low-yielding segregants	3.4	31.6	− 0.52[a]
Cross mean	36.5	31.7	− 0.31

[a]Denotes significance at $p < 0.05$.

ACKNOWLEDGMENTS

We wish to acknowledge the assistance of research associates K. C. Jain, S. C. Sethi, O. Singh, and G. C. L. Gowda, without whom the chickpea breeding program would be unable to function.

REFERENCES

Frey, K. J. (1975). Breeding concepts and techniques for self pollinated crops. In *International Workshop on Grain Legumes*, pp. 257–278. ICRISAT, India.

Hanson, W. D. (1959). The breaking of initial linkage blocks under selected mating systems. *Genetics 44*:857–868.

Helbaek, H. (1970). The plant husbandry at Hacilar. In *Excavations at Hacilar* (Mellart, J., ed.), pp. 189–191. Edinburgh Univ. Press.

Jensen, N. F. (1970). A diallel selective mating system for cereal breeding. *Crop Sci. 10*:629–635.

Ladizinsky, G. (1975). A new Cicer from Turkey. *Notes Roy. Bot. Gard. Edinb. 34*:201–202.

Ladizinsky, G. and Adler, A. (1975). The origin of Chickpea as indicated by seed protein electrophoresis. *Isr. J. Bot. 24*:183–189.

Ladizinsky, G. and Adler, A. (1976). The origin of chickpea *Cicer arietinum* L. *Euphytica 25*:211–217.

Lawrence, P. (1974). Introgression of exotic germplasm into oat breeding populations. Unpublished Ph.D. thesis. Iowa State Univ. Library, Ames, Ia.

Redden, R. J. and Jensen, N. F. (1974). Mass selection and mating systems in cereals. *Crop Sci. 14*:345–350.

Sandhu, T. S., Singh, K. B., and Singh, H. (1975). L550: A new Kabuli gram. *Indian Farm.* *24*:21.

Singh, K. B., and Auckland, A. K. (1975). Chickpea breeding at ICRISAT. In *International Workshop on Grain Legumes,* pp. 3–17. ICRISAT.

Sturtevant, A. H. (1938). On the origin of interspecific sterility. *Quart. Rev. Biol. 13*:333–335.

Van der Maesen, L. J. G. (1972). *Cicer L.–A monograph of the Genus with Special Reference to the Chickpea (Cicer arietinum L.).* Veenman and Zoren, Wageningen, The Netherlands.

Van der Maesen, L. J. G. (1973). Chickpea: Distribution of variability. In *Survey of Crop Genetic Resources in their centres of Diversity.* (O. H. Frankel, ed.), pp. 30–34. FAO, Rome.

Wallace, W. H. (1963). Modes of reproduction. In *Statistical Genetics and Plant Breeding* (Publ. 982). Natl. Acad. Sciences, Washington, D.C.

10

Synthetic Amphiploids in Breeding — Genetic and Evolutionary Studies in Wheat

K. A. Siddiqui

Atomic Energy Agricultural Research Centre
Tandojam, Pakistan

ABSTRACT

Synthetic amphiploids play an important role in breeding programs of wheat and in the genetic and evolutionary studies of the wheat group. One of the most obvious uses of amphiploidy has been the development of hexaploid and octaploid *Triticale*. The utilization of synthetic amphiploids as a means of introducing commercially important features of related species into cultivated wheat is now well documented. The projects to produce hybrid wheat are based on the manipulation of cytoplasms and restorers by means of artificially obtained amphiploids. The amphiploidization of interspecific hybrids by treatment with colchicine results in homozygosity. Therefore, a direct use of synthetic amphiploids for genetic studies has been limited to some extent. More often they were used indirectly, viz. as the initial step in the production of single chromosome addition and substitution lines. Such lines were used for detailed and highly informative genetic analyses and also as sources of alien variation for wheat breeding. Crosses between some of the synthetic amphiploids resembling natural species and the cultivated wheats have been successfully used in the evolutionary studies of wheats.

INTRODUCTION

Ever since the recognition of the action of colchicine on the spindle of dividing cells (Blakeslee and Avery, 1937) the relatively simple production of synthetic amphiploids has been possible. The amphiploids that have been produced have been extensively used both directly and indirectly in theoretical studies and programs for the utilization of their practical potential. The production and exploitation of amphiploids in the wheat group has, perhaps, been greater than in any other group of higher plants.

SYNTHETIC AMPHIPLOIDS IN BREEDING

Perhaps the most obvious use of amphiploidy has been the development of hexaploid and octoploid *Triticale* as a consequence of the doubling of the chromosome number of the hybrids *Triticum turgidum* X *Secale cereale* and *Triticum aestivum* X *Secale cereale,* respectively.

The early work of Pissarev (1963) and Muntzing (1963) clearly indicates the value of amphiploidy and the difficulties of using the derived triticales in breeding programs.

Lines from the extensive breeding program of Zillinsky and Borlaug (1971) apparently resulted from an outcross to hexaploid wheat and thus contained both D and R genome chromosomes. In fact, apparently much of the success of the variety Armadillo may be attributed to the reorganized third genome as a result of the hybridization of the natural amphiploid *Triticum aestivum* and the synthetic amphiploid *Triticale.* Gustafson and Zillinsky (1973) described the identification of the D-genome chromosomes in this complex amphiploid situation. Interestingly, similar reconstructed genomes in deliberate crosses between two amphiploids have been reported by Evans (1964), although Riley and Bell (1958) reported a lack of agronomic success in crosses of this type involving synthetic amphiploids of *T. longissimum,* and *T. dichasians* with *T. turgidum* to cultivated hexaploid wheats. Furthermore, repatterning of the differential genome in crosses between two natural amphiploids with one or another genome in common has been recognized by Zohary and Feldman (1962).

The success of the many other synthetic amphiploids in the Triticinae for the production of "new species" for agriculture has been very limited. Riley and Bell (1958), in summarizing work on synthetic species, state, "Nevertheless, though rarely of direct value, amphiploids may be used to introduce into wheat particular features of related species." This type of synthetic amphiploid use is now well documented, and several commercially useful transfers have been accomplished. The earliest work was that of Sears (1956), who used an amphiploid of *T. dicoccoides* X *T. umbellulatum* as a bridge to introduce a chromosome of *T. umbellulatum* into *T. aestivum.* This material was subsequently irradiated, and a gene that affects disease resistance was translocated onto a wheat chromosome.

More direct use of amphiploidy has been made for the introduction of alien variation in cases in which the alien chromosome is homologous to one of the chromosomes of *T. aestivum. Triticum ventricosum* ($DDM^{v}M^{v}$) carries resistance to eyespot (*Cercosporella herpotrichoides*) and should the resistance be controlled by factors in the D genome it should be possible to incorporate it into the D genome of *T. aestivum* via a synthetic amphiploid AABBDDM^{v}M^v with *T. turgidum*. Kimber (1967) described such a manipulation, whereas Dosba and Doussinault (1973) isolated a derivative from similar amphiploid material which had superior disease-resistance characteristics. Studies of the D genome of *T. ventricosum* in synthetic amphiploids and hybrids by Siddiqui and Jones (1967*a*) and Siddiqui (1972) have shown that this D genome appears to be slightly modified from the D genome of *T. aestivum;* however, apparently this does not prohibit recombination between the two D genomes. A similar case in which disease resistance was recognized in a synthetic amphiploid (*T. turgidum* × *T. tauschii*), and is thus available for direct introduction into cultivated wheat, has been described by Tanaka (1961). Crosses between synthetic amphiploids of diploid and tetraploid wheat to natural hexaploid wheat, which should provide a direct bridge for the introduction of desirable features from the A genome of the wild diploids and the cultivated tetraploids together with genes from the B genome of the tetraploids, were of little agonomic value (Riley and Bell, 1958). Equally lacking in agronomic value, but indicative of the potential use of synthetic amphiploids in the transfer of genes to cultivated types, is the non-homologous transfer of a biochemical marker from *T. ventricosum* to *T. aestivum* (Delibes and Garcia-Olmedo, 1973).

Synthetic amphiploids have been used as the first step in the introduction of alien variation into cultivated wheats, particularly when the alien chromosome is not homologous to any of the wheat chromosomes. The manipulations involve the production of hybrids and their amphidiploidization, followed by the isolation, either as an addition or substitution line, of single alien chromosomes in a wheat background. These lines are then either irradiated (Sears, 1956; Driscoll and Jensen, 1963) or the alien chromosome is induced to pair with its homologs by alterations in the 5B regulation system of chromosome pairing (Riley and Kimber, 1966), or by exploiting the tendency of univalent chromosomes to misdivide and then undergo centromeric fusion (Sears, 1972).

Another use of synthetic amphiploids in wheat breeding is to be found in the manipulation of cytoplasms and restorers used in producing hybrid wheat. Generally, the cytoplasms used to induce sterility as well as the genetic restorers are recovered from hybrids between wheat and its related species; however, Gomaa and Lucken (1973) described the use of a synthetic amphiploid of *T. monococcum* and *T. tauschii* as a source of fertility-restorer factors. Similarly, Lacadena and Perez (1973) used amphiploids of *T. durum* and *S. cereale* to obtain both diploid and tetraploid alloplasmic rye.

SYNTHETIC AMPHIPLOIDS IN GENETIC STUDIES

To some extent, the direct use of amphiploids in genetic studies has been limited, perhaps because all the loci of the initial hybrid become homozygous following colchicine treatment for the induction of the amphiploid. However, analysis of protein by gel chromatography and disc electrophoresis in the parents and synthetic amphiploid of *T. monococcum* X *T. ventricosum* was undertaken by Siddiqui et al. (1972) to indicate the epistatic genetic relationships of the two species.

Perhaps the most common, and certainly the most elegant, use of synthetic amphiploids in genetic studies has been their employment as an initial step in the production of single chromosome additions and substitutions. Many workers have undertaken this type of manipulation; a list of the additions that have been produced has been constructed by Driscoll (1975). The addition lines isolated by this technique have found utilization both directly in unique and extraordinarily elegant genetic analyses and indirectly as sources of alien variation for plant-breeding programs.

Okamoto (1962) used a synthetic amphiploid of *T. monococcum* X *T. tauschii* for the identification of the A- and B-genome monosomics of *T. aestivum*. The monosomics identified by this means have been used together with their derived telocentric lines in the production and identification of other sets of aneuploids and in some of the most precise genetic analyses ever undertaken in higher plants (see Law and Worland, 1972, for review). One use of these monosomics was the production of lines from an amphiploid of *T. turgidum* X *T. tauschii* hemizygous for individual chromosomes, the arm ratio of which could then be measured at meiosis when they were recognized as univalents (Larsen and Kimber, 1973). In this case, the individual chromosomes of both a diploid and tetraploid species were identified and measured, a task that probably would not have been possible with such precision without the production of the synthetic amphiploid.

SYNTHETIC AMPHIPLOIDS IN EVOLUTIONARY STUDIES

The use of amphiploids in genome analysis is limited by the fact that each chromosome is represented twice; thus the pairing of these homologs may obscure the relationships of the chromosomes of the constituent species. However, the synthesis of amphiploids that resemble natural species has been accomplished. One of the earliest such synthetic amphiploids of cultivated species was that of *T. turgidum* X *T. tauschii,* which closely resembled the hexaploid *T. aestivum* var. *spelta* produced by McFadden and Sears (1946). Crosses between this amphiploid and natural *T. aestivum* showed up to the expected 21 bivalents, thereby demonstrating the equivalence of the D genome of *T. tauschii* to the D genome of *T. aestivum*. The synthetic amphiploid of *T. umbellulatum* X *T. dichasians* is morphologically and cytologically equivalent to *T. triunciale* (Sears, 1941; Kihara and Kondo, 1943), whereas the synthetic amphiploid of *T. uniaristata* X *T. tauschii* resembles *T. ventricosum* (Matsumoto et al., 1957).

However, difficulties occur which may limit the usefulness of this type of analysis in cases wherein the amphiploid is crossed with either its natural equivalent or with other species that may contain homologous genomes. One such example is to be found when the synthetic *T. aestivum* (AABBDD) is crossed with the natural amphiploid *T. crassum* ($DDD_2 D_2 M^{cr} M^{cr}$). The hybrid contains three D genomes, yet the mean pairing is only 4.10 bivalents per cell (Siddiqui and Jones, 1967b), clearly inconsistent with even the presence of two D genomes. It is possible that the genetic system located on chromosome 5B of polyploid wheats is in some way influential in regulating chromosome pairing in this type of hybrid (Siddiqui, 1972).

CONCLUSION

Genetic diversity in plants is, of course, fundamental to their commercial exploitation. Studies designed to enhance or investigate this diversity are of clear importance in providing a sound basis for future development and exploitation. In this context, synthetic amphiploidy plays a vital role in exploiting natural variability and in permitting the accumulation of induced variability. Even though the direct use of synthetic amphiploids has been, perhaps predictably, limited to *Triticale,* the use of amphiploids in genetic and evolutionary studies has been extensive. It is anticipated that this use will continue and will be further expanded in future studies.

REFERENCES

Blakeslee, A. and Avery, A. (1937). Methods of inducing doubling of chromosomes in plants. *J. Hered. 28*:293–411.

Delibes, A. and Garcia-Olmedo, F. (1973). Biochemical evidence of gene transfer from the M^v genome of *Aegilops ventricosa* to hexaploid wheat. *Proc. 4th Int. Wheat Genetics Symp., Missouri,* pp. 161–166.

Dosba, F. and Doussinault, G. (1973). Resistance to eyespot (*Cercosporella herpotrichoides*) introduced to bread wheat from *Aegilops ventricosa. Proc. 4th Int. Wheat Genetics Symp., Missouri,* pp. 409–414.

Driscoll, C. J. and Jensen, N. F. (1963). A genetic method for detecting induced intergeneric *Newsl. 21*:16–32.

Driscoll, C. J. and Jensen, N. F. (1963). A genetic method for detecting induced genetic translocations. *Genetics 48:*459–468.

Evans, L. E. (1964). Genome construction within the Triticinae. I. The synthesis of hexaploids (2n = 42) having chromosomes of *Agropyron* and *Aegilops* in addition to the A and B genomes of *Triticum durum. Can. J. Genet. Cytol. 6*:19–28.

Gomaa, A. S. A. and Lucken, K. A. (1973). Male fertility and plant-vigor restoration in common wheat with *Triticum timopheevi* and *T. boeticum* cytoplasms. *Proc. 4th Int. Wheat Genetics Symp., Missouri,* pp. 345–350.

Gustafson, J. P. and Zillinsky, F. J. (1973). Identification of D-genome chromosomes in a 42-chromosome Triticale. *Proc. 4th Int. Wheat Genetics Symp., Missouri,* pp. 225–231.

Kihara, H. and Kondo, N. (1943). Studies on amphiploids of *Aegilops caudata* × *Aegilops umbellulata* induced by colchicine. *Seiken Ziho* 2:24–42.

Kimber, G. (1967). The incorporation of the resistance of *Aegilops ventricosa* to *Cercosporella herpotrichoides* into *Triticum aestivum. J. Agri. Sci. Camb.* 68:373–376.

Lacadena, J. R. and Perez, M. (1973). Cytogenetical analysis of the interaction between *Triticum durum* cytoplasm and *Secale cereale* nucleus at the diploid and tetroploid nuclear levels. *Proc. 4th Int. Wheat Genetics Symp., Missouri,* pp. 355–360.

Larsen, J. and Kimber, G. (1973). Chromosome length and arm ratio of *Triticum turgidum* and *T. tauschii* studied by a new method. *Proc. 4th Int. Wheat Genetics. Symp., Missouri,* pp. 691–696.

Law, C. N. and Worland, A. J. (1972). Aneuploidy in wheat and its uses in genetic analysis. *Annu. Rep. Plant Breed. Inst. Camb.* 25–65.

Matsumoto, K., Shimotsuma, M. and Nezu, M. (1957). The amphiploid M^uM^uDD and its hybrids with *Aegilops ventricosa. Wheat Inf. Serv.* 5:12–13.

McFadden, E. S. and Sears, E. R. (1946). The origin of *Triticum spelta* and its free threshing hexaploid relatives. *J. Hered.* 37:81–89; 107–116.

Muntzing, A. (1963). Cytogenetic and breeding studies in Triticale. *Proc. 2nd Int. Wheat Genetics Symp., Lund. Hereditas [Suppl.]* 2:291–300.

Okamoto, M. (1962). Identification of the chromosomes of common wheat belonging to the A and B genomes. *Can. J. Genet. Cytol.* 4:31–37.

Pissarev, V. (1963). Different approaches in Triticale breeding. *Proc. 2nd Int. Wheat Genetics Symp., Lund. Hereditas [Suppl.]* 2:279–290.

Riley, R. and Bell, G. D. H. (1959). The evaluation of synthetic species. *Proc. 1st Int. Wheat Genetics Symp., Univ. Manitoba,* pp. 161–179.

Riley, R. and Kimber, G. (1966). The transfer of alien genetic variation to wheat. *Rep. Plant Breed. Inst., Camb.* 1964–65:6–36.

Sears, E. R. (1941). Amphiploids in the seven-chromosome Triticinae. *Mo. Agri. Exp. Sta. Bull. 336:* 48 pp.

Sears, E. R. (1956). The transfer of leaf-rust resistance from *Aegilops umbellulata* to wheat. *Brookhaven Symp. Biol.* 9:1–22.

Sears, E. R. (1972). Chromosome engineering in wheat. *Stadler Symp., Columbia, Mo.* 4:23–38.

Siddiqui, K. A. (1972). The influence of the B genome on chromosome pairing in trigeneric *Aegilops* × *Triticum* × *Secale* hybrids. *Hereditas* 70:97–104.

Siddiqui, K. A. and Jones, J. K. (1967a). Cytogenetic studies of intergeneric hybrids involving *Aegilops ventricosa* and species of *Triticum. Can. J. Genet. Cytol.* 9:776–784.

Siddiqui, K. A. and Jones, J. K. (1967b). The D genomes of *Aegilops crassa. Boiss. Bol. Genet. Inst. Fitotec.* 4:29–31.

Siddiqui, K. A., Ingversen, J., and Køie, B. (1972). The inheritance of protein patterns in a synthetic allopolyploid of *Triticum monococcum* and *Aegilops ventricosa. Hereditas* 72:205–214.

Tanaka, M. (1961). New amphidiploids, synthesized 6x-wheats, derived from Emmer wheat × *Aegilops squarrosa. Wheat Inf. Serv.* 12:11.

Zillinsky, F. J. and Borlaug, N. E. (1971). Progress in developing Triticale as an economical crop. *CIMMYT Res. Bull. 17:*27 pp.

Zohary, D. and Feldman, M. (1962). Hybridization between amphiploids and the evolution of polyploids in the wheat (*Aegilops–Triticum*) group. *Evolution 16:*44–61.

11

The Use of Aneuploids in Studies
of Genetics, Breeding, and Evolution in Wheat

G. Kimber

Department of Agronomy
University of Missouri
Columbia, Missouri

ABSTRACT

In wheat a unique series of aneuploids is available, ranging from all 21 possible monosomics to complex types which are simultaneously deficient for one chromosome and duplicate for another. Furthermore, lines with chromosomes from related, alien species either added to or substituted for wheat chromosomes are in common cytological use. This contribution considers the use of this range of material in studies designed to elucidate the evolutionary relationships of the species, investigations of the genetics of a polyploid with cytological diploidization, and in potential breeding manipulations.

INTRODUCTION

The constructive use of aneuploids in any type of study obviously depends on the availability, fertility, and viability of an essentially complete series of aberrant types. In cultivated wheat (*Triticum aestivum,* $2n = 6x = 42$) there are available collections of aneuploids unequaled in any other organism. For example, in the cultivar Chinese Spring, Sears (1954) produced complete sets of nullisomics, monosomics, trisomics, and tetrasomics together with the isolation in various combinations of 41 of the 42 possible telocentrics. Furthermore, many combinations of these aneuploids have been constructed for analyzing specific chromosomal, genetic, and evolutionary situations. Similar but less complete sets of aneuploids in other cultivars have been derived from the Chinese Spring material or have been produced independently. These developments have allowed the investigation of the cytogenetics and evolution of *T. aestivum* with an elegance and precision currently unattainable in any other higher organism. The ramifications of these investigations are seen not only in the evolutionary and genetic framework so constructed, but also in actual and potential practical manipulations now available that allow a precise and often predictable genetic control over introduced diversity in the species.

GENETICS

Monosomic Analysis

Genes are located on chromosomes; it therefore follows that the irregular distribution of a genetically marked monosomic chromosome at meiosis will disturb the genetic segregation ratio observed in euploids. It is this disturbance of segregation ratios that allows genes to be assigned to specific chromosomes of the set, and incidentally provides a most convincing demonstration of the fact that genes are indeed located on chromosomes.

In undertaking monosomic analysis in wheat, use is made of the fact that the female transmission of gametes deficient for the monosomic chromosome is approximately 75%. It is therefore conventional to pollinate the monosomic series with the line or variety being analyzed. Certation mitigates against the use of monosomics as male parents. Hence, the univalent chromosome in the hybrid progeny is, neglecting univalent shift, derived from the male parent. The phenotype of the hemizygous progeny, if the gene is recessive, or the disturbed segregation of the selfed progeny clearly indicates the identity of the critical chromosome(s) involved. The more common segregation patterns are listed in Table I.

Monosomic analysis involves maintaining the 21 lines of the tester series, recognizing their cytological makeup and checking for the absence of univalent shift. This is a time consuming task that requires the skill of a cytologist. Consequently, the use of monosomics in genetic analysis has not been as widespread as would be anticipated from the potential and elegance of the method.

Some examples of the utilization of monosomic analysis for locating genes that affect different attributes are (1) morphological characters (Driscoll and Jensen, 1964); (2) disease resistance (Marcer, 1966); (3) gliadin proteins of wheat endosperm (Shepherd, 1968); and (4) metric characters (Law and Worland, 1972). Maan and Lucken (1966), using a modified monosomic analysis, were able to locate genes that interact with the cytoplasm to produce male sterility.

Table I. The Anticipated Segregation Patterns in *T. aestivum*
When a Complete Set of 21 Monosomics of Recessive Phenotype Is
Pollinated with Euploids of Differing Genetic Constitution

Number of genes	Euploid inheritance	Euploid segregation	Monosomic F_1 segregation	Selfed progeny of F_1 monosomics
One	Recessive	3 : 1	20 lines all with dominant phenotype; 1 critical line with recessive phenotype	
One	Hemizygous ineffective	3 : 1	All 21 lines with dominant phenotype	Monosomics in 20 lines segregate 3 : 1; Monosomics in critical line all with the dominant phenotype
One	Dominant	3 : 1	All 21 lines with dominant phenotype	20 lines segregate 3 dominant : 1 recessive; one line all dominant to zero recessive[a]
Two	Duplicate dominants	15 : 1	All 21 lines with dominant phenotype	19 lines segregate 15 dominant : 1 recessive; two lines all dominant to zero recessive[a]
Two	Independent dominants	9 : 3 : 3 : 1	All 21 lines with dominant phenotype	19 lines segregate 9 : 3 : 3 : 1; two lines segregate 3 : 1[b]
Two	Complementary dominant	9 : 7	All 21 lines with dominant phenotype	19 lines segregate 9 : 7; two lines segregate 3 : 1
Three	Triplicate dominant	63 : 1	All 21 lines with dominant phenotype	18 lines segregate 63 : 1; three lines all dominant to zero recessive[a]

[a]Because of the infrequent recovery of nullisomics, occasional plants with the recessive phenotype will be recorded, less frequently in the case of duplicate dominance and even less frequently in the case of triplicate inheritance.
[b]Because of nullisomy, infrequent plants with the recessive phenotype of the independent character will occur.

By recording the association of nucleoli with the micronuclei derived from the aberrant segregation of univalents at the preceding divisions, Crosby (1957) was able to identify the location of the nucleolar organizer regions with specific chromosomes. Various workers (Waines, 1973; May et al., 1973; Hart, 1970; and others) have used other aneuploids, often nullisomic tetrasomics, in locating biochemical markers in wheat.

Bielig and Driscoll (1971, 1973) described the production of monosomic alien substitution lines (MAS) in wheat as having 20 pairs of chromosomes from wheat and a univalent chromosome from an alien species substituted for a deficient wheat homolog. In each case the alien chromosome carries a genetic marker allowing its identification without recourse to cytology. The use of these lines as the female parent in monosomic analyses or in the production of intervarietal chromosome substitutions reduces the amount of cytology necessary and simultaneously permits detection of univalent shift by genetic means.

Morris (1975) published a list of genes in wheat that have been associated with specific chromosomes mainly by monosomic analysis.

Telocentric Mapping and Analysis

The chromosome complement of *Triticum aestivum* consists of 21 pairs of chromosomes, none of which has terminal or subterminal centromeres. Although this situation causes difficulty in recognizing individual chromosomes by size and arm ratio comparisons, it incidentally provides the background against which misdivision products, such as telocentrics, can easily be recognized.

The fortuitous karyotypic situation coupled with the fertility and stability of almost all lines containing one or more telocentrics makes this type of material particularly valuable in genetic analysis and in studies of evolution.

Sears (1966*a*) recognized that the presence or absence of a telocentric chromosome can be used as a phenotypical character, just as any other marker. It follows that because the segregation of telocentrics (as any other chromosome) depends on which pole the centromere moves to, the frequency of occurrence of a telocentric chromosome in a progeny segregating for genes on that chromosome arm can be used as a means of mapping the distance between the centromere and other linked loci.

The technique of Sears consists of crossing the euploid marker stock with the appropriate ditelocentric stocks and then using the F_1 as a male parent onto homozygous recessive euploid females. The recombination value between the marked locus and the centromere is derived in a conventional manner from the proportion of parental (marked whole chromosomes or unmarked telocentric) and recombinant (marked telocentric or unmarked whole chromosomes) types among the progeny. The original analysis gave the B_2, *Sr11*, and *Ki* loci, respectively, 0.44, 45.1, and 51.3% recombination to the centromere on the long arm of chromosome 6B (Sears, 1966*a*). Other workers have used this or modified techniques, to locate other genes; e.g., Williams and Maan (1973) have mapped genes for disease resistance, and Law and Worland (1972) summarized the analysis of both quantitative and qualitative characters on chromosome 7B of the cultivar Hope. McIntosh (1973) lists linkages of various loci in *T. aestivum* together with 31 examples of linkage to the centromere.

The technique of telocentric mapping may also be applied to alien chromosomes added to a wheat background when both the appropriate telocentrics and marker stocks are available. Chang et al. (1973) in a preliminary analysis mapped the *Hp* (hairy peduncle) gene of rye as more than 50 crossover units from the centromere on the long arm of chromosome 5R. The labor and difficulties associated with this type of analysis of alien chromosomes would often make this experiment prohibitive in cost and time; however, it does demonstrate the power of the technique, which allows the mapping of genes on chromosomes of diploid species where the maintenance of aneuploids is often difficult or impossible.

Gill and Kimber (1974) also took advantage of the fact that telocentric chromosomes can be unequivocally identified in somatic cells when they constructed the Giemsa-banded karyotype of *T. aestivum*. By examining only the banding pattern on the known telocentrics it was possible to synthesize a definitive karyotype involving 41 of the 42 chromosome arms. Following the production of this karyotype it is possible to identify the characteristic patterns of the three genomes and relate these to the putative diploid progenitors. The A and D genomes could be well matched to *T. monococcum* and *T. tauschii*, respectively, whereas the B genome is totally different from any of the species previously proposed as donors. Clearly, this now allows for the search of the B-genome donor through examination of the karyotypes of other diploids.

Another use of telocentric aneuploids was made by Fu and Sears (1973) who demonstrated a 1:1 relationship between chiasmata and crossing over. They recorded the chiasma frequency in a heteromorphic bivalent consisting of a telocentric and a complete chromosome. The telocentric and the corresponding arm of the complete chromosome were heterozygous for genetic markers, and the recombination of these characters was observed in the progeny. Interestingly, the chiasma frequency at metaphase was lower than would have been predicted from the recombination frequency. However, the chiasma frequency at diakinesis did show a clear 1:1 correspondence. The lower frequency of chiasmata at metaphase was attributed to terminalization prior to observation.

Linde-Laursen and Larsen (1974) used double monotelodisomics to identify translocations in *T. aestivum* and thus achieved a precise resolution unobtainable with monosomics alone.

Regulation of Chromosome Pairing

The regular bivalent formation in polyploids has classically been ascribed to differential affinity. That is a preferential synapsis of homologs to the exclusion of pairing between similar (homoeologous) chromosomes from the constituent species of the polyploid. The first clear recognition of the genetic control of the cytological diploidization of polyploids came from studies of aneuploid conditions in wheat and wheat hybrids (Okamoto, 1957; Riley and Chapman, 1958) and inferentially in other polyploid species (Kimber, 1961).

In *T. aestivum* (and by circumstantial evidence in *T. turgidum, T. timopheevii,* and *T. zhukovskyi*) the major gene regulating the normal chromosome pairing pattern is located on the long arm of chromosome 5B some 50 crossover units from the centromere (Wall et al., 1971). When this *Ph* locus is present, even in the hemizygous condition, chromosome pairing is restricted to homologous chromosomes. In aneuploid conditions (e.g., nullihaploid or hybrids deficient for chromosome 5B) in which no homologous chromosomes are present, the pairing of homoeologous chromosomes takes place at a frequency considerably higher than when chromosome 5B is present (Riley and Chapman, 1958; Mello-Sampayo and Canas, 1973). In aneuploid situations in which homologous chromosomes are present but chromosome 5B is absent (e.g., nullisomic 5B or nullisomic 5B tetrasomic 5D), then both homologous and homoeologous chromosomes often pair in very complex configurations (Riley and Chapman, 1958; Riley and Kempanna, 1963).

From studies of chromosome pairing in various aneuploids and aneuploid hybrid situations at low, normal, and higher temperatures, several workers have provided evidence for the action and interaction of loci on both the long and short arms of chromosomes of homoeologous groups 3 and 5. The interaction of loci on both normal and supernumerary chromosomes of alien species with the loci on chromosomes of *T. aestivum* has been investigated by several workers (Dvorak, 1972; Kimber and Athwal, 1972; Dover, 1973; Rubenstein and Kimber, 1976).

From measurements of the distance between two telocentrics in the same somatic cell (Feldman et al., 1966; Avivi and Feldman, 1973), the effect of various aneuploid conditions on the secondary association of chromosomes has been determined.

The evidence concerning the regulation of chromosomal pairing in wheat has been most recently reviewed by Sears (1976).

Intervarietal Chromosome Substitution

Aneuploids have been employed extensively in analyzing quantitative characters of cultivated varieties of wheat. The basic manipulation is the construction, in a common background, of sets of lines in each of which a single unrecombined chromosome is substituted from a donor variety. Thus the effects of single chromosomes, their interactions with an essentially uniform background, and the effects of recombination in single chromosomes may be studied. Gale and Law's contribution to this Volume (Chapter 13) deals with one aspect of wheat aneuploid studies in detail; therefore, this important subject will not be considered further in this chapter.

BREEDING

Introduction of Alien Variation

It is axiomatic that in order to practice selection there must be variability. Equally, the greater the range of variability available, the greater the probability that a breeder will be able to locate and utilize desirable alleles in a breeding program. It is with the aim of increasing the available pool of genetic variability that cytogeneticists have attempted to introduce genetic material from alien, but related, species into wheat. Many cases involve the use of aneuploids.

The original introduction of alien variation into a wheat chromosome using aneuploids was the induced translocation of the $Lr9$ gene of chromosome 6^{Cu} onto chromosome 6B of $T.$ $aestivum$ var. Chinese Spring by Sears (1956). A plant to which was added the long arm of chromosome 6^{Cu} monoisosomically irradiated was just prior to meiosis. Euploid $T.$ $aestivum$ was pollinated with pollen from the irradiated plant, and plants with the $Lr9$ locus were recognized by disease testing. Cytological examination of these resistant progeny allowed the isolation of several translocations, one of which was eventually released as breeders' material and was appropriately named Transfer.

Following the introduction of Transfer several other introductions have been produced by similar manipulation, others by modification of Sears' technique and still others by utilizing both aneuploids and alleles that affect chromosome pairing in hybrids. It has further been recognized that the spontaneous introduction of whole alien chromosomes into wheat varieties has taken place and the substitution lines were only identified and characterized subsequent to their release as cultivars.

Driscoll (1963) devised a technique for introducing alien genetic material into wheat chromosomes, which simultaneously reduces the time-consuming cytological analyses of other techniques. The manipulation requires inducing translocations by irradiation of seed of lines in which an alien chromosome is added disomically to the normal wheat complement. The irradiated seed is grown and selfed. In the next generation ear/row progenies are examined for the segregation of the character being investigated. Segregation of the trait usually occurs for two different and recognizable reasons.

First, if the irradiated parent were an unrecognized monosomic addition, it should segregate so that approximately 75% of the progeny would not show the desired trait. Second, if a translocation has been induced, then depending on the frequency of production, orientation, and segregation of the resultant quadrivalent, a small proportion of progeny would not exhibit the phenotype being investigated. It is from these families that the translocated type may be recovered. The cultivar Transec was developed by this technique by Driscoll and Anderson (1967).

A currently untested technique, which combines features of both Sears' and Driscoll's techniques, was devised by Kimber (1971).

The first successful use of induced homoeologous chromosome pairing in an aneuploid situation to transfer a character to wheat was that of Riley et al. (1968) who transferred resistance to the yellow-rust fungus from $T.$ $comosum$ to $T.$ $aestivum.$ The technique involved crossing a disomic addition of chromosome 2M of $T.$ $comosum$ with a form of $T.$ $speltoides$ which, even in the presence of chromosome 5B, allows homoeologous chromosome pairing to take place. Compair, the cultivar that was eventually isolated, includes a chromosome containing the segment of 2M that carries the allele which conditions resistance, yet with enough chromosome 2D to allow the translocated chromosome to pair normally with chromosome 2D.

Using lines in which *Agropyron elongatum* chromosomes were substituted for wheat chromosomes 3D and 7D and wheat aneuploids deficient for chromosome 5B, Sears (1973) was able to recover numerous 3D/Ag and 7D/Ag transfer chromosomes with the leaf-rust resistance conditioned by the *Agropyron* chromosomes.

Zeller (1973) and Mettin et al. (1973) described the identification of wheat varieties already in cultivation that carried rye chromosome 1R substituted for wheat chromosome 1B or that had wheat/rye-translocated chromosomes. The varieties all originated from material which had been derived from hybrids involving rye.

A similar process is seen to occur in hexaploid *Triticale,* where some of the rye chromosomes can be replaced, usually by chromosomes of the D genome of *T. aestivum.* Gustafson and Zillinsky (1973) described the identification of wheat chromosome 2D (and possibly also 5D) when it is spontaneously substituted for 2R in the hexaploid *Triticale* cultivar Armadillo. Evans (1964) observed similar spontaneous chromosome substitution in crosses between two artificially induced amphiploids.

When chromosomes are hemizygous they frequently misdivide at or near the centromere during meiosis. The resultant telocentrics can, presumably for only a short period of time, reunite either with each other or with any other recently misdivided chromosome. Sears (1972) took advantage of this situation by producing plants that were simultaneously monosomic for a genetically marked wheat chromosome and a rye chromosome that also carried genetic markers. Plants were derived containing chromosomes that had one arm of the rye chromosome and one arm of the wheat chromosome joined by a common centromere.

Hybrid Wheat

The commercial production of hybrid wheat is accomplished by utilization of cytoplasms inducing male sterility and chromosomal genetic restoration factors. Driscoll (1972, 1973) devised a system, using aneuploids, in which male sterility is induced by a recessive gene (or deletion) on a wheat chromosome, and fertility is restored by a corresponding epistatic gene on a homoeologous alien chromosome.

The system involves the production of three lines, designated as X, Y, and Z, each of which is homozygous for the recessive male-sterile locus and carries, respectively, 2, 1, and 0 doses of the alien chromosome carrying the epistatic restoring factor. The X line has 44 chromosomes, makes 22 bivalents, is male and female fertile, and relatively true breeding. The Y line has 43 chromosomes, makes 21 bivalents and one univalent, is male and female fertile, but produces two types of gametes, one with 21 wheat chromosomes and the other with 21 wheat plus one alien. The 21-chromosome pollen grains in the Y line do not contain the epistatic restorer but are viable because the recessive male-sterile locus acts on sporophytic tissue. Because line Y is hemizygous for the epistatic restorer, it can produce both types of pollen. Only the 21-chromosome male gametes function because of certation effects against the hyperploid pollen. The Z line has 42 chromosomes, makes 21 bivalents, and is male sterile.

Following the initial production of small quantities of the Z seed from selfed progenies of the Y line, part of the plants from the Z seed are pollinated by pollen from the X line. The seed produced is all Y type. The bulk of the Y line so produced is used as male parent for the remainder of the Z plants. All the seed produced in this cross is Z in type and can be used as the female parent for hybrid production by crossing with any normal variety. The hybrid seed so produced does not carry the alien chromosome, is fertile, and is potentially a new hybrid variety.

EVOLUTION

One of the early uses of wheat aneuploids in evolutionary studies was in the assignment of chromosomes to the three genomes A, B, and D. Sears (1944) was able to identify the D-genome monosomics by crossing the monosomic set with the tetraploid *T. turgidum*. The hybrids involving the A- and B-genome mono-somics had 13 bivalents and 8 univalents at first meiotic metaphase, whereas the hybrids involving D-genome monosomics had 14 bivalents and 6 univalents. The A-genome monosomics were distinguished from the B-genome monosomics by similar analysis of hybrids involving a synthetic AADD allotetraploid (Okamoto, 1962).

Following the identification of the individual chromosomes, Sears (1966*b*) described the identification of the homoeologous wheat chromosomes. By developing plants that were nullisomic for one wheat chromosome and simultaneously tetrasomic for another chromosome it was possible to observe the interaction of the chromosome dosages so produced. Two major classes were recognized as compensating and noncompensating. In the compensating class the phenotype and fertility were restored to relative normality, whereas the phenotype in the noncompensating class was even more aberrant than either the simple nullisomic or tetrasomic alone, and in many cases the noncompensating combinations were nonviable.

Of particular interest and great significance was the fact that the compensating combinations occurred in seven sets of three. That is, if the tetrasomy of one chromosome compensated for the nullisomy of the second, and the tetrasomy of the second compensated for the nullisomy of the third, then the tetrasomy of the third would compensate for nullisomy of the first. Furthermore, these three chromosomes would then not compensate for any of the remaining 18 in the set.

The compensating chromosomes were recognized as genetically similar and were called homoeologous. It was further recognized that in every homoeologous group there was one chromosome from each of the three genomes, A, B, and D.

The recognition of the genetical similarity of the homoeologous chromosomes by these aneuploid studies has considerable evolutionary significance in illustrating the divergence of the three genomes in *T. aestivum* from a common ancestor; yet it also shows how the individual chromosomes have changed mainly by mutation without obliterating their initial identity. As can be anticipated from this analysis and has been demonstrated by numerous workers, other species in the Triticinae have chromosomes which also presumably diverged from the same archetypical and common ancestor and are therefore also homoeologous to the wheat chromosomes.

The cytological equivalent of the genetic demonstration of homoeology was made by Riley and Kempanna (1963), who induced translocations between chromosomes in the absence of chromosome 5B and then identified the translocation products by telocentric analysis. As all the translocations recovered involved homoeologous chromosomes, it is possible to conclude that only homoeologs are able to pair by deletion of chromosome 5B.

The homoeology of alien chromosomes can be investigated, using aneuploids, by two methods—(1) their genetic compensating ability, and (2) their cytological pairing ability when the regulation of pairing to strictly homologous chromosomes is relaxed.

The genetic analysis can be accomplished by attempting to substitute the alien chromosome for wheat chromosomes, when one alien chromosome will generally substitute for the chromosome of one homoeologous group only. Riley (1965) substituted rye chromosome II of the variety King II for all three chromosomes of group 6, thereby demonstrating the homoeology of the alien chromosome to its wheat counterparts. Chromosome II of the King II addition set is now, of course, designated 6R. Similarly Sears (1968) substituted a single rye chromosome (now designated 2R) for wheat chromosomes 2A, 2B, and 2D. The literature contains many references to other alien chromosome substitutions. However, rye chromosome *3R* shows some homoeology with both group 3 and group 1 (Gupta, 1969; Lee et al., 1969) and 5R substitutes for 4A in addition to group 5 chromosomes (Zeller and Baier, 1973). One possible explanation for these apparent mismatches may be the presence of translocations between rye chromosomes, which make each of them partially homoeologous to two wheat groups.

Establishing the cytological relationships of single alien chromosomes to their wheat homoeologous groups generally involves hybridizing telocentric wheat aneuploids to an addition line and then inactivating the *Ph* locus on chromosome

5B, usually by hybridization with high-pairing forms of *T. speltoides*. Under these circumstances, the wheat telocentric chromosome will pair with the alien chromosome only when the telocentric is homoeologous to the alien. It is also necessary that the alien chromosome be identified cytologically either as a telocentric or from a subterminal centromere position. Johnson and Kimber (1967) and Dvorak (1972) demonstrated the cytological homology of *Agropyron* telocentric chromosomes by this technique, and Athwal and Kimber (1972) showed that chromosome A of *T. umbellulatum*, recognizable as an extreme subterminal, was homoeologous to wheat group 6. By algebraic analysis, Riley and Chapman (1966), also using wheat telocentrics, inferred the homoeology of the chromosome of *T. speltoides* that is similar to the chromosome of wheat group 5.

Kimber and Athwal (1972), Kimber (1973*a,b*), and Gill and Kimber (1974) questioned the relationships of *T. speltoides* to the B genome of *T. aestivum*. This reconsideration was stimulated by the discovery of genotypes of *T. speltoides* that did not suppress the regulating activity of chromosome 5B (Dvorak, 1972; Kimber and Athwal, 1972). The possibility existed that not only did these genotypes suppress the activity of chromosome 5B, but they were either asynaptic or desynaptic; this inhibited homologous chromosome pairing in hybrids also. Rubenstein and Kimber (1976) have shown by analysis of the behavior of the isochromosome that the low-pairing genotypes of *T. speltoides* do not prohibit the pairing of known homologous chromosome arms.

CONCLUSIONS

It was stated in the introduction to this chapter that the constructive use of aneuploids in any genetic study depends on the availability, fertility, and viability of an essentially complete series of the aberrant types. The examples of the use of aneuploids of *T. aestivum* described in this chapter, although obviously incomplete, indicate the analytic power and conceptual elegance of aneuploid analysis.

The geneticist can place genes on specific and recognizable chromosomes and map their position relative to the centromere. The cytologist can investigate the pairing and segregation of specific chromosomes recognizable by their centromere position, and can relate behavior to chemical and physical treatments and chiasma frequency to recombination. Individual chromosomes have been stained by the Giemsa technique and are recognizable in hybrids and aneuploids. The evolutionist has an unequaled range of powerful tools available for phylogenetic investigations. Finally, the breeder is now in the position where the appreciation of his crop is both genetically diverse and detailed; moreover, the use of aneuploids allows the introduction and utilization of new, novel, and otherwise unobtainable variation.

SUMMARY

There is available in wheat a unique series of aneuploids ranging from all 21 possible monosomics to complex types that are simultaneously deficient for one chromosome and duplicate for another. Furthermore, lines with chromosomes from related alien species either added to or substituted for wheat chromosomes are in common cytological use.

This contribution considers the use of this range of material in studies designed to elucidate the evolutionary relationships of the species, investigations of the genetics of a polyploid with cytological diploidization, and in potential breeding manipulations.

REFERENCES

Athwal, R. S. and Kimber, G. (1972). The pairing of an alien chromosome with homoeologous chromosomes of wheat. *Can. J. Genet. Cytol. 14*:325–333.

Avivi, L. and Feldman, M. (1973). Mechanism of non-random chromosome placement in common wheat. *Proc. 4th Int. Wheat Genet. Symp., Columbia, Missouri, pp. 627*–633.

Bielig, L. M. and Driscoll, C. J. (1971). Production of alien substitution lines in *Triticum aestivum. Can. J. Genet. Cytol. 13*:429–436.

Bielig, L. M. and Driscoll, C. J. (1973). Release of a series of MAS lines. *Proc. 4th Int. Wheat Genet. Symp., Columbia, Missouri,* pp. 147–150.

Chang, T. D., Kimber, G., and Sears, E. R. (1973). Genetic analysis of rye chromosomes added to wheat. *Proc. 4th Int. Wheat Genet. Symp., Columbia, Missouri,* pp. 151–153.

Crosby, A. R. (1957). Nucleolar activity of lagging chromosomes in wheat. *Am. J. Bot. 44*:813–822.

Dover, G. A. (1973). The genetics and interactions of "A" and "B" chromosomes controlling meiotic chromosome pairing in the Triticinae. *Proc. 4th Int. Wheat Genet. Symp., Columbia, Missouri,* pp. 653–666.

Driscoll, C. J. (1963). A genetic method for detecting induced intergeneric transfers of rust resistance. *Proc. 2nd Int. Wheat Genet. Symp. Lund Hereditas 2*:460–461.

Driscoll, C. J. (1972). XYZ system of producing hybrid wheat. *Crop Sci. 12*:516–517.

Driscoll, C. J. (1973). A chromosomal male-sterility system of producing hybrid wheat. *Proc. 4th Int. Wheat Genet. Symp., Columbia, Missouri,* pp. 669–674.

Driscoll, C. J. and Anderson, L. M., (1967). Cytogenetic studies of Transec–a wheat-rye translocation line. *Can. J. Genet. Cytol. 9*:375–380.

Driscoll, C. J. and Jensen, N. F. (1964). Chromosomes associated with waxlessness, awnedness and time of maturity of common wheat. *Can. J. Genet. Cytol. 6*:324–333.

Dvorak, J. (1972). Genetic variability in *Aegilops speltoides* affecting homoeologous pairing in wheat. *Can. J. Genet. Cytol. 14*:371–380.

Evans, L. E. (1964). Genome construction within the Triticinae. I. The synthesis of hexaploids ($2n = 42$) having chromosomes of *Agropyron* and *Aegilops* in addition to the A and B genomes of *Triticum durum. Can. J. Genet. Cytol. 6*:19–28.

Feldman, M., Mello-Sampayo, T., and Sears, E. R. (1966). Somatic association in *Triticum aestivum. Proc. Natl. Acad. Sci. USA 56*:1192–1199.

Fu, T. K. and Sears, E. R. (1973). The relationship between chiasmata and crossing over in *Triticum aestivum. Genetics 75*:231–246.

Gill, B. S. and Kimber, G. (1974). Giemsa C-banding and the evolution of wheat. *Proc. Natl. Acad. Sci. USA 71*:4086–4090.

Gupta, P. K. (1969). Studies on transmission of rye substitution gametes in common wheat. *Indian J. Genet. Plant Breed. 29*:163–172.

Gustafson, J. P. and Zillinsky, F. J. (1973). Identification of D-genome chromosomes from hexaploid wheat in a 42-chromosome Triticale. *Proc. 4th Int. Wheat Genet. Symp., Columbia, Missouri*, pp. 225–231.

Hart, G. E. (1970). Evidence for triplicate genes for alcohol dehydrogenase in hexaploid wheat. *Proc. Natl. Acad. Sci. USA 66*:1136–1141.

Johnson, R. and Kimber, G. (1967). Homoeologous pairing of a chromosome from *Agropyron elongatum* with those of *Triticum aestivum* and *Aegilops speltoides*. *Genet. Res. Camb. 10*:63–71.

Kimber, G. (1961). Basis of the diploid-like meiotic behaviour of polyploid cotton. *Nature 191*:98–100.

Kimber, G. (1971). The design of a method, using ionising radiation, for the introduction of alien variation into wheat. *Indian J. Genet. Plant Breed. 31*:580–584.

Kimber, G. (1973a). The relationships of the S-genome diploids to polyploid wheats. *Proc. 4th Int. Wheat Genet. Symp., Columbia, Missouri*, pp. 81–85.

Kimber, G. (1973b) A reassessment of the origin of the polyploid wheats. *Genetics 78*:487–492.

Kimber, G. and Athwal, R. S. (1972). A reassessment of the course of evolution in wheat. *Proc. Natl. Acad. Sci. USA 69*:912–915.

Law, C. N. and Worland, A. J. (1972). Aneuploidy in wheat and its uses in genetic analysis. *Annu. Rep. Plant Breed. Inst. Camb.* 25–65.

Lee, Y. H., Larter, E. N., and Evans, L. E. (1969). Homoeologous relationship of rye chromosome VI with two homoeologous groups from wheat. *Can. J. Genet. Cytol. 11*:803–809.

Linde-Laursen, I. and Larsen, J. (1974). The use of double-monotelodisomics to identify translocations in *Triticum aestivum*. *Hereditas 78*:245–250.

Maan, S. S. and Lucken, K. A. (1966). Development and use of an aneuploid set of male sterile Chinese Spring wheat in *Triticum timopheevii* Zhuk. cytoplasm. *Can. J. Genet. Cytol. 8*:398–403.

Macer, R. C. F. (1966). The formal and monosomic genetic analysis of stripe rust resistance in wheat. *Proc. 2nd Int. Wheat Genet. Symp., Lund Hereditas [Suppl.] 2*:127–142.

May, C. E., Vickery, R. S., and Driscoll, C. J. (1973). Gene control in hexaploid wheat. *Proc. 4th Int. Wheat Genet. Symp., Columbia, Missouri* pp. 843–849.

McIntosh, R. A. (1973). A catalogue of gene symbols for wheat. *Proc. 4th Int. Wheat Genet. Symp., Columbia, Missouri*, pp. 893–937.

Mello-Sampayo, T. and Canas, A. P. (1973). Suppressors of meiotic chromosome pairing in common wheat. *Proc. 4th Int. Wheat Genet. Symp., Columbia, Missouri*, pp. 709–713.

Mettin, D., Blüthner, W. D., and Schlegel, G. (1973). Additional evidence on spontaneous 1B/1R wheat-rye substitutions and translocations. *Proc. 4th Int. Wheat Genet. Symp., Columbia, Missouri*, pp. 179–184.

Morris, R. (1975). Chromosomal locations of genes for wheat characters. *Wheat Newsl. XXI*:34–45.

Okamoto, M. (1957). Asynaptic effect of chromosome V. *Wheat Inf. Serv. 5*:6–7.

Okamoto, M. (1962). Identification of the chromosomes of common wheat belonging to the A and B genomes. *Can. J. Genet. Cytol. 4*:31–37.

Riley, R. (1965). Cytogenetics and plant breeding. *Genetics Today. Proc. XI Int. Congr. Genet. 3*:681–688.

Riley, R. and Chapman, V. (1958). Genetic control of the cytologically diploid behaviour of hexaploid wheat. *Nature 182*:713–715.

Riley, R. and Chapman, V. (1966). Estimates of the homoeology of wheat chromosomes by measurements of differential affinity at meiosis. In *Chromosome Manipulations and Plant Genetics* (Riley, R. and Lewis, K. R. eds.). Olive & Boyd, London.

Riley, R. and Kempanna, C. (1963). The homoeologous nature of the non-homologous meiotic pairing in *Triticum aestivum* deficient for chromosome V (5B). *Heredity 18*:287–306.

Riley, R., Chapman, V., and Johnson, R. (1968). The incorporation of alien disease resistance in wheat by genetic interference with the regulation of meiotic chromosome synapsis. *Genet. Res. 12*:199–219.

Rubenstein, J. M. and Kimber, G. (1976). The genetical relationships of the systems regulating chromosome pairing in hybrids and aneuploids of hexaploid wheat. *Cereal Res. Commun. 4*:263–272.

Sears, E. R. (1944). Cytogenetic studies with polyploid species of wheat. II. Additional chromosomal aberrations in *Triticum vulgare*. *Genetics 29*:232–246.

Sears, E. R. (1954). The aneuploids of common wheat. *Missouri Agr. Exp. Sta. Res. Bull. 572*:59.

Sears, E. R. (1956). The transfer of leaf-rust resistance from *Aegilops umbellulata* to wheat. *Brookhaven Symp. Biol. 9*:1–22.

Sears, E. R. (1966*a*). Chromosome mapping with the aid of telocentrics. *Proc. 2nd Int. Wheat Genet. Symp. Hereditas [Suppl.] 2*:370–380.

Sears, E. R. (1966*b*). Nullisomic-tetrasomic combinations in hexaploid wheat. In *Chromosome Manipulations and Plant Genetics* Riley, R. and Lewis, K. R., eds.), Oliver & Boyd, London.

Sears, E. R. (1968). Relationships of chromosomes 2A, 2B and 2D with their rye homoeologue. *Proc. 3rd Int. Wheat Genet. Symp. Aust. Acad. Sci. Canberra*, pp. 53–61.

Sears, E. R. (1972). Chromosome engineering in wheat. *Stadler Symp., Columbia, Missouri 4*:23–38.

Sears, E. R. (1973). *Agropyron*–wheat transfers induced by homoeologous pairing. *Proc. 4th Int. Wheat Genet. Symp., Columbia, Missouri*, pp. 191–199.

Sears, E. R. (1976). Genetic control of chromosome pairing in wheat. *Annu. Rev. Genet. 10*:31–51.

Shepherd, K. W. (1968). Chromosomal control of endosperm proteins in wheat and rye. *Proc. 3rd Int. Wheat Genet. Symp. Aust. Acad. Sci., Canberra*, pp. 86–96.

Waines, J. G. (1973). Chromosomal location of genes controlling endosperm protein production in *Triticum aestivum* CV. Chinese Spring. *Proc. 4th Int. Wheat Genet. Symp., Columbia, Missouri*, pp. 873–877.

Wall, A. M., Riley, R., and Gale, M. D. (1971). The position of a locus on chromosome 5B of *Triticum aestivum* affecting homoeologous meiotic pairing. *Genet. Res. Camb. 18*:329–339.

Williams, N. D. and Maan, S. S. (1973). Telosomic mapping of genes for resistance to stem rust of wheat. *Proc. 4th Int. Wheat Genet. Symp. Columbia, Missouri*, pp. 765–770.

Zeller, F. J. (1973). 1B/1R wheat–rye chromosome substitutions and translocations. *Proc. 4th Int. Wheat Genet. Symp., Columbia, Missouri*, pp. 209–221.

Zeller, F. J. and Baier, A. C. (1973). Substitution des Weizen-chromosomenpaares 4A durch das Roggenchromosomenpaar 5R in den Weihenstephaner Weizenstamm W70a86 (Blaukorn). *Z. Pflanzenzüchtg. 70*:1–10.

12

Prospects and Perspectives in Mutation Breeding

R. D. Brock

CSIRO Division of Plant Industry
Canberra, Australia

ABSTRACT

Induction of mutations, primarily a method of generating genetic variation, can contribute to plant improvement when combined with selection, or recombination and selection, or with other methods of manipulating genetic variation. As a source of variability, induced mutations supplement naturally occurring variation. When specific mutants are selected following mutagenic treatments it is highly likely that a number of mutational changes will have occurred in the selected genotype. Hence, although most of the mutant varieties released so far have resulted from mutation and direct selection, the future trend will be for increasing use of mutants in association with recombination. Whereas induced mutations are generally regarded as random events, there are suggestions of some mutational specificity in response to different mutagenic agents and treatments. The best immediate prospects for increasing specificity lie in the manipulation of the selection environment. Biochemical selection applied to large numbers of plant cells in culture to locate mutations in specific biosynthetic pathways and the subsequent regeneration of whole plants offers great prospect for reducing the cost of breeding programs and altering the amount or composition of a desired end or intermediate product. Mutations in combination with other techniques of genetic engineering will constitute the tools of the plant breeders of the future. Their present role in plant breeding has been established. They have advantages in certain situations, disadvantages in others. Greater under-standing will lead to their more widespread use.

INTRODUCTION

Once breeding objectives have been defined, plant breeding basically involves three phases of activity—first, assembly of an adequate gene pool and the selection of desirable genes or genotypes either as parental material for further improvement, or for immediate testing as potential cultivars; second, manipula-tion of the selected genes or groups of genes to generate more favorable combinations, followed by further selection; and third, comparative tests to demonstrate the superiority of the selected genotypes, culminating in the release of improved cultivars. These three phases are not necessarily separate and discrete. Depending on the circumstances of reproductive system, plant-breeding method, and selection criteria, they can merge and overlap. Induced mutations have a role in the first and second of these phases. Before any assessment can be made of the future prospects, we need to understand the contribution that mutations have already made and to view this in perspective against what might be expected of the technique and the available alternatives.

Induced mutations are considered here as including induced chromosomal changes as well as deletions and changes at the gene level. Although the nature of the genetic change can be determined with favorable genetic organisms, this is not the case for most crop species. The induction of mutations, primarily a method of generating genetic variability, can contribute to plant improvement when combined with selection, or recombination and selection, or with other methods of manipulating variability.

INDUCED VARIABILITY

Plant breeders are well aware of a need for a large and diverse pool of variability to meet the needs of current and future plant-breeding objectives. These needs are conventionally supplied from the reservoirs of the natural gene pools existing in current and obsolete varieties, primitive varieties, and the wild and weedy relatives of the cultivated species. Induced mutations offer an alternative source of variability. Opinions as to the value of induced mutations vary widely. It has been argued that as all variability stems from spontaneous mutation, there is no need to preserve existing variability. The opposite opinion is that most induced changes are deleterious and are therefore useless. It would be neither prudent nor wise to accept either of these extreme views. Natural variability is the product of spontaneous mutation, but this has been molded by recombination and selection. We can induce any gene mutation that has oc-curred naturally, and probably many that have never occurred spontaneously or else have been lost from the existing population. We can, by applying appropriate selection techniques, retain those mutants suitable for modern agricultural systems, rather than be dependent on those that have survived natural and primitive selection. Therefore, at the level of the single gene, there seems little doubt that we can induce and retain the full range of genetic variability that exists in the natural gene pools and there is no theoretical need for the preservation of natural germ plasm. If the required variability already exists, it will probably be simpler and more economical to transfer it to the desired genotype than to induce it anew.

Is the situation similar for quantitatively inherited characters? Induced mutations can generate useful variation in multigenic characters, and where appropriate selection has been applied improvements in yield, adaptability, maturity time, and numerous other quantitative traits have been obtained. The extent to which induced mutations are a satisfactory alternative to natural variation for the improvement of such traits is largely determined by the importance of linked groups of genes and the degree to which selection has built linked gene complexes which will be of adaptive significance in plant-breeding situations. Where such linked sets of genes occur, they can be transferred to other genotypes, but they are unlikely to be produced as a result of random mutation.

There is genetic evidence for the existence of coadapted complexes of genes, and it is generally believed that they are important in the adaptation of populations of natural races and species (Dobzhansky, 1951). Although it is generally assumed that these gene complexes are important for plant improvement, there is surprisingly little evidence to support this assumption. Until the role of such gene complexes is established, the importance of induced mutations as sources of germ plasm for quantitatively inherited traits remains uncertain. Hence, on grounds of prudence and economy we must regard induced mutations as a supplement, rather than an alternative, to conservation of genetic resources.

Some other factors affecting induced variability should be recognized. Seldom, if ever, is a mutation induced in a single gene without some other genetic change occurring in the treated genotype. Working economics dictate that when a mutagenic treatment is applied with the objective of mutating a specific gene or character, high doses of the mutagen are applied. At these doses there is a high probability of deleting groups of genes or simultaneously mutating other genes. All the mutagens at our command induce essentially random changes to the genotype, and at the treatment levels used to give an appreciable number of visible mutations, considerable variation in quantitatively inherited characters is also induced. Hence, if selection is applied only for a specific mutant phenotype, the selected mutant is very likely to be changed in a number of other subtle but nevertheless important ways. Random mutation, in addition to generating deleterious changes, increases the variance for all quantitatively inherited characters. In the absence of selection, or correlated responses, the mean of the character will shift away from the direction of previous selection. As most agricultural species have already been selected for high performance and adaptability, random mutation will on the average reduce the overall performance. This trend can, of course, be reversed by applying selection for all important characters or by incorporating the selected mutant into a breeding program in which the desired mutant gene can be separated from the unfavorable ones.

As already mentioned, induced mutations are generally regarded as occurring at random throughout the genome. There are reports that indicate that this is not always so. Detailed analyses of a large number of mutants at the *erectoides (ert)* and *eceriferum loci* of barley indicate locus specificity, in response to different physical and chemical mutagens. Mutants occur much more frequently at the *ert a* locus, after treatment with sparsely ionizing radiations (X and γ rays) and with certain chemicals, than after treatment with densely ionizing radiations (neutrons). In contrast, the *ert c* locus is more frequently mutated by neutrons (Persson and Hagberg, 1969). Similar differential responses to different mutagens occur at certain *eceriferum* loci (Lundqvist et al., 1968). Differences occur in the relative frequencies of different types of chlorophyll mutations, and in the ratio of viable to lethal mutations, after treatment with different mutagens (see Nilan, 1972, for review). Certain chemical mutagens induce chromosome breakage at specific regions of the chromosomes, e.g., maleic hydrazide specifically breaks at heterochromatic regions (Kihlman, 1966). Widely varying ratios of chromosome aberrations to mutations are induced by different mutagenic agents. Compared with ionizing radiations, certain chemical mutagens, such as ethyl methane sulfonate, diethyl sulfate, and notably sodium azide, induce a high ratio of mutations to chromosome aberrations (Nilan, 1972). Interpretation of these results is restricted by our incomplete understanding of the mutational processes. Application of the findings to mutation plant breeding is hampered by our lack of knowledge of the mutational change required to produce a particular mutant phenotype. With our present knowledge, the best recommendation is to use more than one highly effective mutagen, e.g., a physical and a chemical mutagen, and concentrate on efficient selection.

The early dreams of chemical mutagens which would recognize and specifically mutate particular genes have been dashed by our present understanding of the organization of the genes as linear sequences of the same four bases. The chance of obtaining a chemical mutagen which will recognize the sequence of a structural gene appears very remote. However, there are other possibilities.

Auerbach (1967) favors control of the mutational process by manipulation of the physical, cellular, or genetic environments, to influence the type and frequency of mutations that are recovered.

Transfer of genetic information between species which do not interbreed is a form of directed mutation. Considerable success has already been achieved in this area via radiation-induced translocations initiated by Sears (1956) in his transfer of disease resistance from *Aegilops umbellulata* to wheat. This work was followed by similar transfers utilizing radiation (Acosta, 1961; Knott, 1961; Driscoll and Jensen, 1963; Sharma and Knott, 1966; Weinhues, 1966) or genetic methods (Riley et al., 1968) to achieve alien gene transfer. Gene transfer is also being attempted by methods of transformation and transduction which will be referred to later.

I have earlier (Brock, 1971) referred to experiments with microorganisms that offer prospects for more direct control of the mutational process, some of which may have implications for crop plants. We are attempting to achieve control through the genetic controlling elements rather than the structural genes. The concept of structural genes and controlling elements is now well established for bacteria and bacteriophages and there is some evidence that similar systems operate in higher organisms. We have shown that the β-galactosidase gene of *Escherichia coli* is more readily mutated by alkylating agents when it is switched on (induced) than when it is switched off (uninduced). Ionizing radiations and base analogs do not show this differential action. A second possibility under investigation is an attempt to utilize the DNA-recognizing property of the regulator protein of an operator–regulator controlling system to carry a mutagen to a specific locus. It should be possible to make the regulator protein mutagenic by incorporating $[^3H]$ amino acids, and operator-constitutive mutants should be induced.

MUTATION AND SELECTION

In conventional plant breeding, once a pool of genotypes has been assembled it is sometimes possible to select directly a particular genotype which is superior to the existing cultivars. Similarly, after the induction of mutations it is sometimes possible to select directly a mutant genotype which is superior to the parental cultivar. Indeed, 80 of the 98 crop varieties that resulted from induced mutations up to 1973 were direct selections (Sigurbjornsson and Micke, 1974).

Success in selecting useful mutants from a segregating population is very much influenced by the number of treated cells that contribute to the population and by the efficiency of the selection system. In assessing the number of treated cells that have to be included in the population to be screened, consideration must be given to the mutation rate and the number of loci that can be mutated to provide a particular phenotype. The mutation rate per locus does not appear to vary substantially in eukaryotic organisms, but the number of loci that can be mutated to give a particular mutant phenotype can vary widely. Furthermore, the phenotypic effects of gross chromosomal changes are difficult to estimate and lead to uncertainties. Brock (1971) proposed the following mutation frequencies as a basis for assessing the number of treated cell progenies to be examined (Table I).

Table I. Number of Cell Progenies to Be Examined for Various
Mutation Rates and Probabilities of Occurrence[a]

Mutation frequency (μ)	Number of cell progenies (n)[b]		Type of mutation
	$p = 0.90$	$p = 0.99$	
1×10^{-2}	233	465	Chromosome changes and quantitatively inherited variability
1×10^{-3}	2,326	4,652	Several recessive genes
1×10^{-4}	23,260	46,520	Single recessive gene
1×10^{-5}	232,600	465,200	Single dominant gene

[a]Brock (1971).
[b]Number of cell progenies, n, equals $\log (1 - p)/\log (1 - \mu)$.

Rédei (1974) reviewed the numerous considerations concerning the size of the progeny from treated seeds that need to be examined for the most efficient detection of recessive mutants; he concludes, in conformity with most other authors, that best economy is achieved by large M-1 populations and small M-2 families. From these considerations it is obvious that a basic requirement of mutation plant breeding is the need for large populations and hence efficient screening techniques.

The new techniques of plant cell culture offer great potential in this respect and two facets are important for mutation breeding. The first is the ability to regenerate complete plants from single cells grown in culture. This is now established for tobacco, rice, carrot, sugar cane, and orchids, and there are recent reports of complete regeneration of rape, wheat, rye, coffee, barley, *Stylosanthes hamata,* and *Petunia hybrida.* This wide range of species suggests that appropriate conditions will be found for the regeneration of complete plants from any species. The second important point is that haploid cells can be cultivated by plant cell culture. These cells provide the opportunity for the direct selection of recessive mutations and after chromosome doubling, which is anyway necessary to restore fertility, homozygous mutant plants become available. The use of plant cell culture, by which the highly differentiated diploid plants can be reduced to a single cell, indeed a single haploid cell, offers the prospect of applying to crop plants many of the highly sophisticated techniques developed in prokaryote genetics, particularly bacterial genetics. These techniques offer obvious prospects for selecting mutants in the biosynthetic pathways with changes to the amount or composition of an end or intermediate product. This is of potential importance in various facets of plant improvement, for example, in the domestication of wild species by the removal of toxins and other compounds deleterious to man or his domestic animals, in the adaptation of plants to special environmental conditions, such as high salt concentration, and in the modification of products from crop plants grown for nutritional, industrial, or medicinal purposes.

Indeed, some progress has already been reported in the combination of mutagenesis and biochemical selection techniques applied to plant cell cultures. Heimer and Filner (1970) selected from tobacco cells exposed to N-methyl-N'-nitro-N-nitrosoguanidine a line capable of growing in concentrations of threonine inhibitory to nonmutant cells. These resistant cells had increased ability to assimilate nitrate in the presence of threonine, indicating that the mutation had occurred in the nitrate uptake system which, in wild-type cells, is sensitive to the level of free amino acids. Mutants of this type could increase seed protein levels in seed protein crops, for the rate of protein synthesis is likely to be limited by the supply of organic nitrogen.

Knowledge of the biochemical pathways and control systems enables selection to be applied with the object of influencing the concentration of intermediate or alternative end products in which branched biosynthetic pathways are involved. This has already been utilized in the microorganism *Micrococcus glutamicus* to greatly increase its capacity to produce lysine in industrial fermentation processes. In this case, a mutant blocking threonine formation resulted in large quantities of lysine being excreted in industrial fermentation (Nakayama et al., 1966). This was possible in *M. glutamicus* because only the aspartate kinase, and not the dihydrodipicolinic acid synthetase, is sensitive to feedback inhibition (Fig. 1). There are suggestions that rice has the same minimal control of lysine formation (D. H. Halsall, personal communication), which might make it particularly suitable for deregulating lysine biosynthesis.

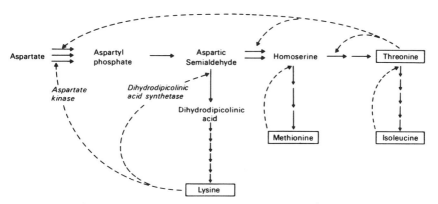

Fig. 1. Feedback inhibition control of biosynthesis of lysine, methionine, threonine, and isoleucine in Escherichia coli.

124   R. B. Brock

A more direct method of decontrolling amino acid biosynthesis is to in-activate the feedback receptor site by mutation. The required mutant can be isolated by selection for resistance to an analogue of the appropriate amino acid. This has frequently been done with bacteria to give overproduction of amino acids. The same technique has been used to deregulate amino acid synthesis in plant cell cultures.

Widholm (1972a,b) selected tobacco and carrot cells in culture for resistance to a tryptophan analog 5-methyltryptophan (5-MT) and obtained resistant cells with markedly increased levels of free tryptophan. In each case it was shown that the anthranilate synthetase from the mutant cells had reduced sensitivity to inhibition by tryptophan or 5-MT (Fig. 2).

In later experiments (Widholm, 1974) further resistant cells were isolated in which the resistance was caused by a decreased uptake of the analog and not by alteration in the anthranilate synthetase. This cell line had only a relatively small increase in the level of free tryptophan compared with the cell lines in which the anthranilate synthetase was mutated.

Carlson (1973a) used a similar technique to select tobacco cells resistant to a methionine analog methionine sulfoximine. Haploid cells in culture were treated with ethyl methane sulfonate, and three resistant calluses were obtained. Diploid progeny were regenerated from these resistant calluses, and in two of them the free methionine concentrations in leaves, stems, and roots were substantially increased.

Chaleff and Carlson (1974) selected diploid rice cells in culture for resistance to the lysine analog, S-(β-aminoethyl)cysteine. Three resistant cell lines were obtained; these had alterations to the free and total levels of a number of amino acids including those derived from aspartate (Fig. 1). As no enzyme studies were made it is not clear whether these were mutations affecting amino acid biosyn-thesis pathways. It was not possible to regenerate plants from these cell lines so no information is available about the possible effects of these mutants on seed storage proteins.

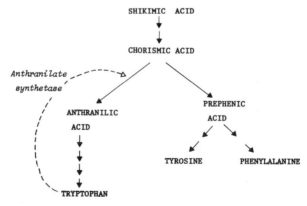

Fig. 2. Tryptophan, tyrosine, and phenylalanine biosynthesis.

Palmer and Widholm (1975) also selected carrot and tobacco cells in culture for resistance to an analog of phenylalanine, p-fluorophenylalanine. They isolated resistant cells in both species but in this case their results suggested that the mutation had altered a general uptake mechanism, rather than a specific enzyme concerned with phenylalanine biosynthesis. The resistant carrot cells had a sixfold increase in the level of free phenylalanine, but the resistant tobacco cells showed no such increase.

An important feature in the success of these experiments has been the ability to apply an extremely efficient selection sieve to large numbers of cells. Although mutants resistant to 5-MT and to methionine sulfoximine occurred at frequencies of 1 in 3×10^5 to 9×10^5 cells, the resistant lines were detected and selected.

Whereas plant-cell culture is of undoubted value in handling such large numbers of mutagen-treated cells, it is not essential. Where cell cultures are not available whole plants can be used. Indeed, in our laboratory 120,000 cell progenies of barley have been screened for resistance to the lysine analog S-(β-aminoethyl)cysteine in search of mutants that overproduce lysine (Brock et al., 1973). This was achieved by harvesting five single ears from each of a large number of M-1 plants treated with ethyl methane sulfonate or γ-rays. Single ears were assumed to represent single-treated cells and M-2 progenies were grown in the presence of the analog without threshing. Progenies from resistant seedlings are now being assayed for free lysine levels.

Efficiency of selection is an obvious requirement for successfully detecting induced genetic variation. This can be improved by modifying the genetic environment as well as the physical environment. Whereas it is sensible to choose a high-yielding, well-adapted genotype as the starting material for a mutation-breeding program designed for the direct selection of useful mutant cultivars, this does not necessarily apply if the object is to provide sources of new variability to be used in subsequent hybridization programs. In such cases it may be most appropriate to start with a genotype for which improvement in the desired characteristic can be most readily expressed (e.g., mutant alleles contributing to increased yield may be most easily selected in a low-yielding genotype or dwarfing alleles in a tall variety).

Before moving to the role of mutations as sources of variation in hybridization programs, brief mention must be made of the use of mutations in those species in which hybridization is not possible (obligate apomicts), or not conventionally practiced because of the long commercial life of individual plants and the highly heterozygous and sometimes chimerical nature of the species (e.g., fruit trees). Improvement of such vegetatively reproduced species is dependent on the chance occurrence of spontaneous mutation (sports). The application of mutagenic treatments which increase variability is of obvious use in providing material for selection. It is surprising that of the 98 cultivars of crop plants released up to 1973, only seven were fruit trees, and one of these involved a self-fertile cherry mutant seedling used in crossing to produce a self-fertile sweet cherry. This low number is supplemented by 47 mutation-induced variants of ornamentals in which the technique has been very successfully used by a small number of breeders.

There are excellent prospects for greater use of induced mutations in these vegetatively reproduced species. The heterozygosity of many horticultural species, which permits the ready expression of recessive mutations, and the value of novelty in floricultural species are special features not often present in agricultural plants.

MUTATION PLUS RECOMBINATION

Although only 18 of the 98 varieties of crop plants emanating from mutations up until 1973 were the result of mutants utilized in crossing programs (Sigurbjornsson and Micke, 1974), a larger proportion can be expected in the future. The latest information published in the International Atomic Energy Agency *Mutation Breeding Newsletters* (Nos. 4–6) and by Gustafsson (1976) reports an additional 21 varieties, 15 of which were hybridized before final selection and two of which were selections from outbreeding species which were likely to have been subjected to some recombination. Only four varieties were the result of direct selection. The average time that elapsed from the end of the mutagenic treatment to the release of the mutant variety was 8.9 years for those which were selected directly, as compared with 18.0 years for those used in crossing programs. These figures suggest that an even larger proportion of the future releases will represent mutants utilized in recombination programs.

Comparison of the time required for the release of mutant varieties with that for varieties from conventional breeding programs is made difficult because of the relatively small number of mutant varieties and the wide range of crop species involved. However, 8.9 years for direct selection is probably somewhat shorter, and 18 years for the mutants incorporated into hybridization programs somewhat longer, than the average time required for the production of a variety by conventional breeding.

These average times, although useful indications of what happened in the early days of mutation breeding, are not necessarily reliable predictions of the future. In addition to the deficiencies of few samples and many species, these data include variables such as the differing requirements of different countries before a variety can be released to commerce.

This glance back into the relatively short history of mutation breeding also demonstrates something which is common in many successful plant-breeding programs, viz., the repeated occurrence of a particular genotype in the pedigree of several successful varieties. Gustafsson (1977) has described the use of the mutant barley varieties Pallas and Mari in recombination breeding programs. Each of these varieties contributed to the pedigree of an additional four varieties. The latest list in the *Mutation Breeding Newsletter* reports three barley varieties, released in Czechoslovakia, all of which had the mutant variety Diamant as a parent. Similar instances are reported in durum wheats (Scarascia-Mugnozza et al., 1972) and oats (Sigurbjornsson and Micke, 1974).

These examples represent an acceptance of induced mutations as a useful source of variability in conventional plant-breeding programs. The future will undoubtedly find more widespread acceptance, for many of the early uncertainties and fallacies regarding induced mutations have been dispelled. Induced mutations have advantages in certain circumstances, disadvantages in others (Brock, 1971). Greater understanding will lead to more general use.

MUTATIONS AND GENETIC ENGINEERING

Genetic engineering is the intentional genetic manipulation of species to produce special forms, and modern plant breeders must be regarded as highly successful genetic engineers. In the broad sense these special new forms are mutants. However, the term genetic engineering is usually restricted to those situations in which major emphasis is placed on the creation of new variability within a species, either by transfer of genes between species that do not normally interbreed or by the creation of "new" variability.

Considerable effort is being applied to the transfer of genetic information. Translocation of chromosome segments between species which have sufficient homology for the chromosomes to coexist in the same cell has been aided by radiation-induced chromosome breakage. Similar exchanges have occurred when special pairing-suppressing genes on chromosome 5B in polyploid wheat were genetically removed and the transfer of yellow-rust resistance from *Aegilops comosa* was achieved (Riley et al., 1968). Selection of genes for pairing suppression is likely to have been a common occurrence during the evolution of polyploid species. Removal of such genes by mutagenic and chromosome-breaking agents should be relatively easy once suitable selection techniques are developed. Once pairing is achieved, crossing over can be enhanced either by the application of external radiation (Henderson, 1970) or more efficiently by the incorporation of [^{3}H] orotic acid (Singh et al., 1974) at the time of meiotic prophase.

The transfer of genetic information between species via purified DNA has been known in bacteria since 1944 (Avery et al., 1944), and there have been a number of attempts to achieve transformation in plants. The results, though not conclusive, are interesting.

Hess (1969*a,b,* 1970, 1972, 1973) extracted DNA from red-flowered genotypes of *Petunia hybrida* and applied this to young seedlings of a white flowered genotype. Up to 25% of the treated plants produced red flowers. Selfing of the red-flowered plants produced progeny with red flowers and no segregation.

Ledoux and his co-workers (1961, 1968, 1971a,b, 1972, 1974a,b) have even more striking claims—that of the transfer and expression of bacterial DNA in plants. Their claims are based on physical and genetic evidence. The physical evidence, the difference in sedimentation density of bacterial and plant DNA, supports the view that the bacterial DNA is covalently linked with the host-plant DNA.

The genetic evidence, the correction of thiamineless mutants of *Arabidopsis thaliana* with bacterial DNA, is more compatible with the bacterial DNA persisting through several plant generations in close association with the host chromosome as an "exosome," as has been proposed for similar observations in *Drosophila* (Fox et al., 1971). Other workers have not been able to repeat the findings of Ledoux and co-workers regarding the covalent linkage of plant and bacterial DNA (Hotta and Stern, 1971; Kleinhoffs et al., 1975; Lurquin and Hotta, 1975).

Virus-mediated DNA transfer (transduction) has been extensively studied in bacteria. Localized transduction is produced by bacterial viruses that insert their DNA into the bacterial chromosomes at specific points. When the phage is excised from the bacterial chromosome it sometimes brings with it a piece of bacterial genome; thus specific bacterial genes can be picked up by particular bacterial viruses (phages) and transferred to new hosts. Doy et al. (1972, 1973, 1975) made use of these phages to transfer genes for lactose and galactose utilization to tomato plant cell cultures which would not grow with either lactose or galactose as sole carbon sources. They were successful in stimulating growth in the tomato callus and used the term "transgenosis" to describe this phenomenon of transfer and expression of genetic information between organisms widely separated in evolution. They claimed to have demonstrated expression of the bacterial genes in the plant cells, but they were unable to demonstrate that the bacterial genes had been incorporated into the plant chromosomes. Two other laboratories have attempted similar experiments. Smith's laboratory at Nottingham (Grierson et al., 1974) reported slow growth of sycamore cells in culture with lactose as the carbon source after treatment with the phage λ *p lac,* but there was no conclusive evidence that the bacterial genes were incorporated or expressed in the plant cells. Carlson (1973b) did obtain expression of two phage genes in barley tissue cultures.

These results of transformation- and transduction-like processes suggest, without finally proving, that genes can be transferred between widely divergent organisms to give new (mutant) forms that could be of great value in plant improvement. We have commenced experiments in an attempt to use the DNA plant virus, cauliflower mosaic virus, as a vehicle to carry foreign genes into plant cells. It is our hope that the plant virus will not only have the ability to penetrate the plant cell, but will have an affinity with the host's system of replication, transcription, and translation.

CONCLUSION

Induced mutations generate genetic variability, which has already been of substantial use in plant improvement. Varieties are in commercial use, the result of the direct selection of mutants, and mutants are being used increasingly in hybridization programs. Once plant breeders have defined their breeding objectives and assessed their sources of variability, they will be in a position to decide whether they should induce mutations. This decision should only be made after a full consideration of the available variation, its genetic nature, the ploidy level and breeding system of the species, the resources they can devote to the program, and the efficiency of selection that can be applied.

If direct selection of mutants as potential cultivars is the chosen approach, the likelihood of changes to the background genotype in characters important to the agricultural suitability of the variety should not be overlooked. These will almost certainly be changed in any mutant genotype selected only for a specific character. If the mutant is to be chosen primarily for use as a parent in recombination breeding, the most favorable physical and genetic environment for the expression of variation should be provided.

In the immediate future there will be more general acceptance and use of induced mutations as sources of variation in sexually reproducing species in which variability is limiting. There will be substantially more use of induced mutations in vegetatively reproduced species. In these species induced mutations will permit faster progress than will reliance on spontaneous mutations and will cause less drastic changes than with sexual recombination. There will be more use of plant cell culture and specific selection techniques as these are developed for crop plants.

The longer-term future is more difficult to predict. Progress in understanding the biosynthetic and genetic systems in plants, increased control of the mutational processes, and the development of specific selection techniques are likely to alter drastically the working economics of mutation-breeding programs. Successful incorporation and expression of alien DNA in crop plants by transformation or transduction techniques will open completely new vistas. The prospects for the future are exciting, but so is the present.

REFERENCES

Acosta, A. (1961). The transfer of stem rust resistance from rye to wheat. Ph.D. thesis, Univ. of Missouri, 56 pp.

Auerbach, C. (1967). The chemical production of mutations. *Science 158*:1141–1147.

Avery, O. T., Macleod, C. M., and McCarty, M. (1944). Studies on the chemical nature of the substance inducing transformation of pneumococcal types. I. Induction of transformation by a deoxyribonucleic acid fraction isolated from pneumococcus type III. *J. Exp. Med. 79*:137–157.

Brock, R. D. (1971). The role of induced mutations in plant improvement. *Radiat. Bot. 11*:181–196.

Brock, R. D., Friederich, E. A., and Langridge, J. (1973). The modification of amino acid composition of higher plants by mutation and selection. *Nuclear Techniques for Seed Protein Improvement (Proc. Symp. Neuherberg, 1972)*, pp. 329–338. IAEA, Vienna.

Carlson, P. S. (1973*a*). Methionine sulfoximine-resistant mutants of tobacco. *Science 180*: 1366–1368.

Carlson, P. S. (1973*b*). The use protoplasts for genetic research. *Proc. Natl. Acad. Sci. USA 70*:598–602.

Chaleff, R. S. and Carlson, P. S. (1974). Higher plant cells as experimental organisms. *Modification of the Information Content of Plant Cells*, pp. 197–214. North-Holland Amsterdam.

Dobzhansky, T. (1951). *Genetics and the Origin of Species*, p. 364. Columbia Univ. Press, New York.

Doy, C. H. (1975). The transfer and expression (transgenosis) of foreign genes in plant cells, reality and potential. *The Eukaryote Chromosome*, pp. 447–458. ANU Press, Canberra.

Doy, C. H., Gresshoff, P. M., and Rolfe, B. G. (1972). Transfer and expression (transgenosis) of bacterial genes in plant cells. *Search 3*:447–448.

Doy, C. H., Gresshoff, P. M., and Rolfe, B. G. (1973). Biological and molecular evidence for the transgenosis of genes from bacteria to plant cells. *Proc. Natl. Acad. Sci. USA 70*:723–726.

Driscoll, C. J. and Jensen, N. F. (1963). A genetic method for detecting intergeneric translocations. *Genetics 48*:459–468.

Fox, A. S., Yoon, S. B., Duggleby, W. F., and Gelbart, W. M. (1971). Genetic transformation in *Drosophila*. *Informative Molecules in Biological Systems*, pp. 313–332. North-Holland, Amsterdam.

Grierson, D., McKee, R. A., Attridge, T. H., and Smith, H. (1974). Studies on uptake and expression of foreign genetic material by higher plant cells. *Modification of the Information Content of Plant Cells* pp. 91–99. North-Holland, Amsterdam.

Gustafsson, A. (1977). Mutations in plant breeding–A glance back and a look forward. *Proc. 5th Int. Congr. Radiat. Res.*, in press.

Heimer, Y. M. and Filner, P. (1970). Regulation of the nitrate assimilation pathway of cultured tobacco cells. II. Properties of a variant cell line. *Biochim. Biophys. Acta 215*:152–165.

Henderson, S. A. (1970). The time and place of meiotic crossing-over. *Annu. Rev. Genet. 4*:295–324.

Hess, D. (1969*a*). Versuche zur Transformation an höheren Pflanzen: Induktion und konstante Weitergabe der Anthocyansythese bei *Petunia hybrida*. *Z. Pflanzenphysiol. 60*:348–358.

Hess, D. (1969*b*). Versuche zur Transformation an höheren Pflanzen: Wilderholung der Anthocyan-Induktion bei *Petunia* und erste Charakterisierung des transformierenden Prinzips. *Z. Pflanzenphysiol. 61*:286–298.

Hess, D. (1970). Versuche zur Transformation an höheren Pflanzen: Mögliche Transplantation eines Gens für Blattform bei *Petunia hybrida*. *Z. Pflanzenphysiol. 63*:461–467.

Hess, D. (1972). Transformationen an höheren Organismen. *Naturwissenschaften 59*: 348–355.

Hess, D. (1973). Transformationsversuche an höheren Pflanzen: Untersuchungen zur Realisation des Exosomen-Modells der Transformation bei *Petunia hybrida*. *Z. Pflanzenphysiol. 68*:432–440.

Hotta, Y. and Stern, H. (1971). Uptake and distribution of heterologous DNA in living cells. *Informative Molecules in Biological Systems,* pp. 176–184. North-Holland, Amsterdam.

Kihlman, B. A. (1966). *Action of Chemicals on Dividing Cells.* Prentice-Hall, Englewood Cliffs, N.J.

Kleinhoffs, A., Eden, F. C., Chilton, M-D., and Bendich, A. J. (1975). On the question of the integration of exogenous bacterial DNA into plant DNA. *Proc. Natl. Acad. Sci. USA* 72:2748–2752.

Knott, D. R. (1961). The inheritance of rust resistance. VI. The transfer of stem rust resistance from *Agropyron elongatum* to common wheat. *Can. J. Plant Sci. 41*:109–123.

Ledoux, L. and Huart, R. (1961). Sur la possibilité d'un transfer d'acides ribo- et desoxy-ribonucleiques et de proteins dans les embryons d'orge en croissance. *Arch. Intern. Physiol. Biochim. 69*:598.

Ledoux, L. and Huart, R. (1972). Fate of exogenous DNA in plants. *Uptake of Informative Molecules by Living Cells,* pp. 254–276. North-Holland, Amsterdam.

Ledoux, L., Huart, R., and Jacobs, M. (1971a). Fate of exogenous DNA in *Arabidopsis thaliana.* I. Translocation and integration. *Eur. J. Biochem. 23*:96–108.

Ledoux, L., Huart, R., and Jacobs, M. (1971b). Fate of exogenous DNA in *Aradibopsis thaliana.* II. Evidence for replication and preliminary results at the biological level. *Informative Molecules in Biological Systems,* pp. 159–172. North-Holland, Amsterdam.

Ledoux, L., Huart, R., and Jacobs, M. (1974a). DNA-mediated genetic correction of thiamineless *Arabidopsis thaliana. Nature 249*:17–21.

Ledoux, L., Huart, R., Mergeay, M., Charles, P., and Jacobs, M. (1974b). DNA-mediated genetic correction of thiamineless *Arabidopsis thaliana. Modification of the Information Content of Plant Cells,* pp. 67–89. North-Holland, Amsterdam.

Lundqvist, U., von Wettstein-Knowles, P., and von Wettstein, D. (1968). Induction of *eceriferum* mutants in barley by ionizing radiations and chemicals. II. *Hereditas 59*: 473–504.

Lurquin, P. F. and Hotta, Y. (1975). Reutilization of bacterial DNA by *Arabidopsis thaliana* cells in tissue culture. *Plant Sci. Lett. 5*:103–112.

Nakayama, K., Tanaka, H., Hagino, H., and Kinoshita, S. (1966). Studies on lysine fermentation. Part V. Concerted feedback inhibition of aspartokinase and the absence of lysine inhibition on aspartic semialdehyde-pyruvate condensation in *Micrococcus glutamicus. Agric. Biol. Chem. 30*:611–616.

Nilan, R. A. (1972). Mutagenic specificity in flowering plants: Facts and Prospects. *Induced Mutations and Plant Improvement,* pp. 141–151. IAEA, Vienna.

Palmer, J. E. and Widholm, J. (1975). Characterization of carrot and tobacco cell cultures resistant to *p*-fluorophenylalamine. *Plant Physiol. 56*:233–238.

Persson, G. and Hagberg, A. (1969). Induced variation in a quantitative character in barley. Morphology and cytogenetics of *erectoides* mutants. *Hereditas 61*:115–178.

Rédei, G. P. (1974). Economy in mutation experiments. *Z. Pflanzenzüecht. 73*:87–96.

Riley, R., Chapman, V., and Johnson, R. (1968). Introduction of yellow rust resistance of *Aegilops comosa* into wheat by genetically induced homoeologous recombination. *Nature 217*:383–384.

Scarascia-Mugnozza, G. T., Bagnara, D., and Bozzini, A. (1972). Mutagenesis applied to *durum* wheat. Results and perspectives. *Induced Mutations and Plant Improvement,* pp. 183–197. IAEA, Vienna.

Sharma, D. and Knott, D. R. (1966). The transfer of leaf rust resistance from *Agropyron* to *Triticum* by irradiation. *Can. J. Genet. Cytol. 8*:137–143.

Sears, E. R. (1956). The transfer of leaf-rust resistance from *Aegilops umbellulata* to wheat. *Brookhaven Symp. Biol. 9*:1–22.

Sigurbjornsson, B. and Micke, A. (1974). Philosophy and accomplishments of mutation breeding. *Polyploidy and Induced Mutations in Plant Breeding,* pp. 303–343. IAEA, Vienna.

Singh, C. B., Brock, R. D., and Oram, R. N. (1974). Increased meiotic recombination by incorporated tritium. *Radiat. Bot. 14*:139–145.

Weinhues, A. (1966). Transfer of rust resistance of *Agropyron* to wheat by addition, substitution and translocation. *Proc. 2nd Int. Wheat Genet. Symp. Hereditas [Suppl.] 2*:370–381.

Widholm, J. M. (1972*a*). Cultured *Nicotiana tabacum* cells with an altered anthranilate synthetase which is less sensitive to feedback inhibition. *Biochim. Biophys. Acta 261*:52–58.

Widholm, J. M. (1972*b*) Anthranilate synthetase from 5-methytryptophan-susceptible and -resistant cultured *Daucus carota* cells. *Biochim. Biophys. Acta 279*:48–57.

Widholm, J. M. (1974). Selection and characteristics of biochemical mutants of cultured plant cells. *Tissue Culture and Plant Science,* pp. 287–299. Academic Press, London.

13

Norin-10-Based Semidwarfism

Michael D. Gale and Colin N. Law

Plant Breeding Institute
Cambridge, England

ABSTRACT

Many short-strawed wheats, including the Norin-10-based semidwarfs now grown in many countries, are characterized by their relative "insensitivity" to gibberellic acid. The nature of this insensitivity, its genetic control, and the relationships between the *Gai* genes and the *Rht* genes, which control height reduction in Norin-10 and Tom Thumb wheats, are described. The role and potential of these genes in agriculture and their relationship to other genes affecting yield, height, and other agronomic features are considered.

INTRODUCTION

During the last 10 years much attention has been focused on the higher yields of bread wheat, *Triticum aestivum,* achieved with the introduction of semidwarf varieties into most wheat-growing countries. Reduction of plant height as a means of increasing yield is not, however, a new idea. In Britain, as in other parts of the world, increases in yield with concurrent decreases in the height of leading varieties have been achieved since the beginning of this century, as shown in Fig. 1. The credit for the increased yields is not all attributable to the breeder—he has simply modified his crop to take full advantage of new improved agricultural practices. The main factor has certainly been the introduction of artificial chemical fertilizers after World War II—a shorter, stronger stem was required to prevent lodging at harvest time after their application. With shorter straw came

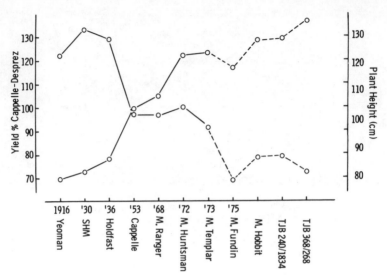

Fig. 1. Relative yields and plant heights of leading British varieties this century. Varieties following Maris Templar are Norin-10-based semidwarfs.

another problem—the new erect-leaved varieties were unable to compete effectively with weeds. The advent of herbicides in the 1950s paved the way to still shorter varieties as other agricultural conditions changed (e.g., in Britain, the reduction in value of the straw itself).

Initially, the breeders achieved reductions in height by producing new combinations of genes already present in their adapted lines. Below the 1-m mark further reductions of this sort were increasingly difficult to obtain. So they turned toward the major genes for semidwarfism in exotic material, in particular, the Japanese variety Norin-10.

NORIN-10 AS A SOURCE OF DWARFING GENES

Norin-10 was imported to North America by Salmon in 1948 (Reitz and Salmon, 1968). During the following year the first crosses were made between adapted varieties and Norin-10 at Washington State University (Vogel et al., 1956). From these crosses emerged the now well-known lines, such as Norin-10—Brevor-14 that have been the genetic base of most semidwarf varieties. The first was Gaines bred by Vogel at Washington State, followed by the Mexican semidwarfs bred by Borlaug at CIMMYT. The first semidwarf varieties, again based on Norin-10—Brevor-14, have now been released in Britain (Fig. 1) and have been bred by Lupton and Bingham at the Plant Breeding Institute, Cambridge.

Although the Norin-10 semidwarfing factors are known to be "major" genes, the variation in final plant height released in crosses with conventional varieties is by no means discrete, as shown in Fig. 2. Whereas the breeders have been able to make major reductions in straw length very rapidly, the genetic analysis of Norin-10 dwarfism has been severely hampered by its essentially quantitative nature.

THE NEED FOR AN UNDERSTANDING OF THE GENETICS OF DWARFISM IN WHEAT

A breeder may exploit variation of the type provided by Norin-10 without any knowledge of the genetic control mechanisms involved. However, especially with variation of the agronomic importance of semidwarfism, genetic analysis can aid a practical breeding program.

First, knowledge of the numbers of genes involved, their effects, and their genetic interactions may be used in selecting suitable parents for crosses and in predicting their outcome in terms of a desired height phenotype. Second, knowledge of the chromosomal locations of the loci carrying the genes may be used to avoid or exploit known linkages and, more importantly, allow their

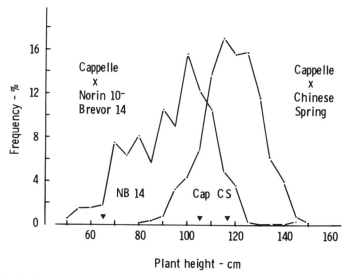

Fig. 2. F_2 plant-height frequency distributions showing continuous variation with or without segregation of the Norin-10 "major" genes.

direct introduction, either singly or together, into any genetic background by employing the now-standard aneuploid techniques available in hexaploid wheat (Law and Worland, 1973). In this way those genetic backgrounds most compatible with one or the other of the genes may be readily recognized. Third, the ability to recognize the presence of the genes in individual plants will permit an understanding of the physiological and developmental mechanisms through which the genes operate. Knowledge of how these mechanisms affect characters other than plant height may allow a rational choice between the use of one or more of the genes in a potential variety.

Such in-depth analysis of height reduction in wheat is only now emerging, which is surprising considering the impact these genes have had on world agriculture.

THE MAJOR GENES FOR HEIGHT REDUCTION IN WHEAT

Even in 1968, seven years after the introduction of Gaines, the number of genes involved in Norin-10 dwarfism was not clear. Then Allan et al. (1968) showed that Norin-10–Brevor-14 carried two genes determining the semidwarf habit and that just one of these genes could give rise to a semidwarf phenotype in varieties such as Suwon-92. The two genes are additive in their effects, and the alleles determining reduced height at each locus are recessive (Fick and Qualset, 1973). These genes have now been assigned the symbols *Rht 1* and *Rht 2*. *Rht 2* has been shown to produce shorter straw than *Rht 1* (Allan, 1970). A third gene, *Rht 3,* which has a larger dwarfing effect than do the Norin-10 genes is carried by the dwarf wheat Tom Thumb (Zeven, 1969). This allele displays little dominance and appears to have arisen several times in different parts of the world.

The chromosomal location of the *Rht* loci has not been easy to ascertain. Because suitable intervarietal chromosome substitution series have not been available, monosomic analysis has generally been applied. The use of F_1 and F_2 monosomic analysis (Sears, 1953) is most efficient in locating dominant genes whose influence on the phenotype is unaffected by monosomy itself. However, both *Rht 1* and *Rht 2* are recessive and almost hemizygous ineffective. Also, plant height is a character affected considerably by monosomy for almost every chromosome of wheat. In such cases, the variation released by allelic differences on a particular chromosome will be confounded with that released by the aneuploid condition of that chromosome. Typical effects of monosomy on plant height are shown by the Bersee monosomics in Fig. 3, which shows that monosomy induces considerable height reduction for the chromosomes in homologous group 2 and lesser reductions for those in groups 4, 6, and 7, whereas height increases are induced in groups 1, 3, and 5. Therefore it is not surprising that many of the possible locations for the *Rht* alleles pinpointed by monosomic

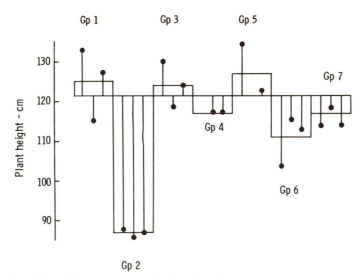

Fig. 3. The effects of monosomy on plant height in the variety Bersee. Each line represents the mean height, relative to Bersee, of monosomics for the A, B, and D genome chromosomes (L–R in each homologous group). The bars represent the mean monosomic family height for each homologous group (data from Law and Worland, 1973).

analyses fall in the homologous groups in which the effects of monosomy mimic those of the height-reducing factors.

Allan and Vogel (1963) found chromosomes 2A, 2B, 2D, 3D, and 4B to be the most probable carriers of the *Rht 1* and *Rht 2* loci. Jha and Swaminathan (1969) pinpointed 2A, 4D, and 6D. Chromosomes 6D (Bhowal, 1970), 1B, and 5D (Singhal et al., 1973), and 2A and 4B (Baier et al., 1974) have also been reported as the critical chromosomes in different semidwarf varieties.

Rht 3, being hemizygous effective, was conclusively located on chromosome 4A by Morris et al. (1972).

Clearly then, in order to establish the location of *Rht 1* and *Rht 2,* a different approach was needed. A method of accurately identifying the genes was required.

INSENSITIVITY TO APPLIED GIBBERELLIC ACID

Relatively early in the investigations of major gene dwarfism, Allan et al. (1959) observed that Norin-10 derivatives and Tom Thumb displayed a much-reduced height response to applied gibberellic acid (GA). Whereas the internode lengths of tall varieties could be almost doubled by injections of GA, those of the dwarfs were relatively unaffected. GA-response individuals can be easily distinguished from GA-insensitive plants by application of a GA solution to seedlings. Figure 4A shows this difference between Chinese Spring (responsive) and Minister Dwarf, an insensitive Tom Thumb-type dwarf.

This seedling GA-response test may be employed to ascertain the number of genes controlling insensitivity in crosses of Norin-10 derivatives and Tom Thumb dwarfs with tall responsive varieties. In Norin-10—Brevor-14, two partially dominant alleles *Gai 1* and *Gai 2* control the character. Fifteen insensitive: one responsive segregations are obtained in F_2 families from crosses of Norin-10—Brevor-14 with tall varieties. Where the segregations of *Gai 1* and *Gai 2* are observed separately, *Gai 1* is seen to display less penetrance and dominance than *Gai 2*. Insensitivity in Tom Thumb dwarfs is controlled by a single, extremely potent and dominant gene *Gai 3*. Typical GA-treated seedlings from the F_2 derived from Chinese Spring × Minister Dwarf are shown in Fig. 4B.

THE RELATIONSHIP BETWEEN SEMIDWARFISM AND GIBBERELLIN INSENSITIVITY IN WHEAT

Differential responses to applied GA have been observed between tall and dwarf forms in several plant species. Genetic dwarfs have been shown to display increased responses, as compared with tall forms, in morning glory (Ogawa, 1962), maize (Phinney, 1961), red bean (Proano and Greene, 1968), rice (Suge and Murakami, 1968), and in wheat (Gale and Law, 1973), whereas decreased responses of dwarf genotypes have been reported in rice (Harada and Vergara, 1971) and in maize (Phinney, 1957). Thus, associations between abnormal GA metabolism and genetic variation in plant height are commonplace.

The genetic association between plant height and insensitivity in dwarf wheat is best demonstrated in segregational tests. For example, F_2 individuals resulting from a GA responsive × insensitive hybrid may be classified for plant height and their *Gai* genotype ascertained exactly by F_3 seedling progeny testing with applied GA. Figure 5 shows the individual plant heights plotted against their derivative F_3 family means for 61 F_2's derived from a Minister Dwarf (*Gai 3*) × April Bearded (*gai 3*) hybrid. Each line has been classified for *Gai 3* genotype. Clearly the two characters are closely associated genetically. This experiment indicates that *Gai 3* and *Rht 3* are either the same locus and that the effects on plant height are mediated by the GA insensitivity mechanisms or that if the two genes are carried at separate loci, they must be closely linked. This result is one of several in which no recombination between *Gai 3* and *Rht 3* has

---

Fig. 4. Variation in GA response. All seedlings after 14 days growth at 18°C in culture solution containing 10 ppm GA_3. (A) L–R, Chinese Spring and Minister Dwarf; (B) seven F_2 seedlings, CS × MD, euploid; (C) seven F_2 seedlings, CS monosomic 4A × MD—the weak GA responsive seedling on the extreme left is a nullisomic, i.e., lacking both 4A chromosomes.

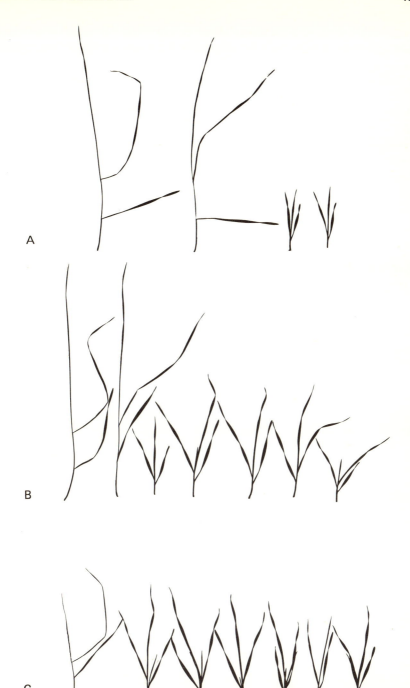

A

B

C

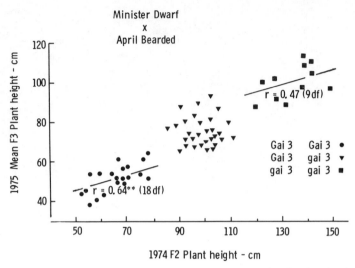

Fig. 5. *The relationship between F_2 plant height and mean F_3 family plant height for F_2 individuals classified for Gai 3 genotype by subsequent F_3 progeny testing.*

been observed; however, Hu (1974) reports segregation at the *Gai 3* locus in lines assumed to be homozygous for the *Rht 3* allele. So the possibility of the existence of two distinct loci must be kept open. In Fig. 5 heritable variation capable of modifying the *Rht 3* phenotype is displayed by the positive correlation between F_2 and F_3 plant heights within the *Gai 3 Gai 3* genotypic group.

The results of a similar F_2 segregational test are shown for Hobbit (*Gai 2 Rht 2*) X Chinese Spring (*gai 2 rht 2*) in Fig. 6. Clearly, the two phenotypes are again highly associated. However, the continuous nature of the variation in plant height within *Gai 2* genotypic groups does not allow a distinction to be made between the alternative hypotheses of pleiotropy or linked genes, as was concluded by Hu (1974) and Konzak et al. (1973). Similar associations between *Gai 1* and *Rht 1* have been demonstrated by Hu.

Other circumstantial evidence appears to favor the hypothesis that insensitivity and height reduction are the products of just three genes, rather than three pairs of closely linked genes. First, the relative potency of each of the *Gai* alleles exactly matches the height-reducing effects of their associated *Rht* alleles, i.e., in potency, *Gai 3 > Gai 2 > Gai 1,* and, in height reduction, *Rht 3 > Rht 2 > Rht 1.* Second, all the Norin-10 derivatives produced at the Plant Breeding Institute, Cambridge and all those from the CIMMYT program in Mexico tested in this laboratory display GA insensitivity. It should be noted, however, that this could indicate that other agronomic advantages are associated with insensitivity resulting in the automatic inclusion of the *Gai* alleles in semidwarf selections.

Genotype   n

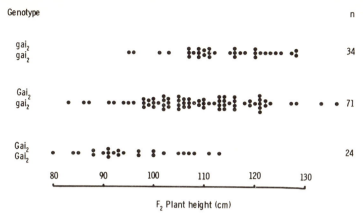

F₂ Plant height (cm)

Fig. 6. Hobbit (Gai 2) × *Chinese Spring (gai 2).* The relationship between F₂ plant height and *Gai 2.*

Nevertheless, it is clear that whatever the nature of the association between the *Gai* and *Rht* genes, the chromosomal locations of the *Gai* genes must be identical with those of the *Rht* genes with which they are genotypically paired.

LOCATION OF *GAI 1* AND *RHT 1*

As a qualitative character, GA insensitivity is well suited for monosomic analysis as monosomy itself has no effect on the classification of insensitive or responsive individuals. The line Sdl, extracted by Allan and Vogel (1968), can be shown to carry *Gai 1*. In monosomic F₂'s from hybrids between the 19 available monosomics of Bersee (Law and Worland, 1973) and Sd1, the three insensitive : one responsive segregation observed in the euploid F₂ was found to be distorted for the Bersee monosomic 4A/Sd1 family. In this family, the relatively few GA-responsive plants were all found to be nullisomic, i.e., lacking both 4A chromosomes (Gale and Marshall, 1976). The location of *Gai/Rht 1* on 4A has been confirmed in a Cappelle-Desprez monosomic/Olsen analysis.

LOCATION OF *GAI 2* AND *RHT 2*

F₁ monosomic analysis was used to locate *Gai 2,* as monosomics in Hobbit, which carries the gene, were available. In this experiment (Gale et al., 1975*b*), in which each of the Hobbit monosomics was crossed with the tall responsive variety Poros, the critical chromosome was identified as 4D. Monosomic F₁'s of the hybrid Hobbit monosomic 4D/Poros were all responsive, whereas euploid F_1's from the same hybrid were found to be insensitive. All other monosomic hybrids were insensitive as expected if chromosome 4D carries *Gai/Rht 2*. The location of *Gai/Rht 2* on chromosome 4D has since been confirmed in Sd2, Ciano-67, and Olsen by various aneuploid techniques.

LOCATION OF *GAI 3* AND *RHT 3*

The location of *Gai 3* was shown to be chromosome 4A in an F_2 monosomic analysis involving the Chinese Spring monosomics and Minister Dwarf (Gale et al., 1975a). The location of *Rht 3* has been shown independently to be chromosome 4A by Morris et al. (1972).

THE GENETIC RELATIONSHIP BETWEEN NORIN-10- AND TOM THUMB DWARFISM

The finding that *Gai/Rht 1* from Norin-10 and *Gai/Rht 3* are both carried on chromosome 4A prompted a reevaluation of the relationship between the two types of dwarfism. Norin-10 and Tom Thumb have been reported to be genetically distinct by Piech (1968), Fick and Qualset (1973), and Chaudhry (1973).

The relationship between *Gai 1* and *Gai 3* on chromosome 4A was first examined in 1600 F_2 seedlings from *Gai 1 Gai 2* X *Gai 3* hybrids. Assuming independent assortment 1/64th (or 25) of 1600 seedlings were expected to be GA responsive. No such individuals were found, which indicates that *Gai 1* and *Gai 3* are either alternative alleles at the same locus or alleles carried at two linked loci. Further investigation of F_3 families from the same hybrids still demonstrated no recombination (Gale and Marshall, 1976). Data from this experiment, although yielding an estimate of zero linkage, reduced the maximum recombination value possible between the loci to 0.7% with 95% confidence. Clearly, this type of experiment can never prove the allelism of *Gai 1* and *Gai 3;* nevertheless, these results strongly support this possibility. If this is the case, a demonstration that the *Rht* loci in Norin-10-type (*Rht 1 Rht 2*) X Tom Thumb-type (*Rht 3*) dwarfs are distinct would indicate that at least one of the *Gai/Rht* gene pairs is carried at separable loci.

However, the basis of such results has generally been the observation of transgressive segregation, i.e., the appearance in the F_2 of individual plants taller than either parent. In the light of what is now known of the locations and relative effects of the *Rht* alleles, transgressive segregation is clearly to be expected, whether *Rht 1* and *Rht 3* are alternative alleles at the same locus or not. The difference between the two hypotheses would lie in that the tallest possible segregants in the former case, i.e., *Rht 1 rht 2* will be shorter than those possible in the latter, i.e., *rht 1 rht 2 rht 3*.

The data shown in Fig. 7 represent the pooled F_2 distributions of two types of cross, in which *Rht 1* and *Rht 2* segregate with *Rht 3* (type 1) and without *Rht 3* (type 2). If *Rht 1* and *Rht 3* were independent, plants as tall as the tallest from type 2 would be expected in type 1—although at a reduced frequency. No such plants were observed among the 655 type 1 F_2 individuals in Fig. 7. This apparent difference between type 1 and type 2 crosses could be caused by the presence of dispersed genes for tallness only in type 2. Although this explanation cannot be excluded, it seems unlikely because Norin-10–Brevor-14 is common to all crosses and the tall parents in type 2, Chinese Spring, and Cappelle-Desprez are only of standard height. Also, similar F_2 height distributions for type 1 and type 2 crosses were obtained by Fick (1971) involving different parents, which indicates that the lack of tall plants is more likely to be caused by allelism of the *Rht* alleles than by the presence of height-promoting gene combinations only in type 2.

It is therefore probable, but by no means substantiated, that the variation controlled by the major dwarfing genes in both insensitive dwarf types, Norin-10 and Tom Thumb, is all carried at two, possibly homologous loci, *Gai/Rht 1* and *Gai/Rht 3,* being alternative alleles at the locus on chromosome 4A and *Gai/Rht 2* at the other on 4D.

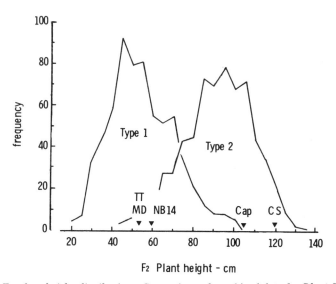

Fig. 7. F_2 plant height distributions. Comparison of combined data for *Rht 1 Rht 2* × *Rht 3* (type 1 crosses) and *rht 3* × *Rht 1 Rht 2* (type 2 crosses). Parents: *Rht 1 Rht 2,* Norin-10–Brevor-14; *Rht 3,* Tom Thumb and Minister Dwarf; *rht 3,* Cappelle-Desprez and Chinese Spring.

VARIETAL CLASSIFICATION

A conventional test-crossing procedure enables GA-insensitive genotypes to be classified for the presence of *Gai/Rht 1, Gai/Rht 2,* and *Gai/Rht 3.* Table I shows the named varieties classified to date.

THE NATURE OF GIBBERELLIN INSENSITIVITY

The first evidence relating to the mechanism of GA insensitivity was provided by Radley (1970) who observed that the tissues of Norin-10 and several semidwarf derivatives contained higher levels of endogenous GA than did some tall varieties. She concluded that insensitivity was caused by a block in the utilization of endogenous hormone. This result was confirmed in Tom Thumb types by Gale and Marshall (1973*a*), who also reported a shift in the proportions of GA_1-like and GA_3-like activity in dwarf tissues, which is again consistent with a block in turnover of the hormone. Evidence is also available that suggests that the high endogenous GA levels are not the result of increased production. GA release from germinating embryos of dwarf wheats was found to be quantitatively similar to that from tall varieties (Gale and Marshall, 1975). Clearly, the evidence favors an effect of the *Gai* alleles on "turnover" of GA in the plant. Furthermore, these genes may be shown to be "active," rather than simply null mutations resulting in the removal of some essential part of the GA metabolic pathway, as nullisomics for chromosome 4A and 4D are GA-responsive (Fig. 4C). It is therefore possible that the genes could act via the production of a GA antagonist, which must operate at the "active sites" of GA

Table I. *Gai/Rht* **Alleles—Varietal Classification**

Gai Rht 1	Gai Rht 2	Gai Rht 1 + 2	Gai Rht 3
Sd1[a]	Hobbit	Norin-10–	Tom Thumb
Jarral 66[a]	Fundin	Brevor-14	Tom Pouce
Mexipak	Ciano 67	Olsen	Minister Dwarf
	Sd2[a]		
	Gaines[a]		
	Coulee[a]		
	Toquifen S[a]		
	Pitic 62[a]		
	Suwon 92/4[a]		
	Sonora 64		

[a]From Hu (1974).

action, and not on the GA molecule itself, as homozygotes for the *Gai* alleles are insensitive even at very high concentrations of applied GA.

Research in progress is producing results concerning the nature of this antagonism. Protein fractions from dwarf peas have been found that selectively bind with biologically active GA's (Stoddart et al., 1974). Preliminary work with Norin-10 semidwarfs indicates that the capacity for such selective binding by similar protein fractions may be positively correlated with the stature of the plant from which the extracts are made (Stoddart, personal communication).

Clearly then, while these results link the physiology of the insensitive reaction with that of height reduction and reinforce the pleiotropy hypothesis, they also indicate that the *Gai/Rht* genes affect a basic change in the metabolism of varieties that carry them. Some pleiotropic effects of these genes on aspects of the plants' development occur well before the achievement of final plant height. High-tillering patterns in dwarf types have been linked with an abnormal tillering response to applied GA (Gale and Marshall, 1973b) and *Gai 3* has been shown to operate in the germinating grain by restricting the release of hydrolytic enzymes, including α-amylase, in response to exogenous hormone (Gale and Marshall, 1975).

THE GENETIC RELATIONSHIP BETWEEN HEIGHT AND YIELD, AND THE EFFECTS OF THE *GAI/RHT* GENES

In the absence of segregation for semidwarfing genes and lodging it appears to be a general rule that plant height and grain yield are positively genetically correlated in wheat (Chaudhry, 1973; Law et al., 1974; Knott and Kumar, 1975), oats (Sampson, 1971), and in barley (Riggs and Hayter, 1975). This correlation has been found under both spaced and normal drilled sowing conditions. Recent investigations have shown that this relationship is probably due to the pleiotropic action of genes affecting both characters. (Law et al., 1977). It should be stressed that this association applies only to segregating generations from individual crosses and need not apply to varietal comparisons, e.g., over the varieties in Fig. 1.

Given this positive genetic association, it is important to determine whether the *Gai/Rht* genes act in a similar manner to give reduced yields. Several reports of strong positive correlations among semidwarfs are available (e.g., Allan, 1970; Joppa, 1973; Stoskopf and Fairey, 1975). However, in this laboratory the correlations from semidwarf × tall crosses, although still generally positive, tend to be weaker than those from semidwarf × semidwarf or tall × tall crosses. Also, in a set of F_1 and F_2 diallel crosses involving semidwarf and standard varieties, the linear regression lines for yield on height of family means of the semidwarf varieties and their hybrids and the tall varieties and their hybrids were found to differ. Although the two slopes were similar and positive, the mean yield for the semidwarf families was higher than that for the tall families (Chaudhry, 1973). These results suggest that the *Gai/Rht* genes are associated with increasing yield rather than the reverse—the more general effect of other height genes. Of course, whether the yield advantage is due to pleiotropy or due to linkage with a gene(s) for higher yield cannot be determined from this evidence.

Up to now investigations concerning any effects of the Norin-10 semidwarf-have been hampered by an inability to exactly define the *Rht* genotype of any individual or line in segregating populations. Hitherto, these genotypes have been assessed on final plant height, except where test crosses have been used, e.g., Allan (1970). For example, in Fig. 6, without the benefit of F_3 seedling GA-response testing, individuals within the range of 100–110 cm could only be classified as having a high probability of being *Rht 2 rht 2* heterozygotes, whereas in fact 18 of the 45 plants were either *Gai/Rht 2* or *gai/rht 2* homozygotes.

In the experiment from which the data shown in Fig. 6 were taken, which consisted of two blocks of field-grown spaced F_2 plants from the cross Hobbit × Chinese Spring, the ear yields, grain numbers, and grain weights were scored for the leading tiller of each plant as well as height at maturity. The data for height and ear yield and their correlations are summarized in Table II. The overall association between height and yield in the F_2 is low, but stronger correlations, typical of semidwarf × semidwarf F_2's grown in the same trial, are obtained within the *Gai 2 Gai 2, Gai 2 gai 2,* and *gai 2 gai 2* groups of plants. Clearly, the strong positive relationship between height and yield is confounded by the effects of *Gai 2,* or genes linked to *Gai 2,* which give rise to the differences in elevation of similar slopes, as shown in Fig. 8. Further analysis showed that the yield differences were mainly the results of grain number rather than grain weight.

Similar results were found for two other F_2 families derived from crosses of Chinese Spring with Maris Bilbo, a *Gai 2* semidwarf bred at this Institute and

Table II. Chinese Spring (*gai 2*) × Hobbit (*Gai 2*), F_2[a,b]

Genotype	n	r	Plant height (cm)	Ear yield (g)	a	b
Hobbit	20	0.14	93.4	3.75		
Chinese Spring	20	0.13	118.2	2.62		
Overall F_2	122	0.10	107.9	3.10	1.93	0.011
Gai 2 Gai 2, F_2	21	0.45	94.9	3.61	−0.19	0.040
Gai 2 gai 2, F_2	67	0.37	108.6	3.08	−0.46	0.033
gai 2 gai 2, F_2	34	0.36	114.6	2.84	−0.89	0.033

[a]Differences between *Gai 2* genotype regressions: Scatter, NS: Slope (b's) NS; Elevation (a's) $p < 0.001$.
[b]Correlation coefficients (r) and linear regression components (a, b) for height and ear yield with *Gai 2* genotypes.

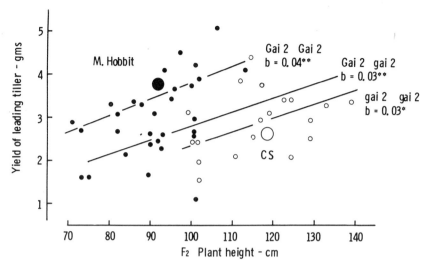

Fig. 8. *The association between* F_2 *plant height and ear yield within groups of plants classified for Gai 2 genotype from the cross Hobbit (Gai 2)* × *Chinese Spring (gai 2).* Individual points for *Gai 2 gai 2* plants are not shown.

Ciano-67, a *Gai 2* semidwarf from the Mexican program, thereby strengthening the argument that the *Gai/Rht* themselves have a beneficial effect on yield. But because all the results were obtained from spaced plants of relatively similar crosses, it remains to be established whether the relationship holds over a wide range of genetic backgrounds under normal agricultural regimes.

Despite these reservations, the results are sufficiently remarkable to propose an operational model (Chaudhry, 1973; Law et al., 1976) from which the consequences of various approaches to semidwarf wheat breeding can be predicted. Given a genetic architecture in which many of the genes for increasing height also increase yield and in which the *Gai/Rht* genes have the reverse effect, the best course of action to achieve higher yield is to fix the semidwarfing factors early in a breeding program while maintaining other variation in the population. Thereafter, selection should be for increased height, rather than for shorter and shorter versions of a dwarf ideotype.

The model, summarized in Fig. 9, also shows that depending on the lodging cutoff point, yield gains can be made even if the dwarfing gene used has a mean negative effect on yield. If, however, the effect of the dwarfing gene on yield is positive, as appears to be the case for *Gai/Rht 2* in Fig. 8, then yield benefits are to be had under all conditions.

Selection for "tall dwarfs" to give increased yields has several advantages, not the least of which is the highly heritable nature of the character height compared with that of yield. Also, by not selecting strongly for shortness, the

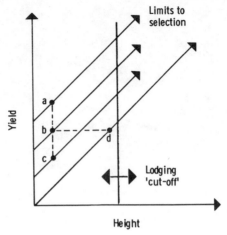

Fig. 9. *A model showing the effects of selection for increased height in populations into which semidwarfing factors have been introduced.* It is assumed that the genes for dwarfism do not affect the positive relationship between height and yield determined by the other genes present in each of the populations. The "lodging cutoff" is the plant height at which losses in yield due to lodging begin to occur—this point is moveable and is determined by environmental and genetic factors. In each case ● denotes the mean of the population carrying a particular allele. (a) Substitution of an allele for dwarfism having a positive effect on yield; (b) substitution of an allele for dwarfism whose effect on yield is neutral or identical to the effect of the allele for tallness on yield; (c) substitution of an allele for dwarfism whose effect on yield is negative; and (d) population carrying the tall allele.

rapid dissipation of much of the variation available for further yield improvement is avoided.

Undoubtedly, other genes affecting yield in ways different from those outlined earlier exist in wheat; some account must be made of these additional genetic constraints in any breeding program. Also genotype–environment interactions may be such as to render the genetic relationships observed in the experiments described above inapplicable under some circumstances. It remains to be seen whether the model presented provides a useful approach in realizing high yields or if it is an oversimplified view of the organization of the genes of economic importance in the wheat crop.

CONCLUSIONS

1. Norin-10–Brevor-14 carries two semidwarfing alleles, *Rht 1* and *Rht 2;* Tom Thumb carries a third, *Rht 3.*
2. Each of these genes is associated with insensitivity to gibberellin.

3. *Gai/Rht 1* and *Gai/Rht 3* are carried on chromosome 4A, *Gai/Rht 2* on 4D.
4. *Gai/Rht 1* and *Gai/Rht 3* are likely to be alternative alleles at the same locus.
5. The *Gai/Rht* alleles effect a basic change in the metabolism of the wheat plant and their effects may be observed throughout development.
6. Limited data suggest that *Gai/Rht 2* has a positive effect on yield via increases in grain number and that maximum yields may be obtained by breeding for "tall dwarfs." This exploits the positive pleiotropic effects of genes that control height and yield in the presence of the Norin-10 dwarfing genes.

REFERENCES

Allan, R. E. (1970). Differentiating between two Norin 10–Brevor 14 semi-dwarf genes in a common genetic background. *Seiken Ziho 22*:83–90.

Allan, R. E. and Vogel, O. A. (1963). F_2 monosomic analysis of culm length in wheat crosses involving semi-dwarf Norin 10–Brevor 14 and the Chinese Spring series. *Crop Sci. 3*:538–540.

Allan, R. E. and Vogel, O. A. (1968). A method for predicting semi-dwarf genotypes in *Triticum aestivum* L. *Agron.* Abst. p.2.

Allan, R. E., Vogel, O. A., and Craddock, J. C., Jr. (1959). Comparative response to gibberellic acid of dwarf, semi-dwarf, and standard short and tall winter wheat varieties. *Agron.* J. *51*:737–740.

Allan, R. E., Vogel, O. A., and Peterson, C. J., Jr. (1968). Inheritance and differentiation of semi-dwarf culm length of wheat. *Crop Sci. 8*:701–704.

Baier, A. C., Zeller, F. J., Reiner, L., and Fischbeck, G̅. (1974). Monosomenanalyse des Langenwachstums der kurzstrohigen Sommerweizensorte Solo. *A. Pflanzenzüchtung 72*:181–198.

Bhowal, J. G. (1970). Location of genes for dwarfing in the wheat variety Sonora 64. *Indian J. Genet. Plant Sci. 30*:170–179.

Chaudhry, A. J. (1973). A genetic and cytogenetic study of height in wheat. PhD thesis, Cambridge University.

Fick, G. N. (1971). Genetic control of plant height and coleoptile length and association with gibberellic acid response and α-amylase activity in short strawed wheats. PhD thesis, Univ. of California, Davis.

Fick, G̅. N. and Qualset, C. O. (1973). Genes for dwarfness in wheat, *Triticum aestivum* L. *Genetics 75*:531–539.

Gale, M. D. and Law, C. N. (1973). Semi-dwarf wheats induced by monosomy and associated changes in gibberellin levels. *Nature 241*:211–212.

Gale, M. D. and Marshall, G. A. (1973a). Dwarf wheats and gibberellins. *Proc. 4th Int. Wheat Genet. Symp. Missouri Agricultural Experimental Station, Columbia, Mo.* pp. 513–519.

Gale, M. D. and Marshall, G. A. (1973b). Insensitivity to gibberellin in dwarf wheats. *Ann. Bot. 37*:729–735.

Gale, M. D. and Marshall, G. A. (1975). The nature and genetic control of gibberellin insensitivity in dwarf wheat grain. *Heredity 35*(1):55–65.

Gale, M. D. and Marshall, G. A. (1976). The chromosomal location of *Gai 1* and *Rht 1*, genes for gibberellin insensitivity and semi-dwarfism, in a derivative of Norin 10 wheat. *Heredity 37*:283–289.

Gale, M. D., Law, C. N., Marshall, G. A., and Worland, A. J. (1975*a*). The genetic control of gibberellic acid insensitivity and coleoptile length in a 'dwarf' wheat. *Heredity 34*: 393–399.

Gale, M. D., Law, C. N., and Worland, A. J. (1975*b*). The chromosomal location of a major dwarfing gene from Norin 10 in new British semi-dwarf wheats. *Heredity 35*(3): 417–421.

Harada, J. and Vergara, B. S. (1971). Response of different rice varieties to gibberellin. *Crop Sci. 11*:373–374.

Hu, M. L. (1974). Genetic analyses of semi-dwarfing and insensitivity to gibberellin GA$_3$ in hexaploid wheat (*Triticum aestivum* L. em Thell). PhD thesis, Washington State University, Department of Agronomy and Soils.

Jha, M. P. and Swaminathan, M. S. (1969). Identification of chromosomes carrying the major genes for dwarfing in the wheat varieties Lerma Rojo and Sonora 64. *Curr. Sci. 38*:379–381.

Joppa, L. R. (1973). Agronomic characteristics of near-isogenic tall and semi-dwarf lines of durum wheat. *Crop Sci. 13*:743–746.

Knott, D. R. and Kumar, J. (1975). Comparison of early generation yield testing and a single seed descent procedure in wheat breeding. *Crop Sci. 15*:295–299.

Konzak, C. F., Sadam, M. I. R., and Donaldson, E. (1973). Inheritance and linkage in durum wheats of semi-dwarfing genes with low response to gibberellin A$_3$. Proc. Symp. Genet. *Breeding of Durum Wheat, Bari*, pp. 29–40.

Law, C. N. and Worland, A. J. (1973). Aneuploidy in wheat and its uses in genetic analysis. *PBI Annual Report*, pp. 25–65.

Law, C. N., Snape, J. W., and Worland, A. J. (1974). *Plant Breeding Institute Annual Report* pp. 129–132.

Law, C. N., Snape, J., and Worland, A. J. (1977). The genetical relationships between height and yield. *Heredity*, in press.

Morris, R., Schmidt, J. W., and Johnson, V. A. (1972). Chromosomal location of a dwarfing gene in 'Tom Thumb' wheat derivative by monosomic analysis. *Crop Sci. 12*:247–249.

Ogawa, Y. (1962). Quantitative difference of gibberellin-like substances in normal and dwarf varieties of pharbitis nil chois. *Bot. Mag. Tokyo 75*:449–450.

Phinney, B. O. (1957). Growth response of single gene mutants in maize to gibberellic acid. *Proc. National Academy of Science 42*:185–189.

Phinney, B. O. (1961). Dwarfing genes in *Zea mays* and their relation to the gibberellins. In *Plant Growth Regulation* (R. M. Klein, ed.), pp. 489–501. Iowa State College Press, Ames, Ia.

Piech, J. (1968). Monosomic and conventional genetic analyses of semi-dwarfism and grass-clump dwarfism is common wheat. *Euphytica [Suppl.] 1*:613–618.

Proano, V. A. and Greene, G. L. (1968). Endogenous gibberellins of a radiation induced single gene dwarf mutant of beans. *Plant Physiol. 43*:613–618.

Radley, M. (1970). Comparison of endogenous gibberellins and response to applied gibberellin of some dwarf and tall wheat cultivars. *Planta 92*:292–300.

Reitz, L. P. and Salmon, S. C. (1968). Origin, histories and use of Norin 10 wheat. *Crop Sci. 8*:686.

Riggs, T. J. and Hayter, A. M. (1975). A study of the inheritance and interrelationships of some agronomically important characters in spring barley. *Theoret. Appl. Genet. 46*: 257–264.

Sampson, D. R. (1971). Additive and non-additive genetic variances and genotypic correlations for yield and other traits in oats. *Can. J. Genet. Cytol. 13*:864–872.

Sears, E. R. (1953). Nullisomic analysis in common wheat. *Amer. Naturalist 87*:245–252.

Singhal, N. C., Singh, M. P., and Kalia, C. S. (1973). Genetics of dwarfing and awning by monosomic analysis in wheat variety Mex. CB116. *Wheat Info. Serv. 36*:14–16.

Stoddart, J., Breidenbach, W., Nadeau, R., and Rappaport, L. (1974). Selective binding of (^{3}H)gibberellin A1 by protein fractions from dwarf pea epicotyls. *Proc. National Academy of Sci. 71*(8):3255–3259.

Stoskopf, N. C. and Fairey, D. T. (1975). Asynchronous tiller maturity—a potential problem in the development of dwarf winter wheat. *Plant Breed. Abst. 45*(8):467–472.

Suge, H. and Murakami, Y. (1968). Occurrence of a rice mutant deficient in gibberellin-like substances. *Plant Call Physiol. 9*:411–414.

Vogel, O. A., Craddock, J. C., Jr., Muir, C. E., Everson, E. H., and Rohde, C. R. (1956). Semi-dwarf growth habit in winter wheat improvement for the Pacific northwest. *Agron. J. 48* (2):76–78.

Zeven, A. C. (1969). Tom Pouce Blanc and Tom Pouce Barbu Rouge, two *Triticum aestivum* sources of very short straw. *Wheat Infor. Serv. 29*:8–9.

14

Evaluation of Branched Ear Derivatives of *Triticum aestivum* L.

Mohammad Aslam and Manzoor Ahmad Bhutta
Department of Plant Breeding and Genetics
University of Agriculture
Lyallpur, Pakistan

ABSTRACT

The branched spikes of *Triticum turgidum* L. have a potential of producing a high number of kernels. Some of the selected lines of *T. turgidum* yielded up to 150 kernels per spike as compared to 60–70 kernels per spike in the common wheat cultivar Chenab-70. The best of these lines were crossed with the common wheats Chenab-70, Mexipak, and C-271. Among the lines obtained by selection from the advanced generations of the *T. turgidum* × Chenab-70 cross, some are similar to Chenab-70 with respect to tillering, plant shape, plant height, and leaf position, but their spikes are branched like those of the *T. turgidum* parent. These lines appear to be fairly homozygous. Chenab-70 produces, on the average, 60 kernels per spike, 34.8 g of grain per plant and has a 1000-kernel weight of 35 g. The number of kernels per spike, the yield of grain per plant and the 1000-kernel weight of the selected hybrid lines ranged from 25 to 133, from 8.5 to 59.6 g, and from 30.0 to 46.0 g, respectively, which shows that the chances of obtaining high-yielding new common wheat cultivars having spikes branched as those of the *T. turgidum* parent fairly good.

INTRODUCTION

Plant breeders have developed an impressive range of techniques to increase variability. The simplest crop improvement program would involve crossing between promising parents and the selection of high-yielding genotypes from the resulting segregating populations. In this quest, efforts have also been directed in most crop plants to resort to interspecific and intergeneric hybridization, and the present-day *Triticales* represent the fruits of such efforts (MacDonald, 1968). In discussing the development of an ideal wheat plant, Donald (1968) observed that a model wheat plant need not be exclusively suited to existing environments but may involve concurrent adaptability to a new set of artificial components of plant environment such as crop density, placement arrangement, nutrient level, and so forth. On the basis of studies carried out by both wheat breeders and plant physiologists, it is rather difficult to attribute the high yield of new dwarf wheat types to any one single factor, but a good wheat variety is considered to possess a relatively short straw, to have comparatively small and erect leaves, and to develop large, well-filled spikes. There is yet much to learn, however, about the contribution made by the number of spikelets per spike or the number of florets per spikelet toward yield. It is a matter of common experience that a plant having many well-developed spikes with numerous fertile florets produces a high yield. So, if we consider the number of fertile florets as one of the traits associated with the amount of yield, it would appear logical to attempt to increase the number of fertile florets and, implicitly, of seeds per spike. Any limitation to yield imposed by the capacity of the spike to produce a certain amount of grain is usually less than the postanthetic capacity for photosynthesis of the shoot that bears it. In particular, the contribution of high floret number must be expressed under competitive stress of a crop community. The meaning of "large spike" in wheat would thus imply an optimal number of florets leading to the most economic use of photosynthates in producing grain yield. With the knowledge of these features, we have made the effort to induce branching habit in *T. aestivum* through crosses with derivatives of *Triticum turgidum* and *T. polonicum* to see if the yield potential of common bread wheat could be increased in this way. A similar project has been undertaken in Italy at Bologna (Bonvicini, 1955) and at Cimmyt, Mexico (personal communication).

MATERIALS AND METHODS

Some wheat material was received through Dr. A. O. Shaw, the leader of a group of American teachers at the University of Agriculture (Lyallpur) in 1969–1970. These materials were planted in 1970–1972. Lines of wheat shown in Table I, the genealogies of which can be obtained from the author, looked promising in stand, resistance to rust, and fertility.

All these plants were mostly segregating. A few promising plants amongst these were crossed with C271, Pitic, Mexipak, and a few other varieties. The F_1 and subsequent generations of the crosses varied a great deal with respect to height, tillering, branching of spike, and fertility. Only the plants that looked

Table I. Lines of *Triticum* with Useful Characteristics

University accession no.	Derived with participation of *Triticum:*	Plant characteristics
AUT 568	*polonicum*	Very late, resistant to stripe and leaf rusts, short thick culms, spikes heavy and branched at base
AU 540	*turgidum*	Very late, thick culms, segregation for branching of spikes, some spikes with 130 seeds
AU 567	*turgidum*	Dwarf, small and branched red spikes of *aestivum* type, seeds shriveled, culms with waxy bloom
UT 570	*polonicum*	Dwarf, branched spikes of *aestivum* type

more like *T. aestivum* and had branched ears were selected, irrespective of the number of grains they contained. During the 1972–1973 crop year, each selected plant had produced a progeny of about 100 individuals. From the entire population, 503 spikes were selected and classified for type of branching (Fig. 1), number of kernels, 1000-kernel weight, and other seed characteristics. During the 1974–1975 crop year, 252 of these spikes were planted in spike to rod row (4.6 m) progenies with plants spaced 15 cm apart. Most of the progenies were observed to be segregating again, but the majority of the plants now had spikes of uniform appearance. One hundred and twelve plants were again selected from this population with *T.-aestivum*-like spikes, which were branching to a varying degree (Fig. 2). The seeds of these plants were, for the first time, subjected to microplot trials with each plant progeny grown in duplicate 2.75-m-long rows and 7.6–10-cm spacing between the plants.

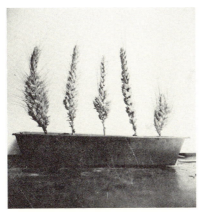

Fig. 1. Branched ear types. Left to right: (1) three-fourths branched, (2) three-fourths branched, (3) one-half branched, (4) unbranched with supernumerary spikelets, and (5) three-fourths branched.

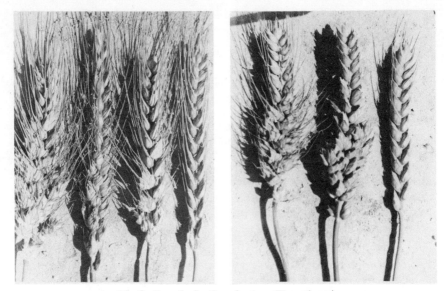

Fig. 2. Branched spike selections (T. aestivum).

RESULTS AND DISCUSSION

Mean values of yield components in some common cultivars are presented in Table II to serve as a basis of comparison of new branched ear derivatives with common types.

A population grown in the 1974–1975 crop year from parent plants selected for high number of seeds per spike and branching had the following composition: 25% of the plants had more than 80 kernels per spike, 39% had between 61 to 80 kernels, and 36% had less than 60 kernels per spike. Comparative figures

Table II. Characteristics of Common Wheat Cultivars (1974–1975 Data)

Variety	Spikelets per spike (average of 30 plants)	Grains per spike	1000-kernel weight (g)
Chenab-70	20.02–23.10	56.00–73.95	30.15–42.65
Lyallpur-73	19.52	49.70	41.47
PARI-73	19.00	48.10	44.15
Najam-3	20.52	51.93	42.40
L.U.-21	19.35	55.58	42.15
C-271	20.75	65.34	45.59

during 1973–1974 were 8%, 31%, and 61%, respectively. A glance at the details given in Table III clearly shows that there was no significant difference between the mean values for number of kernels per spike and 1000-kernel weight between the selected branched ear plants of 1973–1974 and 1974–1975.

The 1975–1976 crop, which is at the present moment in the field, had 47% of plants showing more than 80 grains per spike, 52% with 60–80 grains per

Table III. Comparative Behavior of Branched Spike in Two Years

S. No.	Spike character (branched)	1974		1975		
		Grains/spike	1000-kernel wt (g)	Grains/spike (avg. 5 spikes)	1000-kernel wt (g) (avg. 5 spikes)	
1	–	105	31	70.539	32.715	Seg.[a]
2	–	101	33	81.231	35.985	
3	–	84	27	90.175	34.573	
4	–	125	29	98.167	34.805	
5	–	80	20	117.50	32.34	
6	–	107	35	95.333	34.965	Nonseg.[a]
7	–	105	29	77.50	29.032	Seg.
8	–	106	33	96.364	35.145	
9	–	106	28	83.00	36.145	
10	–	106	28	87.00	36.190	
11	–	123	36	83.00	43.373	
12	–	104	27	100.00	38.750	
13	–	109	29	79.929	26.810	
14	–	97	20	74.00	29.279	
15	–	143	34	95.875	39.113	
16	–	106	32	91.805	33.224	
17	–	94	22	98.071	29.767	
18	–	94	30	64.70	39.09	
19	–	90	26	81.045	29.725	
20	–	89	28	68.571	43.75	
21	–	69	21	78.75	29.84	
22	–	98	22	70.563	26.572	
23	–	76	18	114.00	38.594	
24	–	86	15	100.00	25.333	
25	–	81	23	84.923	24.04	
26	–	85	22	100.00	23.00	
27	–	85	32	98.889	25.76	
28	–	84	15	92.250	32.520	
29	–	131	30	76.714	35.38	
30	–	91	28	99.333	35.570	
31	–	107	35	70.99	33.296	Nonseg.

[a]Seg. = segregating; Nonseg. = nonsegregating.

spike, and only 1% less than 60 grains per spike. As will be evident from Table III, almost all the plants had varying intensity of branching, i.e., from spikes with only basal branching to branching extending to ¾ of the spike. The present crop is just heading and about half a dozen lines show uniformity in branching pattern, though intensity of branching still seems to vary from plant to plant. Four lines in this respect seem to have maintained their branching pattern for the last three years in succession. Kernel size and number of spikelets per spike are also considered components of yield. Therefore, selections are made for kernel weight and high total plant yield, as well as for high number of grains per spike and high kernel weight.

The phenotypic correlations between the various characters were worked out and are given below:

Correlation between 1974 and 1975 crops for number of kernels per spike	0.2
Correlation between yield per plant and tillers per plant	0.657
Correlation between 1000-kernel weight and yield per plant	0.0119
Correlation between grains per spike and yield per plant	0.07

The only significant correlation is that between yield and tillers per plant. The contribution to yield by the number of tillers per plant and also by 1000-kernel weight has already been well established in studies with *T. aestivum* (Engledow and Wadham, 1923).

However, very little work seems to have been done on the development of branched ears in *T. aestivum*. The contribution to yield by a large spike has already been referred to by Donald (1968), but a limitation seems to be imposed by the capacity of the plant to set optimal numbers of effective florets per spike. The habit of the plants with branched spikes to develop a few primary fully branched early culms and late tillers with normal ears needs further investigation. Late tillers with respect to yield seem to be a drag rather than of any use for the plants with branched spikes, as has already been pointed out by Bremner et al. (1963) and Bunting and Drennan (1965). However, there seems to be a good possibility of obtaining strains of wheat with more than 100 grains per spike by selecting types with a few culms bearing branched spikes which would flower simultaneously. Such plants should have a high competitive adaptability. Austin and Jones (1974) have shown that the number of potentially fertile florets in a spike and the number of spike-bearing tillers per unit of cropped area are fully determined before anthesis. The potential number of grains per unit of cropped area, and to a lesser extent the potential yield of grains, are also determined by this time (Lupton et al., 1967; Rawson, 1970). However, many factors intervene to restrict the attainment of the potential. For example, the question why there are normal spikes in some of the culms in a branched-spike plant needs further investigation.

REFERENCES

Austin, R. B. and Jones, H. G. (1974). The physiology of wheat. Part III. *Annual Report,* pp. 20–23. Plant Breeding Institute, Cambridge.

Bonvicini, M. (1955). Nuove caratteristiche genetiche per l'incremento della produzione granaria. *Sementi Elette, 1*:2–7.

Bremner, P. M., Eckersall, R. N. and Scott, R. K. (1963). The relative importance of embryo size and endosperm size in causing the effects associated with seed size in wheat. *J. Agri. Sci. Camb. 61*:139–145.

Bunting, A. H. and Drennan, D. S. H. (1965). Some aspects of the morphology and physiology of cereals in the vegetative phase. In *The Growth of Cereals and Grasses* (Milthorpe, F. L. and Ivins, J. D. (eds.). Butterworth, London.

Donald, C. M. (1968). The breeding of crop ideotypes. *Euphytica 17*:385–403.

Engledow, F. L. and Wadham, S. M. (1923). Investigation on yield in the cereals. I. *J. Agri. Sci. Camb. 13*:390–439.

Lupton, F. G. H., Ali, M. A. M., and Subramanian, S. (1967). Varietal differences in growth parameters of wheat and their importance in determining yield. *J. Agri. Sci. Camb. 69*:111–123.

MacDonald, M. D. (1968). Recent development of hexaploid *Triticales* in Canada. *Euphytica [Suppl.] 1*:185–187.

Rawson, H. M. (1970). Spikelet number, its control and relation to yield per ear. *Aust. J. Biol. Sci. 23*:1–15.

III

Genetic Variability
and Resistance to Disease

15

Artificial Mutagenesis as an Aid in Overcoming Genetic Vulnerability of Crop Plants

C. F. Konzak, R. A. Nilan, and A. Kleinhofs

Department of Agronomy and Soils and Program in Genetics
Washington State University
Pullman, Washington 99163

ABSTRACT

Artificially induced genetic variation is being used effectively to supplement or complement sources of natural origin for practical plant breeding. Thus, creating genetic variation will become increasingly important as crop genetic resources become more difficult to obtain via plant exploration. The artificial induction of useful genetic variation offers important elements that can be used for overcoming genetic vulnerability: (1) new, previously unknown alleles can be induced in crop plant species to broaden the base of variation; (2) useful genetic variation can be induced in modern cultivars helping to shorten breeding time or to extend production "life"; (3) characteristics of existing genetic resource stocks can be improved to make them more useful in breeding; and (4) recombination in crosses may be enhanced. The performance of induced mutant crop cultivars and the successful uses of induced genetic variation in cross breeding indicate that artificial mutagenesis will play an increasingly greater role in plant breeding.

INTRODUCTION

An ultimate goal of artificial mutagenesis is to supplement and eventually succeed plant exploration as the principal means for obtaining new genetic resources for plant breeding. This objective is dictated by cultural developments that are so destroying natural gene resources, the only representatives of primitive cultivars remaining will be maintained by genetic resource centers. The primitive cultivars of the most important crop plants are rarely found in cultivation today. Wild forms of our major crop plants also are being lost from their natural habitats and must be maintained by genetic resource centers. However, the practical use of wild forms often requires very intensive breeding and genetics research to introduce desired genes into modern cultivars.

This chapter summarizes the potential role of artificial mutagenesis in the creation of sources of genetic variation complementary or supplementary to those from plant collections and eventually the major sources for plant improvement and genetic and physiological analyses. This summary has been developed from pertinent facts and ideas about the subject from various publications and from experiences in our own plant-breeding and genetics research.

Some of the important ways artificial mutagenesis might aid in overcoming genetic vulnerability are as follows:

1. Complement and supplement existing germ plasm resources
   a. Create new genetic variability
      i.   New alleles of known genes
      ii. Alleles of previously unknown genes
   b. Create useful genetic variability in modern phenotypes
   c. Improve characteristics of germ plasm sources
      i.   Modify linkages
      ii. Modify character complexes—retain desirable complexes
      iii. Improve agronomic properties, adaptation
   d. Create "isogenic" genetic variants for biochemical, genetic, and physiological analysis
2. Enhance recombination in crosses
3. Extend the useful "life" of successful cultivars
   a. Simple improvement leading to cultivars
   b. Multiline development leading to a "blend" cultivar

These applications of mutagens and mutations are based both on experiences and on certain modern "facts" comparing similarities and differences in the nature and the frequencies of spontaneous and induced mutations, which are reviewed briefly as follows.

1. Mutations of either spontaneous or induced origin are mostly recessive and deleterious. This is now well established (Nilan, 1967; Brock, 1971; Gustafsson, 1975). The frequently voiced impressions of plant breeders that spontaneous mutants are likely to be more useful have no factual support. Spontaneous variation in natural populations appears more useful because natural selective forces have already had their impact and much "plant breeding" has already been done.

2. Dominant and semidominant mutations occur among both induced and spontaneous variants. The dominance of such genes may differ in degree over a seemingly wide range and often may be influenced by epistatic relations with genes affecting the same trait. Some examples will be discussed later.

3. Mutants of either spontaneous or induced origin which are useful for breeding are infrequent or rare. However, as induced mutations can be easily obtained in large numbers, appropriate selection techniques can help identify the few rare useful characters needed. It should be recognized here that recombinant derivatives of mutants often may be more useful for further breeding than the "raw" mutants (Micke, 1962, 1963, 1969; Gaul, 1964; Sigurbjörnsson and Micke, 1974; Gustafsson, 1975; Konzak, unpub. Sigurbjörnsson, 1976).

4. Induced mutants, including useful forms, are more frequent than are those of spontaneous origin. Specific mutant phenotype or genotypes may be induced at about $10^3 - 10^6$ higher frequency than spontaneous (Brock, 1971; Smith, 1971; Nilan, 1967, 1972; Gustafsson, 1975).

5. Induced and spontaneous mutants may have different phenotypic and genotypic spectra. Definitive data on this point are still few for higher plants, especially as regards the range of spontaneous mutation types. However, much evidence indicates that the mutation spectra induced by various artificial mutagens are different. The mutation spectra for physical mutagens appear similar but different from that of chemical mutagens, whereas various chemical mutagens may induce different mutation spectra (Nilan 1972; Gustafsson, 1975).

6. "Pleiotropic" character complexes occur among both induced and spontaneous mutations. Numerous mutants which strongly modify many phenotypic traits are now known. In most cases, these "pleiotropic" character complexes can be modified through selection after recombination breeding. Results of breeding experiments indicate that the difficulties involved are similar for spontaneous and induced mutants (Gaul et al., 1968; Gustafsson, 1972, 1975; Jørgensen, 1976a,b; Konzak, 1976).

7. Alleles of known genes not previously found among natural germ plasm sources may be induced. This is now well established (Lundqvist et al., 1968; Persson and Hagberg, 1969; Lundqvist, 1976) for at least two well-studied phenotypes in barley—erectoides (short straw) and eceriferum (waxless), which are reviewed briefly later.

8. New alleles of previously unknown genes may be induced. This is now well documented for barley and to some extent for wheat and other crop species, especially peas (Gottschalk, 1968, 1969; Blixt, 1974) and sweet clover (Micke, 1962, 1963, 1969; Kleinhofs et al., 1968; Gengenbach et al., 1969). The success here follows results obtained with microorganisms, indicating that the widest range of mutant forms (phenotype and genotype) for any species may be recovered through at least the supplementary use of artificial mutagens.

9. Recombination in crosses may be stimulated by mutagen treatments though the mechanism involved remains unclear (Nilan, 1960, 1972; Powell and

Nilan, 1963). Somatic crossing over appears to be influenced by mutagens in some species at least (Pontecorvo, 1954, 1958; Pontecorvo and Kafer, 1958; Nilan and Vig, 1976), although it is likely that the greatest effect occurs on meiotic crossing over, perhaps as a consequence of induced base pair alterations.

10. The important characteristics of "spontaneous" mutations as used by breeders is their existence in stocks of primitive cultivars obtained from plant explorations and of improved selections and cultivars from plant-breeding programs. Recent spontaneous mutations in such materials are mostly of little practical breeding value. The importance of the spontaneous mutations present in primitive cultivars results from their exposure to natural selective forces over many crop generations, which permits genetic recombination to evolve useful character complexes, including disease resistance, and to select the best for adaptation to ecological niches. These complexes, obtained via natural selection or already constructed in modern cultivars, may have great selective advantage for breeding, because their synthesis is already a fact. Simply inherited variations of rare occurrence, or for which efficient selection procedures are yet unavailable are likewise of great breeding value, whatever their origin. Because selection procedures may never be possible for some desired traits, including those needed to meet newly arisen demands, it is imperative that genetic resource centers acquire, preserve, and maintain a wide diversity of crop plant germ plasm. Storage capacity, documentation, availability of primitive and wild forms, and economic costs are principal limitations.

With relation to the above-mentioned points, some recent results from genetic analyses of certain mutant phenotype groups in barley and in wheat are of interest.

As a specific example of mutants subjected to detailed analysis, a large collection (> 1200) of *eceriferum* or waxless phenotype mutants of barley has been studied by Lundqvist et al. (1968) and Lundqvist (1976). Of these, 988 induced and four spontaneous mutants have been located in the barley genome, to 59 loci scattered over all seven chromosomes. The number of mutants localized to each of the 59 loci differs markedly. At the four most mutable loci, *cer-c, cer-q, cer-u,* and *cer-1,* 144, 114, 114, and 57 mutants have been located, respectively. Different alleles at each locus also occur. These are identifiable not only by slight phenotypic differences, but also through biochemical analysis of the wax composition. Similarly, 26 loci have been identified for the *erectoides* (short straw) trait in barley, with numerous alleles induced at several of the loci (Persson and Hagberg, 1969). For both the *eceriferum* and *erectoides* traits many more alleles have been induced at certain loci by chemicals than by radiations, whereas the reverse occurs for other loci. Loci previously unknown in peas (Gottschalk, 1968, 1969; Blixt, 1974) and in sweet clover (Gengenbach et al., 1969; Kleinhofs et al., 1968; Micke, 1962, 1963, 1969) have also been shown via induced mutations.

Some of the most striking examples of the induction and use of induced genetic variability to counter genetic vulnerability in crop species are those described by Murray (1969) for peppermint, Jain and Pokhiryal (1975) for Pearl millet, and by Awan and Cheema (1976) for rice. In the case of peppermint, the *Verticillium* wilt disease was eliminating economical production of peppermint for oil in the United States. Although resistance to the disease was found in a related species and recombined in cultivated peppermint, Murray (1969) found that the quality and flavor of the oil from the resistant selections were inferior and commercially unacceptable. With considerable determination and the development of systematic screening procedures, Murray then induced by radiation five mutant strains resistant to the wilt. All of these strains retained the oil quality of the original Mitcham mint cultivar. One of these strains has been released and is now widely cultivated under the name Todd's Mitcham.

With Pearl millet in India, a recently developed high-yielding hybrid variety was all but eliminated from commercial production by the appearance of a devastating form of the downy mildew disease. Although resistance might have been found eventually among natural sources and then introduced by backcross breeding, an effort was made to induce resistance by mutagens in the Tift-23 stock which is the cytoplasmic male sterile parent. Within one two-crop season, outstanding resistance was recovered in the male fertile Tift-23 maintainer line and then quickly introduced into the cytoplasmic sterile A line for the hybrid. This resistance permitted rapid return of the high-yielding hybrid (new hybrid Bajra-5) to commercial production (Jain and Pokhiryal, 1975).

In rice, the γ-ray induction of early-flowering mutants in the high-quality aromatic Basmati-370 rice variety will permit the production of two crops per year where only one was possible before. More important, the mutants made it possible to retain the high aromatic properties while improving agronomic potential, a difficult feat to achieve by crossbreeding. Similarly, the induction of an early-flowering mutant in rice permitted the rapid conversion of an unadapted (because of late maturity) but disease resistant cultivar into one of high yield and adaptation to cultivation conditions in Hungary (Mikaelsen et al., 1971).

For mildew resistance in barley, some recent data (Einfeld et al., 1976) indicate that different induced mutants may vary in the phenotypic expressions for their response to disease (Table I). It is of particular interest that genes controlling the seedling-versus-mature plant responses to the disease mutate independently. Some of these resistance expression types apparently were not previously known from natural material (see Wiberg, 1974). The different response types may represent different genotype changes. However, it now appears that the only mildew resistance alleles yet proved to arise as induced mutations are all recessive, all noncomplementing and identified with locus *ml-o*. Locus *ml-o* was first shown via an X-ray mutant (Freisleben and Lein, 1942), but today at least 11 *ml-o* alleles are now known. One of the alleles, found among

Table I. Types of Induced Mildew Resistance in
Barley[a, b]

Mildew reaction	Number of mutants of variety		
	Asse	Bomi	Vada
Highly resistant	9(5)	8(7)	7(3)
Highly susceptible	9(3)	8(2)	3(3)
Resistant mature plant	3(1)	4(2)	6(2)
Susceptible mature plant	6(3)	6(3)	3(2)

[a]Einfeld et al. (1976).
[b]Numbers in parentheses are verified in M-4.

collections from Ethiopia, is of spontaneous origin. In contrast, both sponta-neous dominant and recessive alleles for mildew resistance are known. However, the induced mildew resistance mutants from the more recent research by Einfeld et al. (1976) have not been analyzed genetically, and some of these may prove dominant.

Detailed analyses conducted recently on alleles at the *ml-o* locus illustrate some genetically significant features about mutants (Jørgensen, 1976*a,b*). The *ml-o* phenotype expression is similar for all mutants—typified by necrotic spotting, which occurs even in the absence of the mildew disease. Most impor-tant is that the *ml-o* resistance controls all known races of *Erisiphe graminis*. However, the intensity and severity of spotting apparently varies for the differ-ent alleles. Tests to date show grain yield reduction to be associated with the necrotic spotting (in the absence of disease), and this is "pleiotropically" associated with the resistance.

Genetic recombination studies show that intra-allelic recombination occurs for different mutant alleles, leading to the recovery of mildew susceptible progeny. In carefully controlled studies, Jørgensen (1976*a*) recovered one sus-ceptible plant from among 8200 F_2 progeny of the cross ml-o_1/ml-o_5, and one susceptible from among 5000 F_2 progeny of the cross ml-o_4/ml-o_9. Similar results were obtained earlier by Favret (*pers. comm.,* 1971) from recombination studies among the *ml-o* alleles. The demonstration of intra-allelic recombination proves that the mutant alleles are structurally but not functionally distinct, and that the induced mutational changes have occurred within the *ml-o* locus.

A most important and encouraging result obtained from recent breeding and mass selection studies is that recombinants, carrying the high mildew resistance but less to no necrotic spotting, were recovered (Jørgensen, 1976*a*). These results, based on selection from among large segregating populations, offer hope that the yield-reducing factor(s) have been eliminated from association with the resistance, and suggest clearly that the "pleiotropic" effect either is modifiable through background changes or more likely through recombination involving exchange of gene(s)—closely linked to the *ml-o* locus.

In hexaploid or tetraploid wheat, as in diploid barley, both positive and negative directional mutants are known to occur for a number of traits (Konzak, 1976). Examples include (1) disease resistance to rusts (*Puccinia graminis tritici, P. recondita,* and *P. striiformis*), to *Septoria* (*S. nodorum, S. tritici*: Favret, personal communication, 1971), and to mildew (*E. graminis*); (2) plant height; (3) maturity; (4) vernalization response; (5) herbicide resistance (Dumanovic et al., 1970); (6) protein content (Konzak, 1976); and (7) protein quality. However, genetic analyses of the mutants in wheat are few and still lack the detail of some of the analyses of barley mutants. This is partly because of the more complex genetic structure of wheat, e.g., three times the number of genetic tester stocks are needed for linkage group identification in wheat as compared with barley. In addition, there also has been less intense research on wheat mutants.

Among the genetic studies which show some progress toward detailed analyses of mutants are those from our work with the semidwarfing (now reduced height, *Rht*) genes. A summary of progress in the identification of *Rht* loci (Table II) shows that as of now only the normal and one other allele are known for most loci identified (Konzak, 1976) with the possible exception that *Rht 3* and *Rht 1* may be allelic (Gale and Marshall, 1976). Furthermore, whereas monosomic analyses show that several chromosomes affect plant height expression, mutant loci for reduced height have been associated with only two of the 7 homologous chromosome groups (2 and 4). Many other *Rht* mutants—more than 200—in the Washington State University collection are yet to be studied; most have not been subjected to interallelic test crosses, but the dominance relations of many mutants have been tested in a small number of combinations. The results of the studies to date merely form a base for further development. However, some extremely interesting aspects of the induced vs. spontaneous mutants already have emerged.

1. Dominance expressions differ for different *Rht* genes when used in similar crosses. Epistatic interactions affecting height expressions are extremely common, in many cases reducing the effectiveness of the gene for height reduction. Likewise, combinations of height-reducing factors are generally only partially additive, i.e., total height reduction is less than expected on an additive basis.

2. Negative complexes in "pleiotropic" association with the *Rht* genes are common among both spontaneous and induced forms. Height reduction with the *Rht 1* and *Rht 2* factors, for example, is associated with reduced coleoptile length, and poor emergence from deep seedings. With *Rht 3,* numerous asso-

Table II. Some Sources of Semidwarfing (Reduced Height) Genes in Wheat

Source	Origin[a]	Ploidy (X)	Gene	Dom.[a]	Location	Negative complexes	Ref.[b]
CI13438	S	6	*Rht 1*	D	4A	Coleoptile	(1)
CI13448	S	6	*Rht 2*	D	4D	Coleoptile	(2)
Tom Thumb	S	6	*Rht 3*	D	4A	Multiple	(3)
Burt *ert* 937	I	6	*rht 4*	R	Indep (*Rht 1,2*)	?	(4)
Marfed *ert* 1	I	6	*Rht 5*	D	Indep (*Rht 1,2*)	Multiple	(5)
Sonora 64	S	6	*Rht 2, +*	D	4D, +	Coleoptile	(6,7)
Solo	S	6	2 genes		4B, 2A	?	(7)
Magnif 41 *ert*	I	6	1 gene	D	Indep (*Rht 1,2*)	None ?	(4)
Marfed *ert* 551	I	6	1 gene	R	?	None ?	(4)
Castel Porziano	I	4	1 gene	D	?	None	(8)
Leeds Mut M 131	I	4	1 gene	R	?	None ?	(4)

[a]S, spontaneous; I, induced; D, dominant; R, recessive.

[b]1. Gale, M. D. and Marshall, G. A. (1976). The chromosomal location of Gai 1 and Rht 1, genes for gibberellin insensitivity and semidwarfism, in a derivative of Norin 10 wheat. *Heredity 37:*283–289.

2. Gale, M. D., Law, C. N., and Worland, A. J. (1975). The chromosomal location of a major dwarfing gene from Norin 10 in new British semi-dwarf wheats. *Heredity 35:*417–421.

3. Morris, R., Schmidt, J. W., and Johnson, V. A. (1972). Chromosomal location of a dwarfing gene in 'Tom Thumb' wheat derivative by monsomic analysis. *Crop Sci. 12:*247–249.

   Fick, G. N. and Qualset, C. O. (1973). Genes for dwarfness in wheat, *Triticum aestivum* L. *Genetics 75:*531–539.

4. Konzak, C. F. (1976). A review of semi-dwarfing gene sources and a description of some new mutants useful for breeding short stature wheats. In *Proc. 1st Research Coordination Meeting on the Use of Aneuploids for Wheat Improvement.* International Atomic Energy Agency, Vienna.

5. Woo, S. C. and Konzak, C. F. (1969). Genetic analysis of short-culm mutants induced by ethyl methanesulphonate in *Triticum aestivum* L. In *Induced Mutations in Plants.* (STI/PUB/231), pp. 551–555. International Atomic Energy Agency, Vienna.

6. Jha, M. P. and Swaminathan, M. S. (1969). Identification of chromosomes carrying the major genes for dwarfing in the wheat varieties Lerma Rojo and Sonora 64. *Curr. Sci. 38:*379–381.

   Vogel, O. A., Allan, R. E., Peterson, C. J., Jr. (1963). Plant and performance characteristics of semidwarf winter wheats producing most effectively in eastern Washington. *Agron. J. 55:*397–398.

   Baier, A. C., Zeller, F. J., and Fischbeck, G. (1974). Identification of three chromosomal interchanges in common wheat, *Triticum aestivum* L. *Can. J. Genet. Cytol. 16:*349–354.

7. Baier, A. C., Zeller, F. J., Reiner, L., and Fischbeck, G. (1974). Monosomenanalyse des Langenwachstums der Kurzslrohigen Sommerweigen sorte "Solo." *Z. Pflanz. 72:*181–198.

8. Scarascia-Mugnozza, G. T. and Bozzini, A. (1968). Short straw mutants induced in durum wheat. *Euphytica [Suppl.] 1:*171–176.

Table III. Stripe Rust Reaction of Omar Mutants
and F_1 Hybrids[a]

		F_1		
Designation	Reaction[b]	WA5572 (1/30)	M642085 (3/10)	M6610131 (3/10)
WA5572	1/30 (fleck)[c]	–	2/10	–
M6610131	3/10	–	2/5	–
G680043	5/20	2/10	–	–
G680048	7/40	–	–	3/20
CI13072 (Omar)	8/80	8/40	–	–
M65002-05	6/10	–	1/10	–
M65035-01	5/30	4/40	–	–
M65047-01	5/10	6/20	–	–
M65073-04	5/30	8/50	–	–
M668019	8/80	–	–	7/40

[a] Field reaction, Pullman (1972).
[b] Reaction: Infection type 0–9/severity %.
[c] Fleck also appears in absence of disease.

ciated effects occur, including the short coleoptile, low test weight, possibly poor root development, and so forth. Each of these three *Rht* loci also is linked with low response to gibberellin (GA insensitivity), but different degrees of linkage are involved (Hu, 1974; Konzak, 1976). The use of new semidwarfing genes should help to broaden genetic diversity in future cultivars.

Some other mutants induced in wheat at Washington State University also appear to be of more special interest for breeding toward reduced crop genetic vulnerability. Among these are mutants toward resistance to stripe rust caused by *Puccinia striiformis* (Table III). Although the work with these mutants is as yet preliminary, indications are that several different forms of resistance are present, that the resistances are in some cases additive, show dominance or recessiveness, apparently functioning in every way like those known from spontaneous sources. All these mutants appear to carry a mature plant type of resistance, as all are susceptible in the seedling stage. A way these mutants might be used in variety development will be discussed later.

Mutations that increase the vernalization response in wheat have long been known, and many mutants of little breeding value have been observed in our research at Pullman. However, recent attempts to induce mutants for reduced vernalization response also appear to have been successful, and some of the resulting lines appear to have exceptional breeding value. These results tend to confirm similar experiments on the induction of spring habit mutants in winter wheat (Konzak et al., 1963). The technique for selection is extremely simple: The M-2 population is sown in the field in the spring, late enough to limit possibilities for vernalization. Those plants which flower and produce seed are selected and subjected to further tests. Several spring habit lines isolated from the local soft white winter wheat variety Luke following this procedure appear to have retained much of the winter hardiness, as well as the high yield, good quality, disease resistance, and other agronomic properties of the original line, but can be sown in the spring. Besides providing for easier use in recombination breeding, these selections may be adapted to earlier spring planting and for our region may compete successfully as fall-sown wheats in some areas. The production of facultative wheats should ensure availability of carryover seed stocks for spring replanting of winter-injured stands of genetically vulnerable winter wheats. Moreover, the greater cold tolerance of these facultative wheats should permit earlier spring planting and the trait may be valuable for reducing vulnerability to frost injury of spring wheats in other areas.

Although direct release of these wheat mutants will obviously extend the exposure period of specific genotypes to disease attack, thereby creating a temporary state of greater genetic vulnerability, it is expected that breeding with other germ plasm sources will greatly reduce or modify the likely vulnerable genetic relationships between the new spring habit forms and the original winter wheats. Genetic and physiological studies of the mutants are in progress.

USES OF INDUCED MUTANTS IN BREEDING

Besides serving as often unique germ plasm sources for specific traits of breeding significance, some new approaches in breeding appear to offer new ways to exploit the potential of artificial mutagenesis toward the reduction of crop genetic vulnerability. The most important of these new approaches involves the development of multiline or "blend" varieties. Ordinarily, the many lines required are developed using backcrosses. The procedures require both the search for and identification of numerous different forms of resistance that can be backcrossed into the common parent background and controllably introduced into cultivation as blends. The composition of the blends changes as disease removes any component. The use of induced mutations is perhaps simpler, since the mutant selection process, being phenotype and not genotype dependent, provides a range of genetic variability for the lines in the eventual multiline blend. This approach is currently under study for the control of mildew in barley (Röbbelen, personal communication, 1976).

RECENT DEVELOPMENTS IN SCREENING TECHNOLOGY

The efficiency and usefulness of mutation induction methods for plant improvement is greatly dependent upon the efficiency of selection methods applicable for the desired traits. If mutant phenotypes are readily discernible, as those discussed earlier, e.g., plant height, vernalization response, disease resistance, earliness, and so forth, selection may be relatively easy, and applications in practical breeding can be routine. For the less discernible traits, as those concerned with many biochemical and physiological processes, biochemical or microbiological types of M-2 mass screening procedures often can be applied (Jacobs, 1965). Some examples of traits and detection methods include (1) amino acid quantity via amino acid analog resistance of germinating seeds (Brock et al., 1973), (2) nitrate utilization via resistance to chlorate (Oostinder-Braaksma and Feenstra, 1973) or via leaf tests for nitrate reductase level (Warner, unpublished 1976), (3) herbicide resistance via direct application of herbicide, and (4) pathogen resistance by screening with standardized specific phytoxins.

MOST USEFUL MUTAGENS

Four main types of agents can be distinguished as "most useful mutagens" for research directed toward plant improvement by means of the avenues described earlier (Table IV). Because there is evidence for different mutation spectra for the different artificial mutagenic agents, no one type or specific agent can be singled out as best. The four types of agents differ in mutagenic potency and use hazard. Among the alkylating agents, several other potent chemicals such as ethyleneimine could be included. However, the greater carcinogenicity of these compounds compared with the sulfonates (EMS, iPMS, nPMS) and diethyl sulfate is an important consideration. Methyl nitrosourea, like methyl nitrosourethane and ethyl nitrosourea, appears to be an unusually potent agent, especially for polyploid wheat. Methyl nitrosourea is therefore recommended in

Table IV. Most Useful Mutagens

Agents	Example	Mutagenicity	Useful mutants	Carcinogenicity hazard
Alkylating agents	(EMS, dES)	High	G	Low ?
Nitroso compounds	(NMH)	High	VG	High
Azide	(AZ)	High	?	None ?
Radiations	(X, γ, N)	Low medium	F	Low[a]

[a] Assuming required safety practice.

spite of its extremely hazardous nature. Use of these agents requires special precautions, but such precautions are not difficult to achieve, hence need not deter anyone. Preferably, these potent mutagens should be used with the help of a skilled chemist and under safe laboratory conditions.

In contrast, the newest of the group of potent agents, azide, merits special attention because of its unusual properties, i.e., potency and relatively lower hazard potential (Kleinhofs et al., 1975; Nilan et al., 1973; Sideris et al., 1973; Kleinhofs and Smith, 1976; McCann et al., 1976). Azide is possibly the most potent of all mutagens for higher plants, yet appears to be noncarcinogenic (Ulland et al., 1973). However, whereas azide was proved exceptionally potent as a mutagen for several diploid species—barley, pea, rice, and einkorn wheat— similarly high yields of mutations have not yet been obtained in the polyploid wheats or in oats (Konzak, unpublished, 1976). The work with azide is still too new for an evaluation of the usefulness of the mutants recovered, but indications are that a high proportion of selected mutants will have positive breeding value.

NEW DIRECTIONS AND RESEARCH NEEDS

If artificial mutagenesis is to be an important contribution in alleviating genetic vulnerability of our major crop species and achieve its role in practical plant breeding and genetics research, we see these directions as necessary:

1. Wider, intensive evaluation of artificial mutagenesis methods to already tested problem areas
2. Wider use of induced genetic variation in crossbreeding
3. Intensive genetic and agronomic analyses of mutants
4. Exploration of new problem areas
5. Further improvement of mutagenesis and mass selection technology
6. Increased effort by genetic resource centers to obtain and preserve useful induced mutants and to develop programs to induce useful mutants

CONCLUSIONS

Artificial mutagenesis has already been proved an effective and efficient tool for creating new and useful genetic variability for both practical breeding and genetics studies of crop plants. As with any other single method for creating genetic variation, artificial mutagenesis is no panacea; its role is most likely to be complementary and supplementary to more conventional approaches. Thus, artificial mutagenesis methods should be used wherever and whenever their special attributes will facilitate the achievement of breeding objectives, consider- ing the requirement for efficient mass-scale screening techniques and possibilities for work with large M-2 populations. When time and genetic vulnerability are critical factors, the use of several approaches may be desirable.

ACKNOWLEDGMENT

This information paper is based on projects 1068 and 1568, College of Agriculture Research Center, Washington State University, Pullman.

REFERENCES

Awan M. A. and Cheema, A. A. (1976). Performance of early flowering lines of rice variety Basmati-370. *Mutat. Breed. Newsl.* 7:4–5.

Blixt, S. (1974). The pea. *Handbook of Genetics* (King, R. C., ed.), Vol. 2, Chap. 9, pp. 183–184. Plenum Press, New York.

Brock, R. D. (1971). The role of induced mutations in plant improvement. *Radiat. Bot.* 11:181–196.

Brock, R. D., Friederich, E. A., and Langridge, J. (1973). The modification of amino acid composition of higher plants by mutation and selection. In *Nuclear Techniques for Seed Protein Improvement* (STI/PUB/320), pp. 319–338. International Atomic Energy Agency, Vienna.

Dumanovic, J., Ehrenberg, L., and Denic, M. (1970). Induced variation of protein content and composition in hexaploid wheat. In *Improving Plant Protein by Nuclear Techniques.* (STI/PUB/258), pp. 107–119. International Atomic Energy Agency, Vienna.

Einfeld, C., Abdel-Hafex, A. G., Fuchs, W. H., Heitfuss, R., and Röbbelen, G. (1976). Investigations on resistance of barley against mildew (*Erisiphe graminis*). In *Induced Mutations for Disease Resistance in Plants,* pp. 81–90. International Atomic Energy Agency, Vienna.

Freisleben, B. and Lein, A. (1942). Über die Auffindung einer mehltau-resistenten Mutante nach Röntgenbestrahlung einer anfälligen reinen Linie Von Sommergerste. *Naturwissenschaften 30:*608.

Gale, M. D. and Marshall, G. A. (1976). The chromosomal location of Gai 1 and Rht 1, genes for gibberellin insensitivity and semidwarfism, in a derivative of Norin 10 wheat. *Heredity* 37:283–289.

Gaul, H. (1964). Mutations in plant breeding. *Radiat. Bot.* 4:155–232.

Gaul, H., Grunewaldt, J., and Hesemann, C. U. (1968). Variation of character expression of barley mutants in a changed genetic background. In *Mutations in Plant Breeding II* (STI/PUB/182), pp. 77–95. International Atomic Energy Agency, Vienna.

Gengenbach, B. G., Haskins, F. A., and Gorz, H. J. (1969). Genetic studies of induced mutants in *Melilotus alba*. I. Short-internode dward, curled leaf, multifoliolate leaf, and cotyledonary branching. *Crop Sci.* 9:607–610.

Gottschalk, W. (1968). Simultaneous mutation of closely linked genes: A contribution to the interpretation of 'pleiotropic' gene action. In *Mutations in Plant Breeding II* (STI/PUB/182), pp. 97–109. International Atomic Energy Agency, Vienna.

Gustafsson, Å. (1972). The genetic architecture of phenotype patterns in barley. In *Induced Mutations and Plant Improvement* (STI/PUB/297), pp. 7–12. International Atomic Energy Agency, Vienna.

Gustafsson, A. (1975). Mutations in plant breeding—A glance back and a look forward. In *Biomedical, Chemical and Physical Perspectives* (Nygaard, O. F., Adler, H. I., and Sinclair, W. K., eds.), pp. 81–95. Academic Press, Inc., New York.

Hu, M. L. (1974). Genetic analyses of semidwarfing and insensitivity of gibberellin GA$_3$ in hexaploid wheat (*Triticum aestivum* L. em Thell.). Ph.D. dissertation, Washington State University, Pullman, Washington.

Jacobs, M. (1965). Isolation of biochemical mutants in *Arabidopsis*. In *Arabidopsis Research* (Röbbelen, G. ed.), Vol. 1, pp. 106–112. (Arabidopsis Information Service Suppl.) Institut für Pflanzenbau und Pflanzenzüchtung, Universität Göttingen, Germany.

Jain, H. K. and Pokhiryal, S. C. (1975). Improved Pearl millet hybrids. *Mutat. Breed. Newsl.* 6:11–12.

Jørgensen, J. H. (1976a). Studies on recombination between alleles in the *ml-o* locus of barley and on pleiotropic effects of alleles. In *Induced Mutations for Disease Resistance in Crop Plants*, pp. 129–140. International Atmoic Energy Agency, Vienna.

Jørgensen, J. H. (1976b). Identification of powdery mildew resistant barley mutants and their allelic relationship. In *Barley Genetics III* (Gaul, H. ed.), pp. 446–455. Verlag Karl Thiemig, Munich.

Kleinhofs, A. and Smith, J. A. (1976). Effect of excision repair on azide-induced mutagenesis. *Mutat. Res. 41*:233–240.

Kleinhofs, A., Gorz, H. J., and Haskins, F. A. (1968). Mutation induction in *Melilotus alba annua* by chemical mutagens. *Crop Sci. 8*:631–632.

Kleinhofs, A., Kleinschmidt, M., Sciaky, D., and Von Broembsen, S. (1975). Azide mutagenesis. *In vitro* studies. *Mutat. Res. 29*:497–500.

Konzak, C. F. (1976). A review of semi-dwarfing gene sources and a description of some new mutants useful for breeding short stature wheats. In *Mutations in Crossbreeding, Proc. Advisory Group*, pp. 79–93. International Atomic Energy Agency, Vienna.

Konzak, C. F., Nilan, R. A., Froese-Gertzen, E. E., and Ramirez, I. A. (1963). Physical and chemical mutagens in wheat breeding. *Hereditas [Suppl.] 2*:65–84.

Lundqvist, U. (1976). Lucus distribution of induced *eceriferum* mutants in barley. In *Barley Genetics III*. (Gaul, H. ed.), pp. 162–163. Verlag Karl Thiemig, Munich.

Lundqvist, U., von Wettstein-Knowles, P., and von Wettstein, D. (1968). Induction of *eceriferum* mutants in barley by ionizing radiations and chemical mutagens. II. *Hereditas 59*:473–504.

McCann, J., Choi, E., Yamasaki, E., and Ames, B. N. (1976). Detection of carcinogens as mutagens in the *Salmonella*/microsome test: Assay of 300 chemicals. Part II. *Proc. Natl. Acad. Sci. USA 73*:950–954.

Micke, A. (1962). Eine bitterstofffreie Mutante bei *Melilotus albus* nach Bestrahlung von Samen mit thermischen Neutronen. *Naturwissenschaften 49*:332–333.

Micke, A. (1963). Genetisch-züchterische Arbeiten beim weissen Steinklee. *Z. Acker Pflanz. 116*:354–360.

Micke, A. (1969). Improvement of low yielding sweet clover mutants by heterosis breeding. In *Induced Mutations in Plants* (STI/PUB/231), International Atomic Energy Agency, Vienna.

Mikaelsen, K., Saja, Z., and Simon, J. (1971). An early maturing mutant—Its value in breeding for disease resistance in rice. In *Rice Breeding with Induced Mutations III* (STI/DOC/10/131), pp. 97–101. International Atomic Energy Agency, Vienna.

Murray, M. J. (1969). Successful use of irradiation breeding to obtain *Verticillium*-resistant strains of peppermint, *Mentha piperita* L. In *Induced Muatations in Plants* (STI/PUB/231), pp. 345–371. International Atomic Energy Agency, Vienna.

Nilan, R. A. (1960). Barley research at Washington State University. *Särt. Sver. Utsädesförenings Tidsk., 1–2*:110–118.

Nilan, R. A. (1967). Nature of induced mutations in higher plants. In *Induzierte Mutationen und Ihre Nutzung: Erwin-Baur-Gedächtnisvorlesungen IV* (Gröber, K., Scholz, F., and Zacharias, M., eds.), pp. 6–20. Akademic-Verlag, Berlin.

Nilan, R. A. (1972). Mutagenic specificity in flowering plants: Facts and prospects. In *Induced Mutations and Plant Improvement (STI/PUB/297), pp, 141*n151. International Atomic Energy Agency, Vienna.

Nilan, R. A. and Vig, B. K. (1976). Plant test systems for detection of chemical mutagens. In *Chemical Mutagens. Principles and Methods for Their Detection,* (Hollaender, A. ed.), Vol. 4, Chap. 39, pp. 143–170. Plenum Press, New York.

Nilan, R. A., Sideris, E. G., Kleinhofs, A., Sander, C., and Konzak, C. F. (1973). Azide–a potent mutagen. *Mutat. Res. 17*:142–144.

Oostinder-Braaksma, F. J. and Feenstra, W. J. (1973). Isolation and characterization of chlorate-resistant mutants of *Arabidopsis thaliana. Mutat. Res. 19*:175–185.

Persson, G. and Hagberg, A. (1969). Induced variation in a quantitative character in barley. Morphology and cytogenetics of *erectoides* mutants. *Hereditas 61*:115–178.

Pontecorvo, G. (1954). Mitotic recombination in the genetic systems of filamentous fungi. *Caryologia [Suppl.] 6*:192–200.

Pontecorvo, G. (1958). *Trendes in Genetic Analysis.* Columbia Univ. Press, New York.

Pontecorvo, G. and Kafer, E. (1958). Genetic analysis based on mitotic recombination. *Advan. Genet. 9*:71–104.

Powell, J. B. and Nilan, R. A. (1963). Influence of temperature on crossing over in an inversion heterozygote in barley. *Crop Sci. 3*:11–13.

Sideris, E. G., Nilan, R. A., and Bogyo, T. P. (1973). Differential effect of sodium azide on the frequency of radiation-induced chromosome aberrations *vs.* the frequency of radiation-induced chlorophyll mutations in *Hordeum vulgare. Radiat. Bot. 13*:315–322.

Sigurbjörnsson, B. (1976). The improvement of barley through induced mutation. In *Barley Genetics III* (Gaul, H., ed.), pp. 84–95. Verlag Karl Thiemig, Munich.

Sigurbjörnsson, B. and Micke, A. (1974). Philosophy and accomplishments of mutation breeding. In: *Polyploidy and Induced Mutations in Plant Breeding* (STI/PUB/359), pp. 303–343. International Atomic Energy Agency, Vienna.

Smith, H. H. (1971). Broadening the base of genetic variability in plants. *J. Hered. 62*:265–276.

Ulland, B., Weisburger, E. K., and Weisburger, J. H. (1973). Chronic toxicity and carcinogenicity of industrial chemicals and pesticides. *Toxicol. Appl. Pharm. 25*:446(Abst).

Wiberg, A. (1974) Sources of resistance to mildew in barley. *Hereditas 78*:1–40.

16

Principal Diseases of Major Crops in Pakistan with Reference to Genetic Resistance

C. M. Akhtar

Punjab Agricultural Research Institute
Lyallpur, Pakistan

ABSTRACT

Varietal resistance is reported for the major diseases of wheat, rice, sugarcane, and cotton crops prevalent in Pakistan. In wheat, a number of varieties/lines exhibit resistance to rusts (leaf and stem), loose smut, flag smut, complete bunt, partial bunt, and earcockle diseases. Of the commercial varieties, Blue Silver, Lyallpur-73, PARI-73, and Sandal exhibit different degrees of resistance to rusts, whereas Mexipak-65 and Khushal are resistant to loose smut. Similarly, varieties Lyp-73 and Nayab are resistant to flag smut; Blue Silver, Mexipak, and Potohar are resistant to complete bunt; and Tarnab-69 to partial bunt. In rice, a newly evolved and promising strain, PK-178, exhibits high resistance to blast disease, whereas Basmati-370 shows resistance to Helminthosporium leaf spot; seven varieties/lines exhibit resistance to kernel smut. In sugarcane, varieties/lines exhibit resistance to kernel smut. In sugarcane, varieties/lines exhibit resistance to smut and red rot diseases. In the irradiated material, two varieties exhibit resistance to red rot disease, suggesting mutation has been induced. In cotton, none of the *hirsutum* types available in the country is resistant to bacterial blight disease, while all the approved *arboreum* (local) types are resistant to the disease. No genetic resistance has been observed so far against the root rot disease of cotton.

INTRODUCTION

Wheat is the major winter (Rabi) crop in Pakistan, and rice, sugarcane, and cotton are the major summer (Kharif) crops. Genetic resistance in these crops against major diseases in Pakistan is considered in this chapter. Because these diseases vary from region to region, a land-use map of Pakistan (Fig. 1) and a map of Punjab showing the districts (Fig. 2) are included for purposes of discussion.

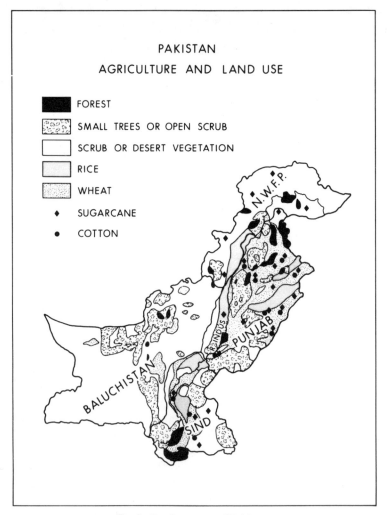

Fig. 1. Land use map of Pakistan.

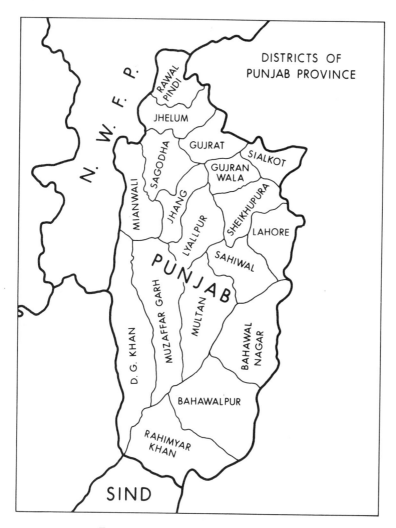

Fig. 2. Map of Punjab showing the districts.

DISEASES OF WHEAT

Wheat occupies a position of paramount importance in Pakistan, both with respect to the extent of the area it covers and to the magnitude of food production. It is the staple food crop and is cultivated over an area of about 15 million acres (with fluctuations in the rainfed areas). The wheat crop in Pakistan is susceptible to a number of plant diseases that bring about heavy losses in the form of lowered yield and quality. Some diseases, such as leaf and stem rusts, are found all over the country, whereas the others are of regional importance. Stripe rust is important in the foothill districts of the Punjab and the Northwest Frontier (NWFP), extending to a lesser extent into the central plains. Complete bunt of wheat is serious in Baluchistan and occurs to some extent in the northern foothill districts of the Punjab and the NWFP. Partial bunt is usually confined to Sialkot and Gujranwala districts of the Punjab, whereas flag smut occurs in Rawalpindi division of the Punjab and parts of the NWFP. Septoria leaf spot and powdery mildew are observed during cool and wet springs. Earcockle disease occurs mostly in Khairpur division of Sind and parts of the Punjab. Loose smut of wheat is prevalent all over the country, the incidence being more in areas where the old, tall varieties are grown. Helminthosporium leaf blight and root rot have been observed in Sind and the central plains of the Punjab, whereas downy mildew has been reported from Sind. Coordinated efforts are in progress for development of desirable varieties resistant to various diseases. Survey and identification of the rust races prevalent in the country and the screening of wheat varieties against individual races of all three types of rust are being carried out at the Central Institute of Cereal Diseases, Murree, whereas screening of the varieties against other diseases is generally being done at the provincial institutes.

Rusts of Wheat

The three rusts of wheat occur in Pakistan—stripe, leaf, and stem rust caused by *Puccinia striiformis tritici, P. recondita tritici,* and *P. graminis tritici,* respectively. Stripe rust appears first at the tillering stage, and is generally confined to the foothill districts of the Punjab and the NWFP, where winter rains favor its development. Occasionally, when the climatic conditions are favorable, it spreads to the central plains. Investigations of the physiological races indicate the presence of races 25, 31, 64(Eo), 67(Eo), 66(E16), and 66(Eo). The varieties Blue Silver, Lyp-73, PARI-73, SA-42, and Sandal are resistant, whereas the varieties Barani-70, Khushal-69, Mexipak-65, Pak-70, and Tarnab-73 are moderately susceptible, and the variety Potohar is susceptible to strip rust (Hasan, 1975).

Leaf and stem rusts occur all over the country in wheat and become serious wherever and whenever weather conditions remain favorable for longer periods. Leaf rust appears first in the coastal region and lower Sind in the last week of January, and with the rise in temperature, leaf rust gradually spreads to the central plains and foothill districts of the Punjab and the NWFP. Stem rust starts about one week later than leaf rust in the coastal areas, spreading similarly to the northern areas with the rise in temperature.

The survey of physiological races of leaf and stem rusts has indicated the presence of races 12, 20, 57, 77, 84, 144, 158, and 184 of leaf rust, and races 9,

11, 15, 15B, 17, 21, 24, 34, 40, 42, and 117 of stem rust, respectively. Of these races, 57 and 77 of leaf rust and 17 and 21 of stem rust are more common.

Among the commercial varieties, Blue Silver, Lyp-73, PARI-73, and Sandal are resistant, whereas the varieties Barani-70, Chenab-70, Khushal-69, Pak-70, Mexipak-65, Potohar, Tarnab-73, and SA-42 are susceptible to the prevalent races of leaf rust. Similarly, the variety Lyp-73 is resistant to the prevalent races of stem rust, whereas Potohar is susceptible. Varieties Blue Silver, Barani-70, PARI-73, SA-42, Tarnab-73, and Sandal are moderately resistant, whereas Chenab-70, Khushal-69, Mexipak, and Pak-70 are moderately susceptible. [See Appendix I for those varieties of wheat which can be used as useful sources of resistance to leaf and stem rusts in Pakistan (Hasan, 1975).]

Loose Smut of Wheat

Loose smut of wheat (*Ustilago tritici*) is next in importance to rusts of wheat in Pakistan. The incidence of this disease is more in the regions where the old tall local varieties are grown. Four physiological races 1, 2, 10, and 12 have been identified (Hasan, 1975). Among the current commercial varieties Barani-70, Chenab-70, SA-42, Pak-70, and PARI-73 are susceptible, while Mexipak-65 and Khushal-69 are resistant to the disease. [See Appendix I for those varieties/lines of wheat which have shown constant resistance to the field collections of loose smut for a number of years, and which provide useful sources of resistance (Akhtar, 1973–1975; Hasan, 1975).]

Flag Smut

Flag smut of wheat (*Urocystis tritici* Koern.) is found in the submountainous tracts of Pakistan. Its incidence has increased recently after the introduction of high-yielding, semidwarf varieties. Preliminary studies on the physiological races indicate the presence of the races 1 and 4.

The current commercial varieties Barani-70, Blue Silver, Chenab-70, Khushal-69, Mexipak-65, Pak-70, PARI-73, Potohar, SA-42, and Sandal are susceptible to the disease, whereas Lyallpur-73 and Nayab are resistant. [See Appendix I for those varieties/lines of wheat which have exhibited resistance to the prevalent races for two years, and which can provide some sources of resistance (Hasan, 1975).]

Complete Bunt of Wheat

Complete bunt of wheat caused by *Tilletia foetida* (Wallr) Liro and *T. caries* (DC.) Tul is an economically important disease in Baluchistan and in the foothills and hilly areas of the Punjab and the NWFP. Three physiological races—L-8, L-9, and L-13—have been identified. Of the current commercial varieties, Barani-70, Chenab-70, Khushal-69, Lyallpur-73, SA-42, and Sandal are susceptible to this disease, while Blue Silver, Mexipak, and Potohar are resistant. [See Appendix I for those varieties of wheat which have exhibited resistance to the prevalent races and field collections for several years, and which provide useful sources of resistance (Hasan, 1975).]

Partial Bunt of Wheat

Partial bunt of wheat caused by *Tilletia indica* (Mitra) Mundkar occurs in the foothill districts of the Punjab and parts of the NWFP. The commercial varieties Barani-70, Khushal-69, Chenab-70, Lyallpur-73, Mexipak-65, Pak-70, and Potohar are susceptible to the disease, whereas Tarnab-69 is resistant. [See Appendix I for those varieties which have remained resistant to the field collections of partial bunt for several years, and which provide useful sources of resistance (Hasan, 1975*a*).]

Earcockle of Wheat

Earcockle disease of wheat caused by *Anguina tritici* occurs in parts of the Punjab and Sind provinces. Among the current commercial varieties, Mexipak-65, Barani-70, Chenab-70, and Blue Silver are susceptible to the disease, whereas Lyallpur-73, Potohar, and Sandal are resistant. (See Appendix I for those varieties/lines which have remained resistant for some years, and which provide useful sources of resistance.)

Root Rot and Leaf Blight

Root rot and leaf blight caused by *Helminthosporium sativum* Pamm, King, and Bakke occurs in parts of Sind and the Punjab plains, especially in poor soils and under water-stress conditions. Of the commercial varieties, Mexipak, Chenab-70, Blue Silver, and SA-42 are susceptible, whereas the varieties Potohar and PARI-73 are resistant to the disease.

DISEASES OF RICE

Rice is a food crop second only in importance to wheat in Pakistan; it is cultivated over about 3.6 million acres, producing about 2.2 million tons annually. It is attacked by a number of plant diseases like blast, helminthosporium leaf spot, stem rot, and kernel smut. Prior to 1964—1965 no epiphytotic outbreak of any rice disease had occurred in this country, and consequently not much attention was paid to research on these diseases. Rice breeders did not even seek any specific resistance of the varieties against any of the prevalent diseases. In 1964 the sudden outbreak of blast disease in the commercial field trials of a newly released variety, C-622, put the rice scientists on the alert. After that, serious attention was given to the development of varieties resistant to the diseases, particularly rice blast. The information available in this respect is briefly given below:

Blast Disease of Rice

Blast disease of rice caused by *Piricularia oryzae* Cav. is known to occur in all the rice-growing countries of the world. The disease is serious in most of the humid rice-growing regions of the world. Previously it was considered to be a minor disease in Pakistan. The 1964 epiphytotic outbreak of the disease in the fields under the newly developed susceptible variety, C-622, not only completely destroyed the crop, but also was instrumental in the widespread distribution of the disease inoculum. Since then, the disease occurs commonly in the Punjab. None of the commercial varieties is resistant to the disease. However, a recently developed high-yielding and promising variety, Pak-178, has been found to exhibit high resistance to the disease. Of the different varieties/lines of rice included in the blast screening nurseries, see Appendix II for those found to provide useful sources of resistance to this disease.

Helminthosporium Blight

Helminthosporium blight of rice caused by the fungus *Helminthosporium oryzae* is worldwide in distribution. In Pakistan it is known to occur in all the rice-growing tracts,·but it normally does not cause severe damage to the crop. Nevertheless, in an epiphytotic outbreak, this disease can cause yield losses up to 90%. Two such epiphytotics—one in Godavari delta in 1918, and the other in Bengal in 1942—have occurred in the Indo-Pak subcontinent. The seedling blight phase of the disease is not common in Pakistan. The susceptibility of the rice plant to the disease increases with its age, and the plant is very susceptible to the disease at the flowering stage. Five pathogenic races of the causal fungus have been identified (Nawaz and Kausar, 1962), of which race 5 is the most virulent. The variety Basmati-370 is resistant to the races 1, 2, and 3, whereas Palmen-246 is resistant to the races 2 and 4. Variety Sathra-278 is resistant to race 4.

Kernel Smut

[*Tilletia barclayana* (Bref), Sacc., and Syd]. Kernel smut of rice, also known as bunt of rice, occurs widely in the major rice-growing countries of the world. In Pakistan it is common in the Punjab and Sind provinces. The incidence of the disease varies from year to year and from variety to variety.

Losses from this disease are directly proportional to the percentage of infected grains, because the entire grain is converted to a black powdery mass consisting of chlamydospores of the causal fungus. All the coarse varieties are susceptible to the disease. Commercial varieties Jhona-349, Sathra-278, Basmati-370, Kangni, and Sada Gulab are susceptible. Continuous large-scale cultivation of these varieties is likely to aggravate this disease problem. Of the 900 coarse and fine varieties/lines of local and exotic origin tested for resistance by artificial inoculations, under field conditions, only the fine varieties, namely 622-B, 66107-B, Imperial Blue Rose, 197-B Jajai, 198-B, and Bengalo exhibited resistance to the disease (Hasan, 1975).

Stem Rot of Rice

Stem rot of rice caused by the fungus *Leptosphaeria salvinii* Catt. (*Sclerotium oryzae* Catt.) is a widespread disease, known to occur in almost all the rice-growing areas of the world. In Pakistan, the incidence of the disease varies from 1 to 25%, prevalent mostly in the districts of the Punjab. None of the 400 varieties/lines tested for resistance against this disease was found to be resistant. Further investigations are needed to locate sources of resistance to stem rot.

DISEASES OF SUGARCANE

Sugarcane is one of the major cash crops in Pakistan and is grown over an area of 1.66 million acres, with an annual production of 20.9 million tons. It is attacked by a number of plant diseases of which smut, red rot, and mosaic are important. The effective, practicable control of these diseases is possible only through the development of resistant varieties. The information available on the genetic resistance to the prevalent important diseases is as follows.

Smut of Sugarcane

Sugarcane smut caused by *Ustilago scitaminea* Syd. occurs throughout the country, in the sugarcane fields. It is more common in the Sind areas, due to favorable climatic conditions. None of the commercial varieties is resistant to the disease. The varieties BL-4*, CoL-29, L-116, CoL-54, and L-118 are moderately susceptible, whereas the variety Co-547 is susceptible to the disease. [See Appendix III for those varieties/lines of sugar cane that have remained free in

*BL: Barbados Lyallpur; CoL:, Coimbatore Lyallpur; L: Lyallpur; Co: Coimbatore (India); F: Formosa.

the screening trials for two years, and which provide very useful sources of resistance to the disease (Akhtar, 1973–1975).

Red Rot of Sugarcane

Red rot of sugarcane caused by *Physalospora tucumanensis* Speg. conidial stage *Colletotrichum falcatum* Went. occurs commonly in Pakistan. This disease is more often found in the districts of Lyallpur, Sheikhupura, Gujranwala, and Sialkot. None of the current commercial varieties is resistant to the disease, but they do vary in degree of susceptibility. Varieties BL-4 and CoL-54 showed comparatively less susceptibility to the disease. Among the 21 promising varieties, Co-547, Co-564, and L-118 are moderately resistant, whereas Co-454, Co-61, and F-134 are moderately susceptible to the disease. All the other varieties are susceptible to the disease. Among 950 varieties/lines tested for resistance to red rot, there were 12 varieties which remained resistant for two years, and which provide useful sources of resistance to the disease (Akhtar, 1973, 1973–1975). (These are listed in Appendix III.)

Induced Mutation through Radiation

Out of 1400 irradiated canes of the high-yielding commercial varieties BL-4 and L-116 tested for resistance against red rot disease, 25 canes of BL-4 and 14 canes of L-116 showed resistance to the disease, indicating a change which we attribute to induced mutation. Material from these resistant canes is being multiplied for further tests.

Sugarcane Mosaic

Sugarcane mosaic caused by the mosaic virus is the third important disease known to occur very widely in nearly all the sugar cane fields in Pakistan. None of the available varieties/lines of sugar cane is resistant. Further work is needed in order to locate sources of resistance to this disease.

COTTON

Cotton is the other major cash crop of Pakistan, grown over an area of about 5 million acres, with an annual production of about 3.5 million bales. The arboreum types are grown on about 0.17 million acres, whereas the hirsutum types are grown in the remaining area. Although a number of plant diseases have been recorded on cotton in Pakistan, only two diseases—bacterial blight and root rot—are of major importance. The investigations made on the varietal resistance and biological control of these diseases are as follows.

Bacterial Blight

Bacterial blight of cotton caused by *Xanthomonas malvacearum* was not known to occur commonly in Pakistan in the past. Its severe incidence was observed in some areas of the Punjab in 1967; since then it has been observed to occur commonly in the cotton-growing areas of Pakistan. Investigations on the genetic resistance to this disease have shown that none of the hirsutum types being grown in the country is resistant to the disease, whereas all the commercial arboreum types, namely, D-9, D-108, D-105, and 231-R are highly resistant to the disease. However, 22 hirsutum-type lines of the recently imported exotic material have exhibited high resistance to the disease and can be used as sources of resistance to the disease (Hussain, 1975). (These are listed in Appendix IV.)

Root Rot

Root rot is one of the most important diseases of cotton in Pakistan. It occurs in patches throughout the cotton-growing areas of the country. The incidence of the disease varies from 1 to 20% in different localities. Recent investigations (Akhtar, 1973) indicate that the disease is caused by the fungus *Rhizoctonia solani.* There is no known source of resistance to this disease in Pakistan. The pathogen involved is established deep in the soil; hence, chemical control of the disease is not practicable. Because of the economic importance of root rot, measures have been investigated to find successful ways of dealing with the disease (Akhtar, 1973–1975).

CONCLUSIONS

There are resistant varieties available to counteract most of the diseases which afflict the major crops of Pakistan (Appendixes I–IV). There are three noteworthy exceptions—stem rot of rice, sugarcane mosaic, and root rot of cotton. The crops, for which resistant varieties exist, need to be upgraded by conventional plant-breeding techniques. For the others, resistant varieties need to be sought or methods of biological control need to be undertaken to lessen the impact of each disease.

APPENDIX I

Varieties of wheat that can be used as useful sources of resistance to leaf and stem rusts in Pakistan:

Lyp-73	Nuri-70	Vicam
PARI-73	Tobari-66	Chris
Bajio	Penjamo-62	FKN
		Pushmore Suprema

Varieties/lines of wheat which have shown constant resistance to the field collections of loose smut for a number of years, and which provide useful sources of resistance:

AU-44

(Ch53 × N10B)Y54

Cajeme-60

Gala

Indus-66

Mexipak-65

Penjamo 62

114B-35 × Nad-63 (Bulk) (V1017)

23584-SA-42; Pk-6145-15-0a. (V1076)

Mexipak × Dwarf 120 Pk-3383-1a-1a-0a
    (V1092)

Nor67(NP876-on × Kalyan-CB479)
    Pk-5939-11a-0a (V1108)

Pk-2858-7a-3a-3a-0a (V1132)

Pk-2858-7a-3a-4a-0a (V1133)

Cno "s"-Gallo. II-27829-19y-2M-4Y-0M
    (V1135)

NP-876-Pj 62 N Cno "s"-Pj 62
    27983-21y-1M-1Y-OM (V1136)

Khushal (V1165)

Mpak × Dwarf 120 Pj-3383-1a-1a-Oa
    (V1172)

(Pi-62-Frond × Pi62-Mance)Mpak
    Pk-2858-7a-3a-1a-0a (V1196)

Pk-2858-7a-3a-2a-0ay (V1197)

Inia × Bb II-26478-80M-2Y-3M-0Y
    (V1200)

Kalyan × Bb II-26992-30M-300Y-3M-501Y
    -500M-)Y (V1203)

Np-876-Pj 62 × Cnl "s"-Pj 62
    II-27987-21y-1M-1Y-0M (V1204)

tn15 × Mpak (V4093)

Mpak × Norin. Ankauc B (V4057)

Kalyan × Ciano "s" (V4098)

HD 832-0n × Kalyan (V1360/L)

MP65.Ciano × Sndus-66 Y 50 (V3091)

Pi Gb × Nai-60 (V1358/L)

Varieties/lines of wheat which have exhibited resistance to the prevalent races of flag smut for two years, and which provide useful sources of resistance:

Agatha	Exchange	Lancer
Cougher	F334-1	Nainari-60
Dular	F430-Lee-Nd-74	Veranopolis
		Wankan

Varieties of wheat which have exhibited resistance to the prevalent races and field collections of complete bunt for several years, and which provide useful sources of resistance:

299	Dular	Yuma
Br-7	Mexipak-65	Yagla-305
Cougher	Selkirk	T. Timopheevi

Varieties of wheat which have remained resistant to the field collections of partial bunt for several years, and which provide useful sources of resistance:

Bovie	FKN	T. Timopheevi
Cougher	Gala	Waban
Exchange	Nainari-60	Wankan
		Yuma

Varieties/lines of wheat which have remained resistant to earcockle for some years, and which provide useful sources of resistance:

114B-35 X Nad63 (Kal 227A/CJE Gb56-GHR)S-64 Y50(E) X TRO Pk-7324-2a
Bb X Mpak. Pk6087-1a-1a
CC-Inia X Bb-Inia. Pk8728-11K-0a

APPENDIX II

Varieties/lines of rice included in the blast screening nurseries, and which provide useful sources of resistance:

Gina	747220	6005
Narian.20	IR424-3-43-PKI-2	2750
Tainaus	5603	6153
Taichung	6071	6119

APPENDIX III

Varieties/lines of sugarcane which have remained free of smut in the screening trials for two years, and which provide useful sources of resistance:

1-29-57	CP-50-9	1-181-54
Co-356	Zmex-54-86	CoL-81
I-242-56	Co-565	CB-36-147
I-39-55	Co-626	I-12-61
Co-549	I-32-56	I-66-61
Co-961	Co-370	POJ-2878
		I395-56

Varieties/lines of sugarcane which remained resistant to red rot for two years, and which provide useful sources of resistance:

I-29-53	Co-565	CoL-81
I-242-56	Co-626	I-12-61
Co-549	Co-370	Co-338
CP-50	I-181-54	I-395-56

Note: I: Ishardi (Bangla Desh); Co. Coimbatore (India) CoL: Coimbatore Lyallpur; POJ: Profstation Oost Java; CB: The variety imported from Kenya (Originally this variety belonged to Brazil. The exact explanation of the letters CB is not known.)

APPENDIX IV

Hirsutum-type lines of cotton which have exhibited high resistance to bacterial blight, and which can be used as sources of resistance:

Bs(67)1470	Hairy Acala 1	HA 10
B2(67)1473	HA 2	HA 10-2
C2(67)577	HA 3	HA 11
C2(69)1485	HA 6	HA 12
UK AC2(67)577	HA 7	Reba B50
UK AB2(69)1456	HA 8	AMA 1-38
UK AB2(69)1440	HA 9	AMS 1-48
		101-102.B

REFERENCES

Akhtar, C. M. (1973–1975). *Annual Report of Plant Pathologist,* P.A.R.I., Lyallpur. (unpublished).

Akhtar, C. M. (1973). Root rot of cotton—A study of the active microflora of the root rot in affected and healthy cotton soils during the active period of the disease and pathogenicity of the predominant isolates. *J. Agr. Res. (Punjab) II*(4):40–48.

Hasan, S. F. (1975a). Wheat diseases in relation to varietal improvement in Pakistan. *1st Workshop for National Task Force Leaders. U.N.D.P./F.A.O. Regional Project & Feed Food Crops, Lahore, Pakistan, March 1975.* (unpublished).

Hasan, S. F. (1975b). Kernel smut of rice in Pakistan, R.C.D. Seminar on integrated pest control in rice, Islamabad, Pakistan. (unpublished).

Hussain, T. (1975). *Annual Report of the Division of Plant Pathology,* Cotton Res. Inst., Multan, Pakistan. (unpublished).

IRRI. (1963). *The Rice Blast Disease Proceedings of a Symposium at the International Rice Research Institute, 1963.*

Nawaz, M. and Kausar, A. G. (1962). Cultural and pathogenic variation in *Helminthosporium oryzae. Biologia 8*(1):35–48.

17

The Measurement of Disease Severity in Cereal Smut

J. V. Groth

University of Minnesota
St. Paul, Minnesota

C. O. Person

University of British Columbia
Vancouver, British Columbia, Canada

and

T. Ebba

Institute of Agricultural Research
Addis Ababa, Ethiopia

ABSTRACT

For smut diseases of cereal crops in which the presence of disease is signaled by the occurrence of diseased culms, the tradition has been developed whereby disease severity is measured in percentages, either of plants or of culms, which show the disease. However, the data that have accrued have contributed relatively little to an understanding of either the disease or host resistance to it. In this study the percentages of infected tillers on diseased plants (within-plant disease severity) were both recorded and were found, on analysis, to be strongly correlated. Although the strong correlation suggested a general identity of genes responsible for among- and within-plant disease severity, other aspects of the analysis suggest that the fungus must pass through two distinct barriers, or thresholds, in order to produce teliospores. If the first threshold is surmounted, the fungus will be able to cause smutting in at least one tiller of the plant (as measured by among-plant disease severity); if the second threshold is also crossed, additional culms will also be smutted (as measured by within-plant disease severity). One can regard the individual culm as having two separate (but not independent) opportunities of remaining healthy following inoculation of the seed. Both are measured and defined in terms of probability.

INTRODUCTION

Common to all studies of plant disease is the problem of measuring the extent to which the disease has developed. The measure may be based on manifestations shown by individual plants (e.g., the type of pustule that is formed) or by populations of plants (e.g., loss in yield). For those smut diseases of cereal crops in which the presence of disease is signaled by the occurrence of diseased culms, the tradition has developed of measuring disease severity in percentages, either of plants or of culms, that show the disease. Although this method of measurement appears to be quantitative, we intend to show in this paper that more often than not it has failed to meet the requirements needed for quantitative precision.

The lack of precision just referred to arises from the fact that usually it is not possible to distinguish, among symptomless plants—(i) those that may have escaped infection; (ii) those that may have resisted infection; and (iii) those that may have resisted disease development following a successful infection. Also, for plants that do show at least one smutted culm, and for which the infection is known to have succeeded, the disease may be expressed by more than one, and, in the extreme case, by all the culms of the diseased plant. The possibility exists that resistance to smutting may involve two genetically determined components, viz. resistance to infection and resistance to disease development following infection, and that symptomless plants of groups (ii) and (iii) are genetically different. In any event, it is clear that where the disease is measured in terms of healthy and smutted plants, those classified as healthy will include the three possible groups listed above, and those classified as smutted will include plants for which the extent of disease development is variably expressed. And where disease is measured in terms of healthy and smutted culms (i.e., without regard to individual plants), no distinction is possible, either between resistance to infection and resistance to disease development following infection, or among smutted plants which may show variable levels of disease expression.

Among 65 papers on smut diseases that we have examined, percentages of smutted plants are recorded in 38, and of smutted culms in 16; in nine papers attempts were made to measure more than simply the percentages of smutted plants or culms, and in the two remaining, different sections of the papers involved different methods of measurement.

Correlations between percentages of smutted plants and of smutted culms are presented in several studies (Briggs, 1926; Tapke, 1929,1931; Welsh, 1932;

Clark et al., 1933; Ruttle, 1934; Churchward, 1937–1938; Reed and Stanton, 1938) and in two of these (Clark et al., 1933; Ruttle, 1934) the correlation is discussed. It must be pointed out, however, that this correlation by itself has no statistical validity. This is because they are not logically independent—except for the unlikely event that the two percentages are negatively correlated, a higher frequency of smutted plants would also mean a higher frequency of smutted culms. The correlation between the percentage of smutted plants (among-plant disease severity) and the percentage of smutted culms on smutted plants (within-plant disease severity) is not necessarily positive, and warrants further investigation. A beginning has been made by Gaines (1923), who determined the proportions of totally bunted wheat plants (designated c), of partially bunted plants (b), and of bunted culms on bunted plants (a), and noted that the latter proportion (a) was smaller for four resistant cultivars than it was for the four susceptible cultivars that were also tested. The values obtained (0.25 and 0.67) provided good qualitative evidence for the existence of a positive correlation among the tested cultivars. In a study involving *Ustilago tritici* and many different wheat cultivars, Oort (1947) showed what appeared to be a close correlation between within- and among-plant disease severity. Oort's sample sizes were rather small, and for most cases the statistical analyses were not presented. Nevertheless, this was the only study found in the literature in which the correlation was investigated as a primary objective.

One feature of the smut diseases on cereals may prove of particular value in future studies—It is the inverse relationship that exists between reproductivities of host and parasite. One smut sorus or one seed will be produced, but not both, and the reproductivities of host and parasite are both easily quantified. A system of this kind may be particularly useful in studies of the populational dynamics of parasitism. But the problem of measuring disease severity must be investigated first. This is the objective of the work described in the following section.

MATERIALS AND METHODS

Twelve barley cultivars and 21 *U. hordei* dikaryons were used in these studies. Only those genotypic combinations which showed smut in at least five percent of inoculated plants were included. The smut dikaryons included representatives of the original 13 physiological races described by Tapke (1945). These were obtained as teliospore samples from North Dakota State University, where they have been maintained. The other eight cultures represent as wide a range of smut biotypes as it was possible readily to obtain. All are from North America except for the three prefixed Et, which are from three separate collections made in Ethiopia.

Of the 21 dikaryons here used, one was derived from the haploids E3a and I4A which have been used in previous work (Welsh, 1932). For the other 20 dikaryons, the constituent haploids were both derived from a single teliospore. These 20 dikaryons were thus produced through "selfing" of two of the four products of 20 tetrads derived from 20 different teliospores. The tetrads were derived in the following way. A thin layer of complete agar was poured into a petri dish. Blocks about 15 mm^2 were cut and each was placed on a 22-mm^2 sterile cover slip. Five-mliter aqueous suspensions of teliospores were prepared in test tubes. After adding to these suspensions a drop of achromycin suspension (10 mg achromycin per mliter H$_2$O), a small drop of the teliospore suspension was transferred to the centre of each agar block with a Pasteur pipette. Depending on the germination rate of the teliospores used, the concentration was adjusted so that from 10 to 100 teliospores were included in each drop transferred. The agar blocks with their teliospores were then incubated at 22°C for about 12 hr (somewhat longer for older samples), by which time most of the 5-10 viable teliospores had germinated. A suitably germinated teliospore, with all four sporidial products accessible for microdissection, was selected on each block. The four primary sporidia were drawn away from the promycelium, one to each of the four sides of the block, using a deFonbrune micromanipulator and an upward-bent fine glass needle. Their position on the promycelium was recorded directly on the cover slip, near the edge. In 3–4 days, visible colonies had formed from the four sporidia. They were transferred singly to fresh plates and, after sufficient growth, were tested for mating-type as described earlier (Groth and Person, 1975). Small amounts of sporidia were put into screwcap tubes containing fine-textured, very dry silica gel for long-term storage. Two of the four cultures of each tetrad were selected at random to form the dikaryons which were used throughout the study.

Seed treatment and inoculation were as described earlier (Groth and Person, 1975).

Considering the size of the overall experiment in relation to the amount of field space and recording time available, the minimum number of smutted plants which would be examined for within-plant severity in each genotypic combination was set at 30. Only plants with three or more culms were included. In order to be reasonably certain of obtaining 30 plants, for those combinations where information was available concerning the amount of smut to be expected, the number of inoculated seeds needed for planting was determined by using the relationship

$$(1 - P)^n = 0.01$$

where P is the percentage of plants showing smut and n, the number of plants needed to be 99% certain of obtaining at least one smutted plant. The net result was that more seeds were planted when, for a particular genotypic combination, it was expected that the smutting percentage would be low.

Inoculated seeds were planted in the field in 4.5-m rows. The rate of seeding varied from 90 to 150 seeds per row, depending on percent viability of the seed and on the amount of tillering exhibited by the cultivar at a given seeding rate. Usually a particular genotypic combination was planted in 1–2 blocks of several rows each.

Data were recorded when all spikes had emerged. Generally, the percentage of plants smutted was based on samples of at least 300 plants. In the few cases in which fewer plants were available, the percentage of plants smutted was high enough so that sample sizes were statistically adequate (Steel and Torrie, 1960). Smutted plants to be examined on a tiller basis were carefully pulled. When time was not limiting and the plants were available, 40–50 plants were examined. Plants with one and two tillers were also recorded, but, for reasons to be given, they were not used in determining the degree of within-plant severity. The arcsin transformations and correlation analyses of smutted head and plant percentages were done by computer.

RESULTS

The work of Tapke (1945) was consulted to determine which combinations of host and parasite genotypes to investigate. As shown by his data, any combination that produced less than 1.0% smut (he used a head-per-row basis) was not included in this study. Thus, many of the negative and low readings in the table for the 13 races, and eight of the barley cultivars (his work did not include Conquest, Gateway, Keystone, or Vantage) are the findings of Tapke. Also, while the practical lower limit in the present work was taken as 5% plants smutted, sufficient data were nonetheless obtained for inclusion in the experiment. Information on expected smutting for some of the other combinations was obtained from earlier work (Ebba, unpublished). If there was no available information about a given combination, 5–8 rows (and more later on, if necessary) were planted.

Before making the correlation analysis, a complication involving variation in plant tillering had to be dealt with first. An inverse relationship between the average number of culms per plant and the percent of smutted culms on smutted plants was discovered. For example, Nepal inoculated with Uh6 was planted both at the University of British Columbia and in California. The latter planting was done on highly fertilized land, and other conditions there were also conducive to extremely high tillering. In British Columbia, smutted plants of this cultivar produced an average of 4.26 culms, 95.2% of which were smutted. In California, where smutted plants produced an average of 12.8 culms, a significantly lower 71.1% of the culms were smutted. There was no significant difference in percent of plants smutted at the two locations. A similar discovery was made when Lion and Uh6 were planted at both locations; only here the percentage of plants smutted was actually significantly higher in California. Whether the data for a combination were obtained at British Columbia or in

California was largely random. Yet the mean percent of smutted culms on diseased plants for the 29 combinations under high-tillering conditions was 44.3 with 13.8 culms per smutted plant being produced, whereas that of the 82 low-tillering combinations was 59.4% with 4.3 culms per smutted plant. Analysis of all 111 points demonstrated a significant negative regression of frequency of smutted culms on diseased plants on average tiller production. When low- and high-tillering plantings were analyzed separately, however, there was no significant regression in either grouping (an average of nine or more culms per plant being considered high-tillering). Division of data into two separate analyses reduced the variation of average culms per plant with each data set, thereby minimizing the effect of this variable on within-plant disease severity. This was thought to be the simplest and most effective way to avoid this complication.

Figure 1A,B shows the within- and among-plant disease-severity scatter diagrams for low- and high-tillering plantings, respectively. In both analyses, the variances of x and y were very close. Hence, scatter diagrams involving units of standard deviation were thought unnecessary. As shall be brought out in the discussion, a strong genetic component in the variance of within-plant disease severity is indicated.

Separate within-cultivar and within-dikaryon correlations were made on low-tillering plantings of five cultivars and three dikaryons. The other combinations did not possess sufficient information (points) or sufficient variation of one or both variables to warrant an analysis. The results are summarized in Table I. Five of the eight correlations were significant. Of the three which were not, $v_1 v_2$ and Odessa can be explained by small sample size and lack or variance, respectively. It is possible that, had sufficient information been available, the correlation would have been found in all within-cultivar and within-dikaryon groupings. In conclusion, there is a strong correlation between disease severity within a barley plant and among barley plants, as measured by amount of smutting.

DISCUSSION

The inverse relationship between within-plant disease severity and the average number of culms produced by the plants has been indirectly and directly noted by others. Woodward and Tingey (1941) observed that higher levels of smutting were obtained with barley *U. hordei* on less fertile soil than were obtained on more fertile soil. Because they measured smutted heads, they were probably observing the increased within-plant disease severity which accompanied the decrease in tillering on poorer soil. Milan (1939) observed that the rate of sowing, which also influences the tillering of plants, did not affect the

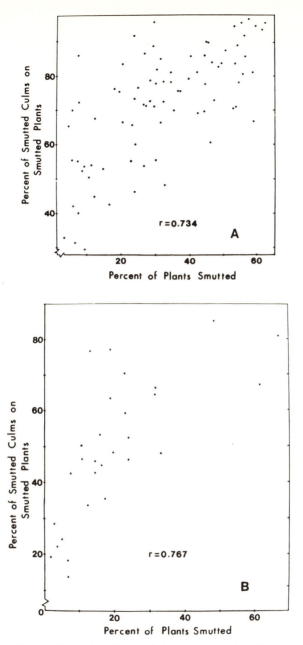

Fig. 1. Scatter diagrams illustrating the correlation of among-plant disease severity, shown on the abscissa, and within-plant disease severity, shown on the ordinate. (A) 82 barley–Ustilago hordei genotypic combinations planted under low-tillering conditions; (B) 29 genotypic combinations planted under high-tillering conditions.

Table I. Common-Cultivar and Common-Dikaryon
Correlations of Between- and Within-Plant
Disease Reactions for Barley–*Ustilago*
hordei Genotypic Combinations[a]

Common cultivar or dikaryon	Number of points[b]	Value of r[c]
Hannchen	10	0.580
Lion	12	0.669*
Nepal	10	0.911*
Odessa	13	0.450
Trebi	10	0.815*
Race 9	7	0.758*
Race 13	8	0.762*
vlv2	9	0.500

[a]All plants were grown under low-tillering conditions.
[b]Number of dikaryons or cultivars with which the indicated
cultivar or dikaryon was associated.
[c]Asterisk indicates a significant correlation at the 5% level.

percentage of inoculated wheat plants smutted by *U. tritici,* but did directly
affect the percentage of culms smutted. A possible explanation for the inverse
relationship, according to Batts and Jeater (1958), is that each infected plant
contains a limited amount of mycelium. Thus, if many tillers are produced by a
plant, a smaller proportion of them will become smutted. They suggested also
that the amount of mycelium varies from embryo to embryo, with the result
that some plants will show a higher frequency of smutted heads than others,
even if other conditions are equal. Unfortunately, the histological work presented by these authors neither supports nor refutes their hypotheses concerning
both limited and variable amounts of mycelium in embryos. The hypotheses are
nonetheless simple and plausible.

Regression analysis of the effect of average tiller production on within-plant
disease severity was made only to determine whether this complication was
important enough to require removal. The analysis was weakened by the fact
that the independent variable, within-plant disease severity, was not distributed
normally. After division of data, however, the distribution in each case appeared
to be closer to normal. Thus, the divided data probably more nearly met the
assumptions for valid regression analysis.

The measures used of within- and among-plant disease severity were chosen
primarily for their simplicity. A refinement of the within-plant measure involves
the fact that one culm of each smutted plant must be diseased and is not free to
vary. Excluding these culms in percentage calculation would have resulted in
disease percentages which are lower than those expressed. Because both correlations are high, such a refinement would not affect the results.

Cultivars such as Odessa, which possessed little among- or within-plant resistance to any of the dikaryons, and Keystone, which generally possessed a high level of both types of resistance, undoubtedly contributed greatly to the correlation. The within-cultivar analyses, however, demonstrated that the correlation is not limited to among-cultivar comparisons. Whereas cultivars that possess a generally high or low level of both of the two types of resistance can be easily picked out, dikaryons do not form such distinct groups. A dikaryon was not found, for instance, which possessed a relatively high among- and within-plant disease-producing ability on all, or even most, cultivars. This leads to the conclusion that, initially at least, studies on the inheritance of host resistance would yield more clear-cut results than studies of the inheritance of pathogen virulence.

The variation shown in within-plant disease reaction is largely genetically determined. Sampling error is around ± 5%. Environmental variation, based on observed smutting differences between locations for identical combinations, is of less importance than genetic variation. Several such combinations were planted in blocks at different locations in the field at Vancouver. Yet variation between replicates was always less than ± 10%. The remaining variation in within-plant reactions must therefore be genetic. An F test established that total variance was significantly greater than residual (environmental + sampling) variance. Earlier studies have established that among-plant disease reactions are largely genetically determined (Thomas and Person, 1965). Thus, the close correlation of this variable to within-plant disease reactions can itself be taken as evidence for the genetic determination of the within-plant disease reaction.

One might expect that the relationship between the two disease-severity measures could be explained, in part, through a simple Poisson relationship. This assumes that the number of culms smutted per plant reflects the "dose" of smut which the plant receives. If the mean number of events is determined, according to the Poisson equation, by the proportion of plants receiving no doses of smut, then an expected frequency of one-dose plants (those with one culm smutted), two-dose plants (those with two culms smutted), etc., can be calculated. When the actual numbers of observed plants in these classes is then found, a good observed/expected fit might indicate that within- and among-plant disease severity are separate facets of the same infection events. When several host–parasite combinations showing high and low disease reactions were thus analyzed, however (J. V. Groth, unpublished), good fits were not obtained. Undoubtedly, an explanation based on Poisson expectations is a gross oversimplification, and several reasons can be conceived why this approach fails to explain the data. Reactions showing high within- and among-plant disease levels were particularly discrepant. The two frequent classes of reaction in such combinations were those showing either no smut or smut in most culms. The intermediate class (i.e., plant with only one culm smutted) was infrequent. The Poisson expectation, in these cases, would give the intermediate class a higher frequency than any other smutted class, and by a wide margin.

Thus, there seem to be two distince thresholds, or stages, through which the fungus must pass in order to produce teliospores. If the first threshold is surmounted, the fungus will be able to cause smutting in at least one tiller of the plant, as measured by among-plant disease severity. If it crosses the second threshold, more culms will be smutted, as measured by within-plant disease severity. One can best think of this second event as taking place separately within each culm. In many plants the fungus does not get beyond the first threshold, i.e., it does not succeed in sporulating. In plants in which the smut does surmount this barrier, it encounters a second barrier as it ramifies through the tissues. Moreover, as the first threshold becomes more difficult to surmount in more resistant cultivars, so does the second. From the standpoint of the host, one can think of the individual culm as having two separate (but not independent) chances of remaining healthy after inoculation of the seed. Both are measured and defined in terms of probability.

The strong correlation between the two measures of disease severity suggests a general identity of genes which govern the two types of disease reaction. Such genes could be in the host, the parasite, or both. Combinations which differ only in their within-plant reactions are noteworthy because they may indicate specific cases of nonidentity of genes governing the two types of resistance. Alternatively, cultivars or dikaryons might differ in environmental sensitivity, although this seems less likely. Both possibilities can be tested by using a proper experimental design.

Because the correlation of the two disease reactions is rather close, it becomes less likely that contrasting phenotypes for genetic studies will be found, each of which possesses only one of the high-disease-reaction types. In particular, there seems to be a lack of host–parasite combinations which show high among-plant reactions and low within-plant reactions. Two possibilities are thus left for genetic study: Cultivars with high within- and among-plant disease reactions can be crossed with those showing low within- and among-plant reactions; or crosses involving varieties which differ only in their within-plant disease reactions can be made. Several examples of each of these were found. The same two classes of phenotypic contrast, examples of which are also available, could be used in genetic studies of virulence in the pathogen.

Fitness of a fungal parasite is highly dependent on, and correlated with, the number of spores produced. The two primary determinants of spore production in smut diseases are identified here. Both within- and among-plant disease severity are highly variable measures, and will certainly account for most variation in spore production. In measuring fitness of smut genotypes, then, the relationship between them must be known. There are other determinants of spore production, as well, whose effects are less important. They have not been quantitatively studied yet, to our knowledge, so we can do no more than call attention to them. Variation exists in number of spores produced per culm. Several reasons for this can be identified. Culms are sometimes only partially smutted, and the frequency seems to depend on the genotype of both host and parasite (J. V. Groth, unpublished). One also must expect to find variation in completely smutted heads. A smutted culm is affected by the genotypes of both organisms. Large differences in smutted culm morphology were noted, particularly when the barley cultivars were highly different (J. V. Groth, unpublished). All these variables will affect fitness. If we wish to understand the exact effect of genes (either in the parasite or host) on parasite fitness, we must be aware of, and account for, all such variables. Host fitness is also made up of components, such as frequency of nonsmutted plants, frequency of nonsmutted culms on smutted plants, degree of tillering, and number of seeds produced per culm, to name a few. Because of the simple relationship in smut diseases between host fitness and parasite fitness, however, the two measurements dealt with in this chapter are of the first two components. In our opinion, they should be of primary importance as host fitness determinants where disease is severe. Thus, by studying the system as a whole, one can get important information pertaining to both host and parasite fitness. This is generally not true for most other host–parasite systems.

REFERENCES

Batts, C. C. V. and Jeater, A. (1958). The development of loose smut (*Ustilago tritici*) in susceptible varieties of wheat, and some observations on field infection. *Brit. Mycol. Soc. Trans. 41*:115–125.

Briggs, F. N. (1926). Inheritance of resistance to bunt, *Tilletia tritici*, in wheat. *J. Agri. Res. 32*:973–990.

Churchward, J. C. (1937–1938). Studies on physiologic specialization of the organisms causing bunt in wheat and the genetics of resistance to this and certain other wheat diseases. *Roy. Soc. N S W 71*:362–384; 547–590.

Clark, J. A., Quisenberry, K. S., and Powers, L. (1933). Inheritance of bunt reaction and other characters in Hope wheat crosses. *J. Agric. Res. 46*:413–425.

Gaines, E. F. (1923). Genetics of bunt resistance in wheat. *J. Agri. Res. 23*:445–480.

Groth, J. V. and Person, C. O. (1975). Estimating the efficiency of partial-vacuum inoculation of barley with *Ustilago hordei*. *Phytopathology 66*:65–69.

Milan, A. (1939). Sensibilità per la *Ustilago tritici* (Pers.) Jens. di alcuni ibridi normali di frumento. *Riv. Pathol. Veg. 29*:71–84.

Oort, A. J. P. (1947). Specialization of loose smut of wheat. A problem for the breeder. *Tijdschr. Plantenziekt. A. 53*:25–43.

Reed, G. M. and Stanton, T. R. (1938). Inheritance of resistance to loose and covered smuts in Markton hybrids. *J. Agri. Res. 56*:159–175.

Ruttle, M. L. (1934). Studies on barley smuts and on loose smut of wheat. *NY Agric. Exp. Sta. Tech. Bull. 221*: 48 pp.

Steel, R. G. D. and Torrie, J. H. (1960). *Principles and Procedures of Statistics*, 481 pp. McGraw-Hill, New York.

Tapke, V. F. (1929). Influence of varietal resistance, sap acidity, and certain environmental factors on the occurrence of loose smut in wheat. *J. Agri. Res. 39*:313–339.

Tapke, V. F. (1931).Influence of humidity on floral infection of wheat and barley by loose smut. *J. Agri. Res. 43*:503–516.

Tapke, V. F. (1945). New physiologic races of *Ustilago hordei*. *Phytopathology 35*: 970–976.

Thomas, P. L. and Person, C. (1965). Genetic control of low virulence in *Ustilago. Can. J. Genet. Cytol.* 7:583–588.

Welsh, J. N. (1932). The effect of smut on rust development and plant vigor in oats. *Sci. Agr. 13*:154–164.

Woodward, R. W. and Tingey, D. C. (1941). Inoculation experiments with covered smut of barley. *J. Amer. Soc. Agron. 33*:632–642.

18

Stabilizing Selection for Pathogenicity in Cereal Rust Fungi

Mohammad Aslam

Agricultural Research Institute
Tarnab, Peshawar, Pakistan

and

L. E. Browder

Department of Plant Pathology
Kansas State University
Manhattan, Kansas

ABSTRACT

Experimental evidence indicates that stabilizing selection for pathogenicity is operative in cereal rust fungi. Similar evidence for other plant parasitic fungi is also presented. Studies on *Puccinia recondita* showed that the number of loci for high pathogenicity in a parasite culture and its relative ability to increase in a mixed population are inversely related. Parasite cultures with fewer number of loci for high pathogenicity exhibited greater longevity *in vitro,* higher infectivity, shorter incubation period, and greater adaptability to varying temperature and light conditions. Based on empirical evidence it is concluded that in a mixed population, in a compatible host:parasite system, low pathogenicity is selected for and high pathogenicity against. In natural populations equilibrium is soon established between low and high pathogenicity provided that the host population is not changed and compatibility is maintained in the host:parasite system. It is proposed that high pathogenicity is the result of a deletion of the locus for low pathogenicity. Possibly, then, a chromosomal segment carrying gene(s) for vital metabolic activity is also removed, thus making the parasite culture unable to compete with other members of the population which do not carry such deletion.

INTRODUCTION

Ever since the publication of Van der Plank's two books (1963, 1968), the concept of stabilizing selection in the evolution of phytopathogenic fungi has aroused considerable controversy. Plant pathologists the world over seem to be divided in their opinions regarding this concept. The importance of this concept becomes even more manifest in view of the search for ways and means to improve the durability and dependability of disease resistance that we are breeding into our crop cultivars. The main cause for the apparent impermanence of resistance has been the appearance, in the parasite population, of new strains that possess the ability to overcome the resistance.

Pathogenicity is a character of the parasite. It has two aspects—one specific pathogenicity and the other aggressiveness, which Aslam (1972) has termed nonspecific pathogenicity. Both specific pathogenicity and aggressiveness are expressed as either low or high. Traditionally, specific low and high pathogenicity have been designated avirulence and virulence, respectively. Corresponding to the parasite character pathogenicity, the host has the character reaction, which is also either specific or nonspecific. Both specific and nonspecific reactions are expressed also as either low or high. In classic terminology, specific low and high reactions have been called resistance and susceptibility, respectively. Aslam (1972), however, distinguished between reaction against the parasite, and resistance against the disease. He further considered that resistance—susceptibility, and avirulence—virulence were not characters in themselves, but rather were expressions of reaction and pathogenicity, respectively.

Working with the flax (*Linum usitatissimum* L.):flax rust [*Melampsora lini* (Ehrenb.) Lev.] host:parasite system, Flor (1959) hypothesized a gene-for-gene relationship between the host and the parasite. The gene-for-gene hypothesis implies that for every gene-conditioning reaction in the host there is a corresponding gene-conditioning pathogenicity in the parasite. Other workers (Samborski, 1963; Williams et al., 1966) experimentally demonstrated similar gene-for-gene relations for the *Triticum:Puccinia* host:parasite systems. Person (1959) presented a model showing that whenever a new gene for low reaction, or resistance, is incorporated into the host, the parasite acquires a corresponding gene for high pathogenicity, or virulence.

On the basis of an analysis of empirical data, Van der Plank (1963) stated that it is axiomatic that the parasite genotype most fit to survive on a "simple" host (one possessing few or no genes for "resistance") was the one with few or no genes for virulence. The concept, which he calls stabilizing selection, implies that in a parasite population only those genes for high pathogenicity are selected for that are essential to overcome the low reaction in the host. In other words, parasite genes for high pathogenicity corresponding to those for low reaction in the host are selected for, whereas all others are selected against.

Flor (1953, 1955) also observed that in the north central United States, races of *M. lini* with "virulence" in excess of that necessary to attack commercial varieties of flax tended to remain in lower frequency in the parasite population. Watson (1958) and Watson and Luig (1961) expressed similar views regarding Australian races of *Puccinia graminis* Pers. f. sp. *tritici,* respectively. Several workers (e.g., Watson, 1942; Loegering, 1951; Hussain, 1956; Kak et al., 1963) have provided experimental evidence showing that certain races of wheat rust fungi tend to predominate over other races while growing in composite or mixed populations.

The frequency of a parasite genotype in a population depends upon its aggressiveness. Aslam (1972) defined aggressiveness as the relative ability of a parasite culture to increase to epidemic proportions in a compatible host/parasite system in a given environment. According to the basic model of gene-for-gene relations in host/parasite systems (Fig. 1), high specific pathogenicity is essential for the survival of the parasite only when the host carries genes for low reaction at the corresponding loci. In the definition of aggressiveness, therefore, high specific pathogenicity in the parasite is precluded as being a requisite for high aggressiveness.

Unlike specific pathogenicity, aggressiveness is a quantitative character. It results from the cumulated expressions of its individual component characters. The component characters of aggressiveness are categorized as infectivity, incubation period, sporulation, longevity *in vitro,* and so forth (Aslam, 1972).

Experimental evidence is available (e.g., Browder, 1965; Bugbee, 1965; Leonard, 1969) to show that cultures and races of *P. graminis* f. sp. *tritici,* and *P. graminis* f. sp. *avenae* with a relatively narrower range of high pathogenicity are more aggressive than are those with a comparatively wider host range. Evidence against the hypothesis of an inverse relationship between high pathogenicity of a parasite culture and its aggressiveness also has been presented (Katsuya and Green, 1966; Brown and Sharp, 1970; Ogle and Brown, 1970; Green, 1971).

HOST REACTION

		LOW R_	HIGH rr
PARASITE PATHOGENICITY	LOW P_	LOW I.T.	HIGH I.T.
	HIGH pp	HIGH I.T.	HIGH I.T.

Fig. 1. Basic model of host:parasite gene-for-gene relationships. Infection types resulting from various reaction:pathogenicity combinations.

The author studied the relationship of the number of genes for high pathogenicity in a parasite culture with the aggressiveness of the parasite culture using three cultures of *P. recondita tritici*. These three cultures, designated UN01-68A, UN01-68B, and 66-763, were chosen because of differences in their pathogenicity toward known genes for low reaction in the host. The cultures were mixed in equal quantities by weight as follows: (UN01-68A)+(UN01-68B), (UN01-68A)+(66-763), (UN01-68B)+(66-763), and (UN01-68A)+(UN01-68B)+(66-763). These mixtures were inoculated in a common host that did not carry any known genes for low reaction. To determine the effect of infection-period temperature on the relative infectivity of these cultures, inoculated plants were kept in the dark at 10°, 20°, and 30°C at near-100% relative humidity for 12 hr. The infection lesions that developed were isolated separately on a short differential set of two near-isogenic lines capable of differentiating between the three cultures. Both differential lines were inoculated with a single pustule. Frequency of each culture in the mixture, after one generation's growth on a common host, was determined by counting the low- and high-infection types produced by each culture on the differential host lines (Table I). It was observed that culture UN01-68B, which carries no known genes for high pathogenicity, exhibited the greatest infectivity at all infection-period temperatures. This culture predominated over cultures UN01-68A, and 66-763, which carry, respectively, one and eight known genes for high pathogenicity. Similarly, culture UN01-68A exhibited greater infectivity than did culture 66-763. Thus, cultures with fewer genes for high pathogenicity showed a higher level of infectivity irrespective of the infection-period temperature. These cultures, therefore, exhibited a tendency to predominate over those with comparatively more genes for high pathogenicity; at least with respect to infectivity.

In another study (Aslam, 1972), cultures of *P. recondita tritici* with different genotypes for pathogenicity were mixed in combinations of two. These mixtures were grown in a common host, through eight generations, under various regimes of temperature/day length. The results supported the view that cultures with fewer genes for high pathogenicity tended to predominate over cultures with comparatively more genes for high pathogenicity. Tests on a common host showed a significantly strong positive correlation between the number of genes for low pathogenicity in the culture and its frequency in the mixture. The increase of the genotype for low pathogenicity over that for high pathogenicity appeared to be independent of the initial frequency of either genotype in the mixture. Similarly, the predominance of one culture over another in the mixture was not affected by the host cultivar, so long as a compatible host:parasite relationship was established. Leonard's (1969) linear model was used for the calculation of the expected proportions of genotypes in the mixture. The expected proportions thus obtained were in a nearly perfect agreement with the observed ones.

Longevity *in vitro,* relative infectivity, adaptability to various temperatures, and sporulation of the three cultures were compared (Aslam, 1972). The results

Table I. The Number of Pustules of Cultures in Mixtures after One Generation in a Common Host at Three Infection-Period Temperatures

Mixture (M)[a]	Infection-period temp. (°C)	Number of pustules isolated	Pustules of cultures in mixture						X^2[b]	
			UNO1-68A		UNO1-68B		66-7.63		Deviation	Heterogeneity
			Number	%	Number	%	Number	%		
M1	10	15	5	33	10	67	—	—		
	20	25	9	36	16	64	—	—		
	30	20	7	35	13	65	—	—	5.400[c]	0.020
M2	10	18	11	61	—	—	7	39		
	20	25	16	64	—	—	9	36		
	30	25	16	64	—	—	9	36	4.765[c]	0.005
M3	20	32	—	—	20	62	12	38		
	30	20	—	—	15	75	5	25	3.115	3.885[c]
M4	10	10	3	30	5	50	2	20		
	20	30	9	30	14	47	7	23		
	30	27	6	22	15	56	6	22	9.343[c]	0.657

[a]M1 = (UNO1-68A) + (UNO1-68B); M2 = (UNO1-68A) + (66-763); M3 = (UNO1-68B) + (66-763); M4 = (UNO1-68A) + (UNO1-68B) + (66-763).
[b]The X^2 values were calculated on the assumption of equal numbers of pustules of cultures in the mixtures.
[c]$p < 0.05$.

are consistent with the hypothesis that the culture with the least genes for high pathogenicity had the greatest longevity when the uredospores were stored in glass vials. Longevity was observed to decrease as the number of genes for high pathogenicity in the culture increased. The culture with the narrowest range of high pathogenicity also exhibited greater adaptability to different temperature regimes, as measured by the germ-tube length. A strong positive correlation was observed also between the length of incubation period and the range of pathogenicity of the culture. Cultures with a wider range of high pathogenicity had relatively longer incubation periods.

The number of spores produced per pustule appeared to be inversely related to the pathogenicity spectrum of the culture. A similar correlation was observed between the pathogenicity range of the culture and its infectivity. In a compatible host:parasite relationship, the culture with the narrowest pathogenicity spectrum exhibited higher infectivity when measured as percentage of spores producing pustules.

These observations indicate that as a parasite culture gains in the number of loci for high pathogenicity, its competitive ability decreases. Uredospore longevity is of great importance in the long distance transport of cereal rust fungi. A culture with lessened spore longevity would be less competitive than one having greater spore longevity. Similarly, adaptability to varying temperatures, infectivity, and incubation period are all of paramount importance in the epidemiology of cereal rusts. Cultures with greater adaptability to varying temperatures or light conditions, or both, would have a better survival value under natural conditions. This, coupled with high infectivity and a short incubation period, increases the ability of a culture to attain epidemic proportions relatively earlier than the culture(s) less fit in regard to these characters.

Differences in the component characters of aggressiveness (infectivity, incubation period, and sporulation) of any two cultures contribute to the differences in their respective reproductive potentials in a mixed population. The difference K in the reproductive potential of any two cultures is directly related to the ability of one culture to predominate over the other when the two are growing in a composite. A high value of K indicates a greater ability of one culture to predominate over another. As the predominance of one culture over another is related to the number of genes for low pathogenicity in the culture (Aslam, 1972), the value of K would be high if there were a great difference between the number of genes for low and high pathogenicity in any two cultures.

A recent survey (Aslam, 1975) of the *P. recondita tritici* populations in the Northwest Frontier Province (NWFP) of Pakistan also showed that pathogenicity groups with a broad spectrum of high pathogenicity were less frequent in the population, whereas those with a relatively narrow range of high pathogenicity were more frequent.

Both experimental evidence (Aslam, 1972), and survey data (Samborski, 1971; Aslam, 1975) indicate that in a mixed parasite population growing in a compatible host:parasite system, the genotype for low pathogenicity is selected for, and the genotype for high pathogenicity is selected against. If the two genotypes are growing together in a compatible host/parasite system, genes for high pathogenicity that are not required to affect compatibility tend to be eliminated from the parasite population. In a compatible host:parasite system, the genotype for low pathogenicity would be selected for until the parasite population stabilizes and the various genotypes for pathogenicity reach a state of equilibrium.

It has been proposed that high pathogenicity is the result of a deletion of the genetic locus for low pathogenicity (Schwinghammer, 1959; Flor, 1960). It is therefore possible that mechanism(s) controlling some vital metabolic activity in the parasite is also lost as part of this deletion. In such a situation, therefore, the parasite culture with a wide range of high pathogenicity would be less fit to compete in a mixed population without such a deletion.

It has been suggested (Jackson, 1931) that in Uredinales the parasitic mode of life was acquired at a very early stage in the phylogenetic history of the group. It also seems that the obligate parasites evolved in association with their hosts. It therefore appears that the genetic systems of the host and the parasite were established in response to two opposing types of selection pressure—(i) that of the host on the parasite, and (ii) that of the parasite on the host. The relation between the host and the parasite is one of coexistence. The host:parasite population as a whole must, therefore, remain in a state of equilibrium. It could be assumed that in the early stages of their coevolution neither the host nor the parasite carried any genes for low reaction or high pathogenicity, respectively. Later, as the host acquired genes for low reaction, the parasite responded by acquiring high pathogenicity. Deployment of host genes for low reaction in a way that they are not accumulated in one host line might stabilize the parasite population with regard to pathogenicity. In a compatible host:parasite system, equilibrium between the host and the parasite would soon be established as a result of elimination of unwanted genes for high pathogenicity from the parasite population.

REFERENCES

Aslam, M. (1972). Aggressiveness in *Puccinia recondita* Rob. ex Desm. F. sp. *tritici.* I. Concepts and terminology. II. Predominance of one culture over another in composites. III. Components of aggressiveness. Ph.D. dissertation, Kansas State Univ., Manhattan, Ks., 90 pp.

Aslam, M. (1975). Pathogenic specialization in *Puccinia recondita* f. sp. *tritici* in NWFP. *Agri. Pakistan* 26(2):171–175.

Browder, L. E. (1965). Aggressiveness in *Puccinia graminis* var. *tritici.* Ph.D. dissertation. Kansas State Univ., Manhattan, Ks., 111 pp.

Brown, J. F. and Sharp, E. L. (1970). The relative survival ability of pathogenic types of *Puccinia striiformis* in mixtures. *Phytopathology* 60:529–533.

Bugbee, W. M. (1965). Studies on the aggressiveness of Race 15B and Race 56 and progenies from crosses of these races of *Puccinia graminis* var. *tritici*. Ph.D. dissertation, Univ. of Minnesota, St. Paul. 70 pp.

Flor, H. H. (1953). Epidemiology of flax rust in the North Central States. *Phytopathology* 43:624–628.

Flor, H. H. (1955). Host–parasite interaction in flax rust–its genetic and other implications. *Phytopathology* 45:680–685.

Flor, H. H. (1959). Genetic controls of host–parasite interactions in rust diseases. In *Plant Pathology–problems and Progress* 1908–1958 (Holton et al., eds.) pp. 137–144. Univ. of Wisconsin Press, Madison.

Flor, H. H. (1960). The inheritance of X-ray induced mutations to virulence in uredospore culture of race 1 of *Melampsora lini. Phytopathology* 50:603–605.

Green, G. J. (1971). Physiologic races of wheat stem rust in Canada from 1919 to 1969. *Can. J. Bot. 49*:1575–1588.

Hussain, S. M. (1956). Studies on competitive ability in certain races of wheat leaf rust. M. S. thesis, Oklahoma State Univ., Stillwater, Ok., 33 pp.

Jackson, H. S. (1931). Present evolutionary tendencies and the origin of life cycles in the Uredinales. *Mem. Torr. Bot. Club 18*:1–108.

Kak, D., Joshi, L. M., Prasada, R. and Vasudeva, R. S. (1963). Survival of races of *Puccinia graminis tritici* (Pers.) Erikss. and J. Henn. *Indian Phytopathol. 16*:117–126.

Katsuya, K. and Green, G. J. (1966). Reproductive potentials of race 15B and 56 of wheat stem rust. *Can. J. Bot. 45*:1077–1091.

Leonard, K. J. (1969). Selection in heterozygous populations of *Puccinia graminis* f. sp. *avenae. Phytopathology 59*:1851–1857.

Loegering, W. Q. (1951). Survival of races of wheat stem rust in mixtures. *Phytopathology 41*:56–65.

Ogle, H. J. and Brown, J. F. (1970). Relative ability of two strains of *Puccinia graminis tritici* to survive when mixed. *Ann. Appl. Biol. 66*:273–279.

Person, C. O. (1959). Gene-for-gene relationship in host:parasite systems. *Can. J. Bot. 37*:1101–1130.

Samborski, D. J. (1963). A mutation in *Puccinia recondita* Rob. ex Desm. f. sp. *tritici* to virulence on Transfer, Chinese Spring X *Aegilops umbellulata* Zhuk. *Can. J. Bot. 41*:475–479.

Samborski, D. J. (1971). Leaf rust of wheat in Canada in 1970. *Can. Plant Dis. Surv. 51*:17–19.

Schwinghammer, E. A. (1959). The relation between radiation dose and frequency of mutations for pathogenicity in *Melampsora lini. Phytopathology* 49:260–296.

Van der Plank, J. E. (1963). *Plant disease Epidemics and Control,* 349 pp. Academic Press, New York.

Van der Plank, J. E. (1968). *Disease resistance in Plants,* 206 pp. Academic Press, New York.

Watson, I. A. (1942). The development of physiological races of *Puccinia graminis tritici* singly and in association with others. *Proc. Linn. Soc. N.S.W. 67*:294–312.

Watson, J. A. (1958). The present status of breeding disease resistant wheats in Australia. *N. S.W. Dept. Agri. Gaz. 69*:630–660.

Watson, I. A. and Luig, N. H. (1961). Leaf rust on wheat in Australia: A systematic scheme for the classification of strains. *Proc. Linn. Soc. N.S.W. 86*:241–250.

Williams, N. D., Gough, F. J., and Rondon, M. R. (1966). Interaction of pathogenicity genes in *Puccinia graminis* f. sp. *tritici* and reaction genes in *Triticum aestivum* ssp. *vulgare* "Marquis" and "Reliance." *Crop Sci. 6*:245–248.

19

Development of Disease-Resistant Chickpea

Abdul Ghafoor Kausar
Department of Plant Pathology
University of Agriculture
Lyallpur, Pakistan

ABSTRACT

The development of high-yielding, disease-resistant varieties of chickpea (*Cicer arietinum*) is one of the urgent needs of agriculture in Pakistan. Major problems include nonavailability of good sources of resistance to prevalent diseases, and combination of resistance to prevalent or major diseases with desirable characters, including high yield and desirable agronomic and acceptable technological characters. Despite inherent problems, some progress has been made in developing varieties of chickpea which combine reasonably high yield with moderate resistance to blight and wilt. Varieties of chickpea with moderate to high resistance to blight and suitable for cultivation in blight-affected areas are available. However, selections with high resistance to blight proved susceptible to wilt. Only a few combine resistance to both blight and wilt, and these are only moderately resistant. Resistance to blight appears to be associated with the intensity and distribution of glandular hair on various malic acid-secreting plant parts. In general, varieties resistant to blight produce higher quantities of acids, including malic acid, particularly in early stages of growth and in the rainless period. A better understanding of the nature of resistance in chickpea to the prevalent diseases should be helpful in a program of developing varieties of chickpea resistant to diseases.

INTRODUCTION

The cultivated chickpea (*Cicer arietinum* L.) is an important grain legume with high protein content. It is grown extensively in the Near East, Southeast Asia,

213

Southern Europe, and Mexico, and forms a major source of protein in animal feed as well as human diet, particularly among the low-income groups. Because of its high protein and lysine content, the chickpea is valuable as a supplement to those who depend on cereal diets. Because it is a relatively inexpensive source of protein and is accepted and consumed as part of a staple diet, it would seem that increased production of the chickpea would be one of the easiest and least expensive approaches to meeting the deficiency of protein of low-income populations.

A major disadvantage is that chickpea production is uncertain and erratic, mainly because of diseases that limit production and contribute to a depressed yield. Epiphytotics of blight constitute a hazard that can upset chickpea production with catastrophic suddenness. Wilts reduce yield, particularly in rainfed areas, especially in years of drought, or even when rainfall is simply low. Virus diseases are becoming increasingly more common.

One of the easiest and least expensive means of reducing losses caused by these major diseases is the development of high-yielding, disease-resistant varieties of chickpea. In the present chapter, an attempt has been made to identify problems, assess progress, and discuss prospects for developing disease-resistant varieties of chickpea, with special reference to conditions existing in Pakistan.

PRESENT STATUS OF CHICKPEA DISEASES

The diseases of chickpea include blight, wilts, Stemphylium leafspot, stem and crown blight, rust, and virus diseases.

Blight caused by *Ascochyta rabei* is a typically epiphytotic disease and has been known for its ravages since the days of Theophrastus and Pliny (Comes, 1891). It is particularly serious in Pakistan, parts of India (Punjab), Iran and Southern Europe (Sattar, 1933; Kausar, 1960, 1965; Kaiser, 1972). Blight generally appears in epiphytotic proportions in Pakistan in areas and years receiving > 15 cm (6 in.) of rainfall during the growing season (Sattar, 1933; Kausar, 1965).

The incidence of blight in Pakistan is positively correlated with winter rainfall received during the growing season; it is negatively correlated with summer rainfall preceding the chickpea crop; thus, forecasting of epidemics may be possible (Kausar, 1964, 1965).

In contrast, wilt and root-rot diseases are favored by dry weather, and are generally serious in chickpea-growing countries in years in which < 8.9 cm (3.5 in.) of rain falls during the chickpea-growing season. There are areas in Pakistan in which these two diseases coexist. Blight is serious in years of high rainfall, and wilt is serious in years of low rainfall. Even in a single year the two diseases may coexist in these areas. This occurs when blight is serious during months of high rainfall and wilt is serious during months of low rainfall, particularly in seedling and flowering stages of chickpea plant (Luthra et al., 1943; Kausar, 1968; Kaiser, 1972).

Wilt of the chickpea has been attributed to *Fusarium orthoceras* var. *ciceri* in the Indo-Pakistan subcontinent (Prasad and Padwick, 1939). Subsequently, a new name, *Fusarium lateritium* f. *ciceri,* has been proposed (Erwin, 1958). The disease has also been attributed to certain physiological, agronomic, and soil factors (Bedi, 1945, 1946). In India, root rot from *Operculella padwickii* causes wilting of tip leaves (Kheswala, 1941); *Fusarium* sp. and *Operculella padwickii* have been isolated from wilted chickpea plants (Williams et al., 1968).

Nematodes are also associated with wilt of the chickpea, particularly Fusarium wilt. *Fusarium* sp. penetrates through punctures caused by the nematodes (Rasheed, 1971).

Fusarium wilt due to *Fusarium lateritium* f. *ciceri* is serious in California (Erwin, 1958). Verticilium wilt caused by *Verticilium albo-atrum* also has been reported from California (Erwin, 1957). Chickpea wilt has also been attributed to *Fusarium oxysporum* (Echandi, 1970). The chickpea was reported to be a new host of *Fusarium solani* f. *pisi* (Kraft, 1969). Five fungi, *Fusarium oxysporum* f. *ciceri, F. solani* f. *pisi, Pythium ultimum, Rhizoctonia solani,* and *Macrophomina phaseoli* are also responsible for chickpea wilt in California (Westerlund et al., 1974). Chickpea wilt is apparently a complex disease attributable to a number of organisms in different countries.

Aphid-transmitted bean yellow mosaic, pea enation, and alfalfa mosaic viruses have been reported in chickpea in California (Erwin and Snyder, 1958). Four aphid-transmitted viruses—alfalfa mosaic, bean yellow mosaic, cucumber mosaic, and pea leaf roll—are known to infect the chickpea in Iran (Kaiser and Danesh, 1971*a,b*).

Losses attributable to Stemphylium leafspot caused by *Stemphylium sarciniforme,* stem and crown blight caused by *Sclerotinia sclerotiorum,* and virus diseases have been reported from Iran and India (Bedi, 1956; Das and Gupta, 1961; Prasad et al., 1969; Kaiser and Danesh, 1971*a,b*; Kaiser, 1972). Rust caused by *Uromyces ciceris arietini* has been reported from India, Pakistan, and countries bordering the Mediterranean and Balkans (Mehta and Mundkur, 1946). These diseases are becoming increasingly more common and have the potential of becoming serious in favorable environments among susceptible varieties (Kaiser and Danesh, 1971*a,b;* Kaiser, 1972).

PROGRESS IN THE DEVELOPMENT OF CHICKPEA VARIETIES RESISTANT TO BLIGHT AND WILT

Out of a collection of 392 chickpea varieties from parts of the Indo-Pakistan subcontinent and elsewhere, three varieties were reported as being resistant to blight (Luthra et al., 1941). The severe blight epiphytotics of the late 1930s brought out clearly the extreme susceptibility of local chickpea varieties, whereas three foreign chickpea introductions showed themselves to be highly resistant.

Among foreign resistant chickpea varieties (F8, F9, and F10) F10 and F8 were superior to F9 in their resistance to blight. Type F8 gave the highest yield and had seed characteristics similar to the best local chickpea variety in cultivation. The cultivation of F8 was taken up in the blight-affected areas (Luthra et al., 1941). However, it proved susceptible to wilt in the drought year of 1940–1941. Type F8 proved a failure in localities other than those affected by blight because chickpea wilt now became a problem. Nevertheless, it was found that this type could replace the local chickpea varieties susceptible to blight in blight-affected areas (Luthra et al., 1943).

Type F8 resisted blight admirably, but its yielding capacity was not as high as that of the best local (but susceptible) type, Punjab-7, in blight-free years. Moreover, F8 required more moisture at the time of its sowing and for its growth. During years of low rainfall, which is unfavorable for blight anyway, F8 gave a lower yield than the local chickpea types (Luthra et al., 1943). Nevertheless, F8 was a boon for the farmers during blight years, and its cultivation made the production of chickpea possible in the worst blight-affected localities.

Hybridization of F8 with the local varieties was taken up for the selection of suitable hybrids, in order to combine high resistance to blight and wilt with high yield. As a result, C12/34 and C-612 were evolved as blight-resistant varieties in 1947 and 1952, respectively. These hybrids yielded more than Pb-7 was able to produce in blight years, but less than Pb-7 could yield in blight-free years.

The search for high-yielding, blight-resistant varieties was continued after the release of C-612 for general cultivation. A screening of available breeding material during recent severe epiphytotics resulted in four chickpea selections with high resistance to blight and another three with moderate resistance to blight. These seven selections had significantly higher yields than the blight-resistant variety C-612 (Kausar and Ahmad, 1967). One of these selections (C-727), which combined moderate resistance to blight with high yield, was approved by the Pakistan Department of Agriculture to replace C-612 for cultivation in blight-affected areas.

Because of the importance of wilt and its coexistence with blight in certain chickpea-growing areas in Pakistan, a study was made of the reaction of blight-resistant selections to wilt and their performance in blight-affected and wilt-infested areas (Kausar, 1968). The highly blight-resistant selections gave significantly lower yield in wilt-infested localities, but they did well in blight-affected localities. These selections gave higher yields during years of high rainfall or under conditions less favorable for the development of wilt and more favorable for the development of blight. One of these selections, (C-727), having a potential for high yield and a moderate resistance to blight, was found to be also moderately resistant to wilt.

Consequently it was suitable for cultivation in blight-affected and wilt-infested areas during years of high intensity of wilt and blight. The performance of the other two moderately blight-resistant selections was more or less intermediate in this respect.

Promising selections of chickpea have been grown in the wilt nursery for the last 15 years. Seeds of plants surviving in the wilt nursery are being planted year after year to study their reaction to wilt. Hopefully, natural selection in surviving populations may help in the selection of genotypes resistant to the disease. This is being attempted because of the nonavailability of appropriate sources of resistance to wilt, although chickpea varieties resistant to wilt have been reported (Dastur, 1928; Plymen, 1933; Ayyar and Iyer, 1936).

High resistance to Fusarium wilt was found in one selection from California and three selections from Ethiopia. Unfortunately, selections from Ethiopia have undesirable agronomic characters (Erwin, 1958).

Resistance to blight was shown by 11 out of 167 types of chickpea in France (Labrousse, 1931). A Bulgarian variety of chickpea was reported to be immune to blight (Solel and Kostrinski, 1964). Eleven varieties of chickpea resistant to blight were reported from Punjab, India (Aujla and Bedi, 1967). Recently, black-seeded chickpea lines proved more resistant to blight than white-seeded types in Iran, and one black-seeded type from Israel proved to be highly resistant to blight (Kaiser, 1972).

A large number of the collection of chickpea varieties has been screened for major diseases of the crop in Iran, India, and Pakistan. This program is being continued.

PROBLEMS ENCOUNTERED IN CHICKPEA BREEDING FOR RESISTANCE TO BLIGHT AND WILT

Certain problems were encountered during the program of developing chickpea varieties resistant to blight and wilt. The major problems were the nonavailability of good sources of resistance, and the difficulty in combining resistance to these diseases with desirable agronomic traits.

The cultivation of varieties resistant to certain diseases and susceptible to others is known to change the status of the disease complex, which has to be studied continuously to make necessary adjustments in a program of developing disease-resistant varieties (Stakman, 1946, 1947).

For the development of blight-resistant varieties, F8 with seed characteristics similar to the best local chickpea was used in preference to F10, which has black seeds. However, F10 excelled F8 in resistance to blight. The black seed color was a problem. However, black-colored chickpea varieties are accepted in certain parts of Pakistan.

The breeding method mostly used was the classic single cross between the high-yielding susceptible parent and the low-yielding resistant parent. The use of backcrosses with the high-yielding susceptible parent and selection for resistance, desirable quality, and high yield could probably have given better results.

A certain amount of infection on highly blight-resistant plants, particularly on pods suggests special care for the multiplication of the seed of blight-resistant varieties. This is particularly essential on account of seed infection through infection on pods of the resistant plants in favourable weather. On account of the seed-borne nature of blight, infection of seed year after year can result in a high proportion of infected seed.

A program of raising basic seed every year from only disease-free selfed plants grown on a plot subjected to high artificial infection of blight is suggested. In further multiplications of these seeds, roguing out of the infected plants or pods and obtaining seed from disease-free pods of disease-free plants appears essential to maintain the purity and resistance potential of the resistant varieties.

FUTURE PROSPECTS

The development of disease-resistant varieties of chickpea is one of the most urgent needs of agriculture in Pakistan and other chickpea-growing countries. Because of hazards of pesticides and increasing emphasis on pest management, particularly by biological methods, the development and use of varieties with built-in mechanisms for resistance to diseases has assumed enhanced significance. Because of a large number of small land holdings in these countries, the use of disease-resistant varieties is the easiest and least expensive method of controlling chickpea diseases. In spite of inherent problems in developing disease-resistant varieties of chickpea, there is a possibility of using this method of disease control as the main strategy for the improvement of chickpea yields.

Based on the problems encountered in the development of chickpea varieties resistant to blight and wilt, and experience in developing disease-resistant varieties elsewhere (Stakman, 1946, 1947), certain lessons have been learned. These lessons and principles should be taken into account in breeding for resistance programs.

The cultivation of chickpea varieties susceptible to disease prevalent in a country is dangerous. The continuous use of susceptible varieties is known to aggravate the disease situation, and to raise minor diseases to the status of major ones (Stakman, 1946; Kausar, 1960).

There is much more to be learned about the nature of resistance in chickpea to various diseases. The basis of resistance to blight has been studied to some extent. A greater amount of malic acid is secreted by resistant varieties than by the susceptible ones. Malic acid is considered to be detrimental to germination of conidia and germ-tube growth, and was considered thus to contribute to resistance. Chickpea plants of resistant varieties F8 and F10 less than 40 days old were as susceptible as those of susceptible variety Pb-7, but had developed resistance after 40 days. Thus, these resistant varieties were considered to have escaped blight in early stages of growth (Hafiz, 1952).

A later study of malic and other acids produced on chickpea plants indicated that five resistant varieties generally produced higher quantities of the acid than the susceptible variety, particularly in the early stages of growth and in a rainless period. The quantity of the acid produced on susceptible and resistant varieties was reduced by rains but increased again after the rain (Khan, 1973).

So far, natural variation within the cultivated *Cicer arietinum* has been used for the development of disease-resistant cultivars, combining high yield with desirable agronomic and technological characters. The natural diversity in these characters does not appear to have been fully exploited. However, the recent discovery of *Cicer reticulatum* (Laduzinsky, 1975) with the same diploid number as that of *Cicer arietinum* and *Cicer echinospernum* indicate future potentialities, if better sources of resistance are found in these wild species. Studies of the characters of these species, particularly *Cicer reticulatum,* including resistance to diseases of chickpea, should prove rewarding.

REFERENCES

Aujla, S. S. and Bedi, K. S. (1967). Relative reaction of different varieties of gram to blight disease incited by *Phyllosticta rabiei* (Pass.) Trot. in the Punjab. *J. Res. Ludhiana 4*:214–216.

Ayyar, V. R. and Iyer, R. B. (1936). A preliminary note on the mode of inheritance of reaction to wilt in *Cicer arietinum. Proc. Indian Acad. Sci. B 3*:438–443.

Bedi, K. S. (1945). Progress report of the gram wilt scheme for the year ending 30th June, 1943. Govt. Print. Press, Lahore.

Bedi, K. S. (1946). Progress report of the gram wilt scheme for the year ending 30th June, 1946. Govt. Print. Press, Lahore.

Bedi, K. S. (1956). A simple method for producing apothocia of *Sclerotinia sclerotiorum* (Lib.) de Bary. *Indian Phytopathol. 9*:39–43.

Comes, O. (1891). *Crittogamia agraria.* Naples.

Dastur, F. J. (1928). Annual report of the mycological section for the year ending 31st March, 1927. Rept. Dept. Agr. Central Provinces and Berar, 1926. *27*:36–37.

Das, G. N. and Sen Gupta, P. A. (1961). A Stemphylium leaf spot disease of gram. *Plant Dis. Rept. 45*:979.

Echandi, E. (1970). Wilt of chickpeas or garbonzo beans (*Cicer arietinum*) incited by *Fusarium oxysporum. Phytopathology 60*:1539.

Erwin, D. C. (1957). Fusarium and Verticilium wilt disease of *Cicer arietinum. Phytopathology 47*:10.

Erwin, D. C. (1958). *Fusarium lateritium* f. *ciceri,* incitant of Fusarium wilt of *Cicer arietinum. Phytopathology 48*:498–501.

Erwin, D. C., and Snyder, W. C. (1958). Yellowing of garbonzo beans. *Calif. Agr. 12*:6,16.

Hafiz, A. (1952). Basis of resistance in gram to Mycosphaerella blight. *Phytopathology 42*:422–424.

Kaiser, W. J. (1972). Occurrence of three fungal diseases of chickpea in Iran. *FAO Pl.Pr.Bull. 20*:73–78.

Kaiser, W. J. and Danesh, D. (1971*a*). Biology of four viruses affecting *Cicer arietinum* in Iran. *Phytopathology 61*:372–375.

Kaiser, W. J. and Danesh, D. (1971*b*). Etiology of virus induced wilt of *Cicer arietinum. Phytopathology 61*:453–457.

Kausar, A. G. (1960). Fifty years of agricultural education and research at Agricultural

College and Research Institute, Lyallpur. Vol II. Chapter XI. Plant Diseases. Ripon Press, Lahore.

Kausar, A. G. (1964). Possibility of forecasting gram blight epidemics. *Abst. Proc. Pak. Assoc. Adv. Sci. Conf. Agri. Sect.* 1964:157.

Kausar, A. G. (1965). Epiphytology of recent epiphytotics of gram blight in West Pakistan. *Pak. J. Agr. Sci. 2*:185–195.

Kausar, A. G. (1968). Performance of blight-resistant gram selections in wilt nursery and at six locations. *Pak. J. Agr. Sci. 5*:264–273.

Kausar, A. G. and Rashid Ahmad. (1967). Reaction of gram selections to blight during recent epiphytotics. *Pak J. Agr. Sci. 4*:108–120.

Khan, Bashir Ahmad. (1973). Studies on the biology of gram blight in West Pakistan. M. Sc. thesis. Univ. of Agriculture, Lyallpur.

Kheswala, K. F. (1941). Foot rot of gram (*Cicer arietinum*) caused by *Opercullela padwickii. Indian J. Agr. Sci. 11*:316–318.

Kraft, J. M. (1969). Chickpeas, a new host of *Fusarium solani* f. sp. *pisi. Plant Dis. Rept. 53*:110–111.

Labrousse, F. (1931). Observations sur quelques maladies des plants maraichères. *Rev. Path. Ent. Agr. 18*:286–289.

Laduzinsky, G. (1975). A new Cicer from Turkey. *Notes Roy. Bot. Gard. Edinb. 34*:201–202.

Luthra, J. C., Sattar, A., and Bedi, K. S. (1941). Determination of resistance to the blight disease, *Mycosphaerella rabiei* Kovaceveski–*Ascochyta rabiei* (Pass.) Lab. in gram types. *Indian J. Agr. Sci. 11*:249–264.

Luthra, J. C., Sattar, A., and Bedi, K. S. (1943). Further studies on the control of gram blight. *Indian Farm. 4*:413–416.

Mehta, P. R., and Mundkur, B. B. (1946). Some observations on the rust of gram (*Cicer arietinum* L.). *Indian J. Agr. Sci. 16*:186–192.

Plymen, F. J. (1933). Reports on the working of the Department of Agriculture of the central provinces for the years ending 31st March, 1932, and 31st March, 1933. 36 pp.

Prasad, H., Haider, M. G. and Prasad, K. D. (1969). Blight disease of gram. *Indian Phytopathol. 22*:405–406.

Prasad, N., and Padwick, G. W. (1939). The genus Fusarium II. A species of Fusarium as a cause of wilt of gram (*Cicer arietenum* L.). *Indian J. Agr. Sci. 9*:371–380.

Rasheed, T. (1971). Studies on the role of nematodes in the causation of gram wilt diseases. M. Sc. thesis, Univ. of Agriculture, Lyallpur.

Sattar, A. (1933). On the occurrence, perpetuation and control of gram (*Cicer arietinum* L.) blight caused by *Ascochyta rabiei* (Pass.) Labrousse, with special reference to Indian conditions. *Ann. App. Biol. 20*:612–632.

Solel, Z. and Kostrinski, J. (1964). The control of *Ascochyta* anthracnose of chickpea. *Phytopathol. Medit. 3*:119–120.

Stakman, E. C. (1946). Plant pathologist's merry-go-round. *J. Hered. 37*:259–265.

Stakman, E. C. (1947). International problems in plant disease control. *Proc. Amer. Phil. Soc. 91*:95–111.

Westerlund, J. V., Campbell, R. N. and Kimble, K. A. (1974). Fungal root rots and wilt of chickpea in California *Phytopathology 64*:432–436.

Williams, F. J., Grewal, J. S. and Amin, K. S. (1968). Serious and new diseases of pulse crops in India in 1966. *Plant Dis. Rept. 52*:300–304.

IV

Genetics of Quantitative Characters

20

Coadaptation in Plant Populations

R. W. Allard

Department of Genetics
University of California
Davis, California, 95616

ABSTRACT

One of the important questions of plant breeding is whether alleles at different loci act independently or whether the population genotype is structured so that favored combinations of alleles occur more frequently than expected under randomness. Studies employing allozyme loci as markers have demonstrated that the distribution of alleles in both natural and experimental populations of inbreeding plants is closely correlated with environment on both micro- and macrogeographic scales. Multilocus analyses have also revealed the occurrence within local populations of striking gametic phase disequilibrium (linkage disequilibrium). These observations demonstrate that selection acts to organize the population into sets of highly interacting coadapted gene complexes that promote high fitness to the local environment.

INTRODUCTION

The notion of coadaptation is discussed by Frankel in Chapter 3 of this volume; it has subsequently appeared either explicitly or implicitly in several other research efforts (see Chapter 6, 9, and 12, this volume). It was stated by Brock (Chapter 12) that the notion of coadaptation, not being supported by adequate data, is conjectural. The issue of the existence of coadaptation is an important one with implications in several aspects of plant breeding. Thus, for example, it bears on the manner of collecting and conserving genetic variation in plants

(Chapter 3, this volume) because coadaptation implies that the combination of alleles found in different ecogeographical regions will be nonrandom and correlated with the local habitat. Coadaptation also bears on selection schemes because of the nonrandomness of associations of alleles that it implies. Standard selection schemes assume additivity, and theory makes it clear that the behavior of interacting multilocus systems cannot, in general, be predicted from such schemes. In addition, the issue of the existence of coadaptation bears on the choice of plant breeding methods. Breeding methods that are appropriate to improving existing varieties with respect to one or a few specific traits generally will not be adequate development for higher-performing genetic systems featuring novel coadapted systems of favored alleles (Chapter 12). This extemporaneous discussion concerning the existence of coadaptation will be based mainly on published works of the author and his co-workers (Allard et al., 1972a,b), which can be consulted for details.

ANALYSIS OF THE PROBLEM

The question to be analysed is: What is required to take the notion of coadaptation away from conjecture and establish that coadaptation does in fact occur in populations of plants? To identify the issues clearly it is appropriate to discuss the theory of coadaptation briefly prior to considering experimental procedures required to establish whether or not the genetic structure of populations features coadaptation.

The simplest model on which we can discuss the genetic basis of coadaptation is one involving two loci, each having two alleles. Assume that the gametic combinations $A^{(1)} B^{(1)}$ and $A^{(2)} B^{(2)}$ yield homozygotes and a heterozygote superior in reproductive capacity, and that the other two gametic combinations $A^{(1)} B^{(2)}$ and $A^{(2)} B^{(1)}$ produce selectively inferiour genotypes. During the life cycle from zygote formation to reproductive maturity selection will favor individuals that carry the 11 and 22 combinations of alleles, causing their frequency to increase from early stages in the life cycle to the reproductive stage. If the two loci are unlinked, free recombination will occur at gametogenesis, which will break up the favored combinations of alleles produced by selection. Thus, the segregation and recombination that occur during reproduction will undo the work of selection. If, however, the loci are linked, the suppression of recombination caused by the linkage will tend to bind the concordant allelic complexes together. Theoretical studies (review in Turner, 1967) have shown that when the crossover value is small enough relative to the intensity of selection, stable nonrandom associations of alleles can develop and persist in the population; and if the linkage is very tight and selection sufficiently strong, the genetic variability will become so organized that only two among four possible gametic types, and only three among nine possible genotypes, will occur in the population. Thus, correlations among loci will be complete, and D (the gametic phase disequilibrium parameter) will take its maximum value. Population fitness will also be maximized with respect to these two loci.

Theoretical studies have shown that any factor that restricts recombination will have an effect similar to linkage in binding concordant nonalleles together and that positive assortative mating in particular can lead to sharp restriction of recombination (Jain and Allard, 1966; Weir and Cockerham, 1973). The way in which this works can be illustrated by considering two individuals with genotypes AABB and aabb in a predominantly selfing population. Owing to predominant selfing, these individuals will produce only *AABB* and *aabb* progeny generation after generation and the *AB* and *ab* alleles will remain correlated within both lineages, just as if they were linked. But when hybridization occurs between the two lineages, producing the *AaBb* heterozygote, there will be a burst of segregation and recombination for a few generations during which the *Ab* and aB gametic types will be produced and the association will be broken. When such intercrosses between lineages occur only once in 50 generations or more, as is the case in many plant species, it is obvious that the frequency of heterozygotes will be very low and hence that recombination will be severly restricted because effective crossing over occurs only in heterozygotes and not in homozygotes.

It would be helpful to have a quantitative measure of the restriction of recombination that is caused by linkage on the one hand and by mating system on the other hand, and for present purposes the rate at which D, the linkage disequilibrium parameter, converges to zero for neutral alleles is convenient. For two loci this rate is given by Weir and Cockerham (1973)

$$1 - \frac{1}{2}\left\{\frac{1 + \lambda + s}{2} + \left[\left(\frac{1 + \lambda + s}{2}\right)^2 - 2s\lambda\right]^{\frac{1}{2}}\right\}$$

where λ is the amount of linkage $(0 > \lambda > 1)$ and s is the probability $(0 > s > 1)$ that an individual chosen at random in any generation is the offspring of a single individual in the previous generation $(t = 1 - s$ is the probability that it had two parents). Note that λ and s enter this expression in the same way and that the magnitude of their effect on rate of decay of D is equal. With random mating $(s = 0)$ and no linkage $(\lambda = 0$, or $c = 0.5$, where c is the crossover value), one-half of any disequilibrium is lost in the next mating cycle. With random mating but tight linkage $(\lambda = 0.98$ or $c = 0.01)$ only 1% of the disequilibrium is lost per generation. This is the well-known result that the asymptotic approach of D to zero for neutral alleles under random mating is at the geometric rate of $(1 - c)$ per generation so that D in any generation t is given by $D_{(t)} = (1 - c)^t D_{(0)}$. With no linkage but 98% self-fertilization, the rate of decay of D is also 1% per generation, or one-fiftieth as large as with random mating and no linkage. And, of course, when tight linkage is combined with heavy selfing, recombination is reduced to the point where little selection is required to hold favorable combinations of alleles together.

It is important to note that there is a difference in the effect of restriction of recombination caused by linkage and that caused by inbreeding. Linkage prevents breakup of favorable combinations of alleles involving loci that are physically close on the same chromosome; but it does not so protect concordant allelic combinations for loci located on different chromosomes. Inbreeding, in contrast, restricts recombination between all loci, whether on the same or different chromosomes. Theory therefore predicts that inbreeding is capable of binding the entire genotype together and hence that it may be a very efficient mechanism for organizing the whole of the gene pool into an integrated system. It also follows that inbreeding populations should be favorable ones for investigating coadaptation experimentally. This is because all loci behave as if they are linked, and it is consequently unnecessary to search for hard-to-find closely linked loci on which to base experiments designed to detect nonrandom associations of alleles.

This brings us to the question of experimental procedures that will provide the type of objective evidence required to elevate the notion of coadaptation above the level of conjecture. One approach to this problem is to classify each of the individuals in a population unambiguously with respect to genotype so that a precise multilocus Mendelian formula can be written for each individual as well as D, the disequilibrium parameter calculated as an estimate of nonrandomness. This has recently become possible as a result of the introduction of electrophoretic techniques into population genetics. I shall now illustrate the results of electrophoretic analysis of population structure with two cases, the first involving natural populations of wild oats (*Avena barbata*) and the second two experimental populations of barley (*Hordeum vulgare* L.).

COADAPTATION IN *AVENA BARBATA*

Avena barbata was introduced into California from the Mediterranean basin during the Spanish period and has since become established as a prominent component of grassland and oak savanna communities in climatic Regions I and II of the state (Durrenberger, 1960). Region I is the Mediterranean warm summer zone (mean temperature of the warmest month exceeds 22°C); Region II is the Mediterranean cool summer zone (mean temperature of the warmest month below 22°C). In addition to mean temperature these two regions differ in rainfall and many other climatic factors. They also differ topographically. Region I, which includes the extensive semiarid grasslands of the lower foothills bordering the central valley and much of Southern California, is much more uniform environmentally than Region II, which includes the topographically diverse coastal range and higher foothills of the Sierra Nevada mountains.

Surveys (Clegg and Allard, 1972; unpublished) of allelic variability at five enzyme loci (esterase loci E_4, E_9, E_{10}; phosphatase locus P_5; peroxidase locus APX_5) and two loci governing morphological variants [black versus gray lemma (B,b), hairy versus nonhairy lemma (H,h)], show that all populations in Region I are monomorphic for all seven loci. Moreover, all populations in this region are monomorphic for the same allele at each enzyme locus, i.e., $E_4{}^{(1)}$, $E_9{}^{(2)}$, $E_{10}{}^{(2)}$, $P_5{}^{(2)}$, and $APX_5{}^{(1)}$ (superscripts 1 and 2 denote the alleles producing the slower and faster migrating isozymes, respectively), and each population is also fixed for the black and hairy lemma morphs. These surveys also show that this same genotype (abbreviated 1221BH) is the exclusive one in the most xeric habitats in Region II, such as those occupying steeper slopes with western exposure. In contrast, populations that occupy the most mesic habitats in this region (e.g., shaded bottomland areas with deep dark soil) are monomorphic and fixed for the genotype carrying the balanced opposite set of alleles, i.e., $E_4{}^{(2)}$, $E_9{}^{(1)}$, $D_{10}{}^{(1)}$, $P_5{}^{(1)}$, $APX_5{}^{(2)}$, b, and usually h. However the great majority of habitats in Region II are intermediate between these extremes, and populations occupying these intermediate habitats are polymorphic for these loci. Furthermore, gene frequencies in the polymorphic populations are closely correlated with degree of xerism. It should be noted that this pattern does not hold on margins of the distribution of the species where populations are often found in sites environmentally atypical for *A. barbata*. Different alleles are found at the enzyme loci in these atypical habitats, and the associations among nonalleles tend to be unique for each population.

In the topographically diverse Mediterranean cool summer region, changes from mesic to xeric habitats frequently take place over very short distances; to determine whether the remarkable correspondence between allelic frequencies that occurs over most of California is repeated on a microgeographic scale, detailed studies were made of some populations that span transitions from mesic to xeric vegetational associations in distances of 100 m or less (Allard et al., 1972a; Hamrick and Allard, 1972). The results showed a consistent pattern of change in allelic frequencies correlated with environment. A typical result was obtained on a hillside transect, designated CSA, located in the Napa Valley. In a distance of about 100 m, the habitat on this hillside changes from highly mesic on the valley floor at the bottom to highly xeric on the steep west-facing slope at the top of the hillside. The one exception to the steady increase in xerism occurs partway up the slope where a well-watered depression occurs in the hillside. It was found that allelic frequencies tracked the environmental almost exactly on this hillside transect—"mesic" alleles decreased steadily from the mesic bottom to the xeric top, except for the depression where mesic alleles were frequent. Correlation coefficients between alleles at pairs of loci are all of the order of 0.90 and significant statistically. Therefore, as any one allele changed in frequency a similar change in frequency occurred in alleles at other loci, and these changes in allelic frequency reflected changes in degree of xerism with remarkable precision.

A more detailed study of one of the parts of the CSA site showed that this microgeographic differentiation extends down to an even finer scale. An area approximately 8 m wide by 18 m long at the bottom of the CSA site was divided into plots 2.6 × 2.6 m from which samples of about 100 individuals were taken (Allard et al., 1972a). Electrophoretic analysis demonstrated that frequencies of the mesic alleles were very high (> 0.9) in the middle of this area and that their frequencies decreased in correlated fashion to very low values (< 0.2) on the margins of the area. Close inspection showed that the plots in which mesic alleles were in high frequency were located in the bottom of a shallow swale, which constitutes a local drainage area, whereas the plots with lowest frequencies of mesic alleles were located on the sides of the swale about 30 cm higher in elevation. Plots with intermediate frequencies were intermediate in elevation, and also in soil type, which became progressively more shallow and rocky up the sides of the swale. Thus, correspondence between allelic frequencies and visible features of the environment clearly extends down to a very fine microscale, and the correlated changes in allelic frequencies over loci suggests that natural selection acts on these loci as a unit.

To determine the extent to which these loci are inherited as a unit requires that sufficiently large samples be taken from individual populations to permit comparisons of observed five-locus gametic frequencies with expected frequencies computed as products of observed single-locus frequencies. When such studies were made in polymorphic populations, it was found that two among the 32 possible five-locus gametic types were in great excess over expectations based on single-locus allelic frequencies. These were the 12221 and 21112 gametic types characteristic of xeric and mesic habitats, respectively. There was, of course, a corresponding deficiency among the remaining five-locus gametic types, and it is interesting that this deficiency tended to be greatest for the more extreme recombinants relative to the two favored types. The relative gametic phase disequilibrium parameter (D'), averaged over pairs of loci, usually took more than 50% of its maximum possible value, showing that these five loci are highly correlated in their inheritance. Allozyme frequencies for the same five loci have been examined in Mediterranean populations of *A. barbata* and the two complexes found in California have not been found. Thus, the patterns of coadaptation, correlated with environment, that are found in California have developed since the introduction of this species two centuries ago.

Electrophoretic variants have also been used to study multilocus organization in *Avena fatua*, another highly self-pollinated species, which like its relative *A. barbata* was also introduced to California during the Spanish period. Highly significant gametic phase disequilibrium has been found in each of the five populations of this species that have been studied in detail. However, the alleles associated are sometimes different in different populations, and there is no indication from this limited sample that widely successful complexes parallel to the mesic–xeric pair of *A. barbata* exist in *A. fatua.* Massive gametic phase disequilibrium has also been found in *Festuca microstachys,* a highly self-pollinated grass endemic to western North America. In this species, as in *A. fatua,* each of the populations studied has shown unique multilocus organization. Thus, highly developed multilocus organization, involving both linked and unlinked loci, has been found in every population of predominantly self-pollinated plants that has been studied in detail, indicating that it is a widespread phenomenon.

DEVELOPMENT OF COADAPTATION IN EXPERIMENTAL POPULATIONS

I will now consider briefly studies of two experimental populations of barley which give an idea of the rapidity with which coadaptation can build up in populations (Clegg et al., 1972; Weir et al., 1972, 1974). The two experimental populations to be considered are Composite Crosses II and V (abbreviated CCII and CCV). CCV was synthesized from 30 barley varieties representing the major barley growing areas of the world. These varieties were crossed in pairs, the resulting F_1 hybrids were again pair-crossed, and this cycle was repeated until a single grand F_1 hybrid was obtained. The F_2 seed from the grand F_1 hybrid was used to initiate the first generation of CCV in 1941, and the population has since been propagated in large plots each year under normal agricultural practice without conscious selection. CCII differs from CCV in parentage, method of synthesis, and time of synthesis. The population was initiated in 1929 by pooling equal numbers of F_1 hybrid seeds from the 378 intercrosses among its 28 parents, which, like the parents of CCV, included a wide sample of the world-wide diversity of cultivated barley. Population size and cultural practices were, however, the same as for CCV.

Four esterase loci were scored in the parents and also in various generations of both CCII and CCV. Analysis of the data involved designating the two initially most frequent alleles at each locus alleles 1 and 2, and the remaining less frequent alleles were combined into a composite synthetic allele designated allele 3. Examination of the gametic input of the parental varieties into both populations showed that alleles of the four loci were associated at random (aside from minor sampling effects associated with the limited number of parents) in the initial generation of both populations, as expected in populations synthesized from random samples of world barley varieties. However, by the fourth generation in CCV and the seventh generation in CCII (the earliest for which viable seed is now available) highly significant gametic phase disequilibrium had developed in both populations. In subsequent generations $|\bar{D}'|$ values increased steadily in both populations until they reached about 50% of the maximum possible value in generation 26 of CCII and about 80% in generation 41 of CCII. As $|\bar{D}'|$ increased, a few among the 81 possible four-locus triallelic gametic combinations became much more frequent, and the great majority of the gametic types became less frequent, than expected on the basis of single-locus frequencies. The three most favored gametic types came to account for more than 40% of the gametic pool in generation 26 of CCV and for nearly 80% of the gametic pool in generation 41 of CCII. It should be noted that the two most favored gametes, 1221 and 2112, which are perfectly complementary over all four loci, were identical in both populations. The development of the same genetic organization in both populations provides strong evidence that selection operating on the linkage blocks marked by the four loci is the primary force responsible for the development of parallel coadapted allelic complexes in these two populations. It should also be noted that both CCII and CCV increased steadily in fitness (measured as grain yield) over generations, in step with the development of gametic disequilibrium.

CONCLUSION

Demonstrated development of coadapted allelic complexes correlated with environment gives substance to the belief of many plant breeders that they must take the entire genotype into account when they select; also, major progress in breeding results from the development of genetic systems featuring novel favorably interacting complexes of genes.

REFERENCES

Allard, R. W., Babbel, G. R., Clegg, M. T., and Kahler, A. L. (1972a). Evidence of coadaptation in *Avena barbata. Proc. Natl. Acad. Sci. USA* 69:3043–3048.

Allard, R. W., Kahler, A. L., and Weir, B. C. (1972b). The effect of selection on esterase allozymes in a barley population. *Genetics* 72:489–503.

Clegg, M. T. and Allard, R. W. (1972). Patterns of gene differentiation in the slender wild oat species *Avena barbata. Proc. Natl. Acad. Sci. USA* 69:1820–1924.

Clegg, M. T., Allard, R. W., and Kahler, A. L. (1972). Is the gene the unit of selection? Evidence from two experimental populations. *Proc. Natl. Acad. Sci. USA* 69:2474–2478.

Durrenberger, R. W. (1960). *Patterns on the Land.* Roberts Publ. Co., Northridge, Calif.

Hamrick, J. L. and Allard, R. W. (1972). Microgeographical variation in allozyme frequencies in *Avena barbata. Proc. Natl. Acad. Sci. USA* 69:2100–2104.

Jain, S. K. and Allard, R. W. (1966). The effects of linkage, epistasis, and inbreeding on population changes under selection. *Genetics* 53:633–659.

Turner, J. R. G. (1967). On supergenes. I. The evolution of supergenes. *Amer. Naturalist* 101:195–221.

Weir, B. S., Allard, R. W., and Kalher, A. L. (1972). Analysis of complex allozyme polymorphisms in a barley population. *Genetics 72*:505–523.

Weir, B. S., Allard, R. W., and Kahler, A. L. (1974). Further analysis of complex allozyme polymorphisms in a barley population. *Genetics 78*:911–919.

Weir, B. S. and Cockerham, C. C. (1973). Mixed selfing and random mating at two loci. *Genet. Res. 21*:247–262.

21

Estimation of Genotypic and Environmental Variation in Plants

V. A. Dragavtsev

Institute of Cytology and Genetics
Siberian Branch of the USSR Academy of Sciences
Novosibirsk, USSR

and

J. Pešek

Agricultural Institute
Troubsko near Brno, CZSSR

ABSTRACT

The frequency of genotypes with the desired degree of expression of economically important quantitative characters within a hybrid or mutant population is usually very low. Therefore, the early identification and selection of such genotypes involves the analysis of very large populations. Because the breeding values of individuals in a population are masked by environmental, competitional, and ontogenic noises, special quantitative–genetic methods of analysis have to be used in order to eliminate their disturbing effects. The present chapter deals with a new approach to such an analysis by using either a simple background character or a background index obtained as a linear function of two, or more than two, background characters. It is believed that the use of this approach would greatly increase the efficiency of selection and shorten the time needed to produce improved new crop cultivars. As the analyses require the handling of large amounts of measurement data, plant breeders must use computer facilities.

INTRODUCTION

Humanity's requirements for foodstuffs, and particularly for grains, are continuously increasing, whereas the cultivable land areas in the world remain the same. Consequently, plant breeders more than ever have to concentrate their efforts on breeding new cultivars capable of producing higher grain yields of acceptable quality. The genetics of yield and of other economically important traits is generally rather complicated. Most, if not all, are probably polygenically controlled; therefore, the genetic improvement would depend on a particular recombination of genes. A simple calculation shows that with many segregating loci the probability of occurrence of a particular true-breeding recombinant in the first segregating generation of a cross is very low. The selection of such a recombinant directly from a hybrid F_2 population is practically impossible because its character expression depends not only on its genotype but also on the nongenetic agencies. There are various approaches to the separation of genotypic variation from the nongenotypic one. What the plant breeders are mostly interested in is the genotypic variance, i.e., that part of the total or phenotypic variation on which the success of selecting new cultivars depends. The present chapter is devoted to the problem of separating variances attributable to different causes.

THE TREATMENT OF THE PROBLEM

The genotypic and nongenotypic variances are usually denoted as σ_g^2 and σ_e^2. On the assumption that the genotypic and nongenotypic contributions to the phenotype are mutually independent, the phenotypic variance σ_{ph}^2 is simply the sum of the two variances, viz. $\sigma_{ph}^2 = \sigma_g^2 + \sigma_e^2$.

Separation of Variances

The σ_g^2 and σ_e^2 constituting σ_{ph}^2 can be separated by means of the following four methods.

Method of Uniform Environment

In a uniform, artificially produced environment, $\sigma_e^2 = 0$; therefore, it follows that $\sigma_g^2 = \sigma_{ph}^2$.

Method of Standards

This method consists of growing the genetically heterogeneous population to be studied together with a related, genetically homogeneous, population used as a standard. The total, or phenotypic, variance within the genetically hetero-geneous population is $\sigma_{ph}^2 = \sigma_g^2 + \sigma_e^2$, whereas that within the homogeneous population is $\sigma_{ph}^2 = \sigma_e^2$. Consequently $(\sigma_{ph}^2)_{het} - (\sigma_{ph}^2)_{hom} = \sigma_g^2$. This method is well known and is widely used, especially with annual and biennial plants.

Method Based on the Estimation of Soil Heterogeneity

This method (Smith, 1938; Shrikhande, 1957) obtained the estimates of σ_g^2 and σ_e^2 directly from the genetically heterogeneous population itself, i.e., with-out using any homogeneous population (e.g., clones, homozygous strains) as a standard. This method is of interest in the case of perennial plants, and particularly in the case of natural populations of such plants.

Method of Background Characters

The main feature of this method is the identification in plants of some background characters (BC) for which the genotypic variance in the population is practically zero (Dragavtsev, 1963, 1969). Consequently, all the variation for such a character is mostly nongenotypic, i.e., $\sigma_{ph}^2 = \sigma_e^2$. BC and the character of interest for selection SC are usually affected similarly by the environmental agencies and, as such, are correlated. As shown in a previous paper (Dragavtsev, 1972), in the case of a BC with $\sigma_g^2 \simeq 0$, and implicitly, $\sigma_{ph(BC)}^2 \simeq \sigma_{e(BC)}^2$, we have

$$r_{e(BC,SC)} = Cov_{e(BC,SC)}/\sigma_{e(BC)}\sigma_{e(SC)} \simeq 1$$

$$r_{e(BC,SC)}^2 = Cov_{e(BC,SC)}^2/\sigma_{e(BC)}^2\sigma_{e(SC)}^2 \simeq 1$$

and consequently

$$\sigma_{e(SC)}^2 \simeq Cov_{e(BC,SC)}^2/r_{e(BC,SC)}^2\sigma_{e(BC)}^2$$

Since $\sigma_{g(BC)}^2 \simeq 0$, then $Cov_{g(BC,SC)} \simeq 0$ and, therefore, $Cov_{e(BC,SC)} \simeq Cov_{ph(BC,SC)}$. By appropriate substitutions and restatements, ultimately we obtain

$$h^2 \simeq 1 - r_{ph(BC,SC)}^2/r_{e(BC,SC)}^2 \qquad (1)$$

as the heritability of the character of interest for selection.

The advantages of the method of background characters are that (a) it estimates σ_g^2 and σ_e^2 and the respective covariances and correlation coefficients directly from F_2 or M_2 populations without recourse to related homogeneous standard populations; (b) it permits the evaluation of individual plants on the basis of their genetic derivation from the population mean, which is of greater importance to the plant breeder than the general population parameters h^2 and σ_g^2; and (c) it is the only method which can eliminate not only environmental background noises but also those resulting from the effects of competition within the population.

The background noises in a plant population can be partitioned as (a) noises masking the genotypic deviations of individuals from the population mean, and (b) noises masking the additive–genetic deviations of individuals from the population mean. The first group of background noises consists of environmental noises expressed by the nongenetic variance σ_e^2, of competition noises expressed by the genotypic and environmental variances of competition, i.e., by $\sigma_{g(com)}^2$ and $\sigma_{e(com)}^2$, and of ontogenic noises expressed in terms of temporal increments of genetic variance $(\Delta\sigma_g^2)$ ascribable to gene sets controlling the character expression at a given time or stage of its development. The second kind of background noises is associated with the maternal effect as well as the aftereffects of environment and age. This group of noises manifests itself particularly in perennial plants.

When the various background noises in the population are taken into account, the quantitative–genetic expression

$$Cov_{PO} = \tfrac{1}{2}\sigma_A^2$$

becomes

$$Cov_{PO} = \tfrac{1}{2}\sigma_A^2 + Cov_{Ae} + Cov_{Me} + Cov_{ag}$$

and the expression

$$r_{PO} = Cov_{PO}/V_PV_O = \tfrac{1}{2}\sigma_A^2/\sigma_P\sigma_O$$

becomes

$$r_{PO} = \frac{1}{2}\ \frac{[\sigma_A^2 + 2(Cov_{Ae} + Cov_{Me} + Cov_{ag})]}{(\sigma_{gP}^2 + \sigma_{gP(com)}^2 + \sigma_{eP}^2)^{1/2}(\sigma_{gO}^2 + \sigma_{Ae}^2 + \sigma_{Me}^2 + \sigma_{ag}^2 + \sigma_{eO}^2)^{1/2}}$$

where Cov_{Ae}, Cov_{Me}, and Cov_{ag} are covariances of environmental aftereffect, maternal effect, and age aftereffect, respectively; σ_{gP}^2, $\sigma_{gP(com)}^2$, and σ_{eP}^2 are genotypic, genotypic–competitional, and nongenotypic parental variances, respectively; and σ_{gO}^2, σ_{Ae}^2, σ_{Me}^2, σ_{ag}^2, and σ_{re}^2 are genotypic, environmental aftereffect, maternal effect, age aftereffect, and residual offspring variances, in that order.

Let us consider the genotypic variance (σ_g^2) of grain yield in cereal crops, for instance. The best genotypes in a mixed population, let us say in F_2 generation of a cross, produce high yields per plant either because of their ability to utilize effectively small areas or because of their competitiveness in occupying larger areas of the total area on which the population grows. Consequently, two genotypes having the same potential for high yield of grain per plant will be classed as more productive and less productive if judged by the amount of grain produced per unit area.

If it is assumed that the genotypic variance for yield consists of variances of productivity ($\sigma^2_{g(u)}$) and competitive ability ($\sigma^2_{g(com)}$), then neglecting the ontogenic noises, we can write

$$\sigma^2_g = \sigma^2_{g(u)} + \sigma^2_{g(com)} \tag{2}$$

and

$$\sigma^2_{ph} = \sigma^2_{g(u)} + \sigma^2_{g(com)} + \sigma^2_{e(com)} + \sigma^2_r \tag{3}$$

where σ^2_r is the residual part of total phenotypic variance. Judging by Gerasimenko's results (personal communication) obtained after two years of field and laboratory experimentation on diallel crosses of wheat at the Institute of Cytology and Genetics of the Siberian Branch of the USSR Academy of Sciences, the $\sigma^2_{g(u)}/\sigma^2_{g(com)}$ ratio for weight of grain per head was 1/7 in 1974 and 1/12 in 1975.

Of the four methods of separating σ^2_g from σ^2_e in σ^2_{ph}, the first three partition σ^2_{ph} as

$$\sigma^2_{ph} = [\sigma^2_{g(u)} + \sigma^2_{g(com)}] + [\sigma^2_{e(com)} + \sigma^2_r] \tag{4}$$

whereas the fourth one, i.e., the method of background characters, does it as

$$\sigma^2_{ph} = \sigma^2_{g(u)} + [\sigma^2_{g(com)} + \sigma^2_{e(com)} + \sigma^2_r] \tag{5}$$

The background characters BC may be molecular–biochemical, physiological, and morphological. Although very convenient, in practice it is rather difficult to find a morphological character with

$$\sigma^2_{g(BC)} = Cov_{g(BC, SC)} = 0$$

i.e., a perfect background character.

The Background Index

Since the probability of the occurrence of a perfect background character in practice is very low, we have to use a background index, which is such a linear combination of several subperfect or semibackground characters that it estimates only the environmental variability. Let y_i be the phenotypic value of the ith background character such that $y_i = x_i + e_i$, where X is the genotypic value and e is a randomly distributed variable reflecting the environmental fluctuations. With a set of such background characters, the background index is obtained as

$$I = \Sigma_i b_i y_i$$

where b is the vector of coefficients of the index. This vector is estimated from the matrix equation

$$b = P^{-1}(1)$$

where P is the matrix of phenotypic variances (p_{ii}) and covariances (p_{ij}) of the background characters and (1) is a vector of ones.

In the case of two background characters, the coefficients b_1 and b_2 are obtained as

$$b_1 = (p_{22} - p_{12})/(p_{11}p_{22} - p_{12}^2)$$

and

$$b_2 = (p_{11} - p_{12})/(p_{11}p_{22} - p_{12}^2)$$

The use of the background index

$$I = \Sigma_i b_i y_i$$

eliminates the environmental and competitional noises and leaves $\sigma_{g(u)}^2$, the genotypic variance for high yield per unit area in this case. This isolation of $\sigma_{g(u)}^2$ from the σ_{ph}^2 allows for a more effective use of the genetic potential of the population when selecting for high-yielding lines.

The background index is mathematically similar to the selection indices (Smith, 1936; Smoček and Sigmundova, 1967; Pešek and Baker, 1969, 1970). However, in the biological sense it is different. The purpose of a background index is to minimize σ_g^2 and maximize r_e with the character of interest for selection.

The use of a perfect

$$\sigma_{g(BC)}^2 = 0, \quad Cov_{g(BC,SC)} = 0$$

or imperfect

$$\sigma_{g(BC)}^2 > 0, \quad Cov_{g(BC,SC)} \neq 0$$

background character in the selection of the best genotypes from the population is graphically presented in Fig. 1, where BC and SC are on x and y axes, respectively. The regression line of unit slope $(b_{e(SC/BC)} = 1)$ implies a complete positive correlation between BC and SC. The points of intercept (x,y) for the individual plants B and C lie on the regression line, whereas that for plant E lies above the line in the region of low BC expression. For the mean background character expression $(\bar{x})$, point E is expected to move to E', i.e., to the right and parallel to the regression line. In the case of a perfect BC, the deviations of B and C from the population mean $(\bar{y})$ have to be ascribed to nongenetic causes. If BC is imperfect, these deviations may be considered partly genetic in origin. No matter whether or not BC is perfect, the individual E has to be considered superior to other individuals with regard to its performance for SC. In other words, for selection purposes, it is necessary and sufficient that the environmental correlation between SC and BC be high.

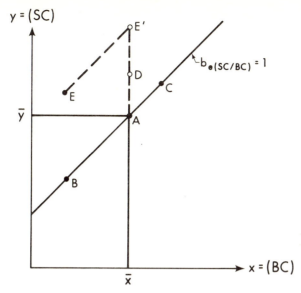

Fig. 1. Pattern of plant selection using background characteric (BV) for obtaining maximum yield per unit area.

CONCLUDING REMARKS

The breeding of productive new crop varieties necessitates, especially during its early stages, the measurement of character expressions on numerous individuals of a large population. The evaluation of measurement data requires the formulation of adequate methods of analysis and a heavy load of computational work. With the development of electronic computers, the calculations can be performed rapidly and efficiently and, as such, do not present a problem. Provided that the approach to the character structure is realistic and logical, it seems to be possible today to select promising progenitors of new varieties from early hybrid generations ($F_{G = 2}$, say) and/or from populations with artificially induced mutations ($M_{i = 2}$, say), and thus reduce both the work load of the plant breeder and the time of producing new varieties. Properly used, the analysis of early-generation measurement data by means of simple background characters or by means of background indices appears to be one of the efficient methods of selection.

REFERENCES

Dragavtsev, V. A. (1963). Phenogenetical analysis of variability in plant populations. *Proc. Acad. Sci. Khasakh SSR 10*:35–42.

Dragavtsev, V. A. (1969). On the possibility of eliminating the environmental component of the between-individuals variance when evaluating the coefficient of repeatability in plants. *Genetika 5*:30–35.

Dragavtsev, V. A. (1972). Experimental comparison of three principles in the estimation of genotypic variability of quantitative characters in plant populations. *Genetika 8*:28–34.

Pešek, J. and Baker, R. J. (1969). Desired improvement in relation to selection indices. *Can. J. Plant Sci. 49*:803–804.

Pešek, J. and Baker, R. J. (1970). An application of index selection to the improvement of self-pollinated species. *Can. J. Plant Sci. 50*:267–276.

Shrikhande, V. J. (1957). Some considerations in designing experiments on coconut trees. *J. Indian. Soc. Agr. Stat. 9*:82–99.

Smith, H. F. (1936). A discriminant function for plant selection. *Ann. Eugen. 7*:240–250.

Smith, H. F. (1938). An empirical law describing soil heterogeneity in the yields of agricultural crops. *J. Agr. Sci. 28*:1–23.

Smoček, J. and Sigmundova, J. (1967). Selection indexes and their use in predicting highest yielding winter wheat genotypes. *Savremena poljoprivreda 15* (N12,: 933–942.

22

Heritability Estimates from Four Generations of a Diallel Cross of Common Wheat

Barkat Ali Soomro

Department of Botany and Plant Breeding
Cotton Research Institute
Sakrand, Sind, Pakistan

ABSTRACT

The heritabilities of 10 quantitative characters were studies in F_1, F_2, backcross, and selfed backcross generations of a five-parent diallel cross of common wheat grown at two locations. From this study it was found that (a) most of the characters in question were highly heritable, (b) the heritabilities estimated by regression and variance component methods were more or less the same ($r = 0.84**$ to $0.95**$), and (c) the heritability of some characters was affected by location or by generation; in one case only (1000-kernel weight) was the heritability of the character affected by both.

INTRODUCTION

The response to selection for a metric trait depends on the heritability of the trait. Heritability is that part of the total variance in a segregating population which is attributed to the average gene effects; it expresses the degree of reliability of the phenotypic values of individuals as a guide to their breeding values. With respect to a particular character, the relative effects of heredity and environment on the phenotype indicate the advance to be expected from selection. In a broad sense, heritability is the ratio of total genetic variance to phenotypic variance; in a narrow sense, it is the ratio of additive genetic variance

241

to phenotypic variance. The method of estimating the heritability of a character depends on the kind of relationship among the individuals considered for analysis. The question of heritability of metric traits in wheat has been considered by several research workers.

Fonseca and Patterson (1968) studied the heritability of six quantitative characters in F_1 and F_2 generations of a seven-parent diallel cross of winter wheat sown in hillplots and in customary nursery yield plots over two years. They found that irrespective of the generation and method of seeding, the heritability estimates were more or less the same. They also found that the estimated heritabilities were high for earliness, plant height, number of heads, and number of kernels per head, and moderate or low for kernel weight and grain yield. Baker et al. (1971) conducted a comprehensive study of heritabilities of several quantitative characters in hard red spring wheats grown in 15 locations for five years. The results obtained showed that bushel weight, 1000-kernel weight, ash, and protein contents of grain had consistently high heritability estimates, whereas the heritability of quality traits appeared to vary from environment to environment. Khadr et al. (1972) compared the heritability of several quantitative characters in three populations derived from six wheat crosses. They reported that the heritabilities (in percentage) estimated by means of variance components were higher than those obtained by the parent–offspring regression method. Khadr and Morsy (1973) have obtained moderate heritability values for five quantitative characters in eight wheat crosses and reported the expected gain from selection for three of them.

The present study reports on heritability estimates for 10 quantitative characters in four generations of a five-parent diallel cross of common wheat (*Triticum aestivum* L.) as obtained by means of parameters from diallel cross analyses and by variance components and parent–offspring regression methods.

MATERIALS AND METHODS

The F_1, F_2, backcross, and selfed backcross generations of a complete five-parent diallel cross of wheat were grown in 1972 at two locations in Canada, viz. at Ellerslie and at Parkland farms of the University of Alberta, Edmonton, Alberta. The experimental design used was a 15×15 partially balanced triple lattice. The parents were the Canadian cultivars Marquis and Chinook, the Pakistani cultivar Khush-Hal, and the Mexican cultivars Ciano and INIA. The characters studied were onset-of-heading, final heading, heading span, plant height, number of tillers per plant, number of spikelets per spike, weight of seeds per spike, 1000-kernel weight, and yield of grain per plant. The details of the experiment were presented and discussed by Soomro (1974, 1975). The diallel matrix of data of each generation was tested for the validity of the assumptions underlying the analysis (Hayman, 1954). The tests were generally found to be satisfactory (Soomro, 1974). The array variances, the covariances between arrays of crosses, and the parental array and the array means provided the basis for calculating the other second-degree statistics from which the genetic parameters D, H_1, H_2, and F were computed. Heritability estimates in the broad and narrow sense were obtained by means of these parameters following the method of Mather and Jinks (1971). Heritability estimates by regression and variance-component methods were obtained following Liang et al. (1969).

RESULTS AND DISCUSSION

The heritabilities of the 10 characters studies and their coefficients of variation based on total mean-squares of the respective analyses of variance are given in Tables I–IV. Tables I and II pertain, respectively, to the heritabilities in the broad and narrow sense, estimated by means of parameters, or components of variability, from diallel cross analyses; Tables III and IV pertain to heritabilities obtained by parent–offspring regression and variance-component methods, in that order. As expected, the broad-sense heritability values were generally higher than those of narrow-sense heritability, and, with some exceptions, had lower coefficients of variability (CV). The heritability values obtained by parent–offspring regression were generally comparable to those in the narrow sense but, with the exception of heading span and final heading, they had higher coefficients of variation. The heritabilities estimated by the variance components method were lower than those obtained by means of diallel cross parameters and by parent–offspring regression for heading traits; they were higher for the characters related directly to yield, but not for yield itself. Hence, for some of the characters the situation was similar to that reported by Khadr et al. (1972). The highest heritability values were obtained for the characters: plant height, earliness (onset-of-heading and final heading), number of seeds per spike, and 1000-kernel weight (Tables I– IV). These findings are in agreement with those reported by Fonseca and Patterson (1968). The heritabilities of the remaining characters were lower. The estimates of the heritability of grain yield per plant ranged from 14% to 72% at one location (Ellerslie) and from –42% (which does not make sense) to 13% at the other (Parkland), a fact reflected by the very high CV% values. Because of this high variability, the results of the analysis of variance of heritability estimates for this character (see Tables I–III) cannot be considered statistically valid. Nevertheless, these results are indicative of the high sensitivity of the character in question to the external and possibly internal agencies of variation. On the average, the heritability of grain yield per plant was $\simeq 20\%$, which is in agreement with the findings of several researchers (Weibel, 1956; McNeal, 1960; Kronstad and Foote, 1964; Johnson et al., 1966; Paroda and Joshi, 1970a,b).

Significant location effects on heritability estimates were found for the characters final heading (Tables I and III), and weight of seeds per spike (Table II). Significant generation effects on heritability were detected for number of

Table I. ANOVA of Broad-Sense Heritabilities ($h^2\%$) of Characters Studied in Four Different Generations Obtained from Diallel Cross-Components of Variation

Character	Mean h^2	CV%	Source of variation	DF	MS	F
Onset of heading	95	1.5	Generations	3	1.458	ns[a]
			Locations	1	6.125	ns[a]
			Gen. × Loc.	3	1.125	
			Total	7	1.928	
Final heading	95	2	Generations	3	0.458	ns
			Location	1	21.125	18.778[b]
			Gen. × Loc.	3	1.125	
			Total	7	3.696	
Heading span	55	18	Generations	3	24.458	ns
			Locations	1	120.125	ns
			Gen. × Loc.	3	157.125	
			Total	7	94.982	
Plant height	97	1.2	Generations	3	2.333	ns
			Locations	1	0.500	ns
			Gen. × Loc.	3	0.833	
			Total	7	1.429	
Number of tillers per plant	55	27	Generations	3	37.125	ns
			Locations	1	1176.125	13.656[b]
			Gen. × Loc.	3	86.125	
			Total	7	220.839	
Number of spikelets per spike	67	30	Generations	3	609.333	ns
			Locations	1	84.500	ns
			Gen. × Loc.	3	329.833	
			Total	7	414.571	
Number of spikelets per spike	78	16	Generations	3	288.125	ns
			Locations	1	1.250	ns
			Gen. × Loc.	3	87.458	
			Total	7	161.125	
Weight of seeds per spike	62	14	Generations	3	103.458	ns
			Locations	1	120.125	ns
			Gen. × Loc.	3	40.125	
			Total	7	78.696	
1000-kernel weight	73	6	Generations	3	32.667	ns
			Locations	1	4.500	ns
			Gen. × Loc.	3	11.167	
			Total	7	19.429	
Yield of grain per plant	23	159	Generations	3	918.125	ns
			Locations	1	6216.125	31.481[b]
			Gen. × Loc.	3	197.458	
			Total	7	1336.125	

[a] ns = $p > 0.05$.
[b] $0.01 < p \leqslant 0.05$.

Table II. ANOVA of Narrow-Sense Heritabilities ($h^2\%$) of the Characters Studied in Four Different Generations as Obtained from Diallel Cross-Components of Variation

Character	Mean h^2	CV%	Source of variation	DF	MS	F
Onset of heading	83	6	Generations	3	31.000	ns[a]
			Locations	1	2.000	ns
			Gen. × Loc.	3	27.670	
			Total	7	25.429	
Final heading	81	7	Generations	3	34.333	ns
			Locations	1	112.000	ns
			Gen. × Loc.	3	13.000	
			Total	7	36.286	
Heading span	29	55	Generations	3	192.458	ns
			Locations	1	1128.125	48.69[c]
			Gen. × Loc.	3	23.167	
			Total	7	253.571	
Plant height	95	1.5	Generations	3	2.833	ns
			Locations	1	0.000	ns
			Gen. × Loc.	3	1.667	
			Total	7	1.929	
Number of tillers per plant	46	34	Generations	3	24.070	ns
			Locations	1	91.125	ns
			Gen. × Loc.	3	528.180	
			Total	7	249.696	
Number of spikelets per spike	67	18	Generations	3	320.458	10.19[b]
			Locations	1	6.125	ns
			Gen. × Loc.	3	31.458	
			Total	7	151.696	
Number of seeds per spike	74	23	Generations	3	502.792	ns
			Locations	1	3.125	ns
			Gen. × Loc.	3	149.458	
			Total	7	279.982	
Weight of seeds per spike	61	20	Generations	3	121.125	ns
			Locations	1	630.125	28.48[b]
			Gen. × Loc.	3	22.125	
			Total	7	151.411	
1000-kernel weight	71	13	Generations	3	118.458	48.193[c]
			Locations	1	276.125	112.337[c]
			Gen. × Loc.	3	2.458	
			Total	7	91.268	
Yield of grain per plant	23	88	Generations	3	268.167	ns
			Locations	1	1800.000	19.081[b]
			Gen. × Loc.	3	94.333	
			Total	7	412.500	

[a] ns = $p > 0.05$.
[b] $0.01 < p < 0.05$.
[c] $p \leqslant 0.01$.

Table III. ANOVA of Heritabilities ($h^2\%$) of the Characters Studied in Four Different Generations as Obtained by Parent–Offspring Regression Method

Character	Mean h^2	CV%	Source of variation	DF	MS	F
Onset of heading	81	18	Generations	3	222.458	ns[a]
			Locations	1	3.125	ns
			Gen. × Loc.	3	265.792	
			Total	7	209.696	
Final heading	81	6	Generations	3	6.458	ns
			Locations	1	78.125	5.531[b]
			Gen. × Loc.	3	14.125	
			Total	7	19.982	
Heading span	26	23	Generations	3	49.833	ns
			Locations	1	32.000	ns
			Gen. × Loc.	3	24.667	
			Total	7	36.500	
Plant height	93	2.5	Generations	3	8.792	ns
			Locations	1	6.125	ns
			Gen. × Loc.	3	1.792	
			Total	7	5.411	
Number of tillers per plant	36	39	Generations	3	75.333	ns
			Locations	1	1012.500	19.788[c]
			Gen. × Loc.	3	51.167	
			Total	7	198.871	
Number of spikelets per spike	45	40	Generations	3	329.667	ns
			Locations	1	264.500	ns
			Gen. × Loc.	3	326.167	
			Total	7	318.857	
Number of seeds per spike	62	30	Generations	3	534.333	ns
			Locations	1	2.000	ns
			Gen. × Loc.	3	261.000	
			Total	7	341.143	
Weight of seeds per spike	38	41	Generations	3	237.833	ns
			Locations	1	4.500	ns
			Gen. × Loc.	3	323.167	
			Total	7	241.071	
1000-kernel weight	60	15	Generations	3	97.458	ns
			Locations	1	210.125	14.876[b]
			Gen. × Loc.	3	14.125	
			Total	7	77.839	
Yield of grain per plant	18	103	Generations	3	115.458	8.579[b]
			Locations	1	2016.125	149.805[c]
			Gen. × Loc.	3	13.458	
			Total	7	343.268	

[a] ns = $p > 0.05$.
[b] $0.01 < p \leqslant 0.05$.
[c] $p \leqslant 0.01$.

Table IV. Heritability Values (h^2%) Obtained by the
Variance Components Method for the Characters
Studied

No.	Character	Heritability (%)
1	Onset-of-heading	72
2	Final heading	76
3	Heading-span	40
4	Plant height	82
5	Number of tillers per plant	66
6	Number of spikelets per spike	55
7	Number of seeds per spike	73
8	Weight of seeds per spike	59
9	1000-kernel weight	64
10	Yield of grain per plant	10

spikelets per spike (Table II). The heritability of 1000-kernel weight was significantly affected by location, or by both location and generation (Tables II and III). Very-low-to-low location, generation, generation within location, and, implicitly, location within generation effects have to be presumed for the heritability estimates of the characters plant height, onset-of-heading, and final heading (see CV% in Tables I–III). High heritability estimates of these characters and their relative stability across generations and locations, except for final heading, are predictive of a positive response to selection. Good prospects with regard to response to selection may also exist for 1000-kernel weight.

The coefficients of simple correlations given in Table V show that the heritabilities estimated in different ways for the characters in question are closely related, and that the discrepancies among them, except for their relative magnitude, could be ascribed to some shortcomings in the experiment and to chance fluctuations.

Table V. The Coefficients of Correlation
between the Heritability Values Obtained by
Different Methods for the Characters Studied

No.[a]	1	2	3	4
1	1	0.94^b	0.95^b	0.88^b
2		1	0.95^b	0.91^b
3			1	0.84^b
4				1

[a](1) Narrow-sense heritability (diallel), (2) broad-sense heritability (diallel), (3) heritability by regression, and (4) heritability by variance component.
[b]$p \leqslant 0.01$.

REFERENCES

Baker, R. J., Tripples, K. H., and Campbell, A. B. (1971). Heritabilities and correlations among quality traits in wheat. *Can. J. Plant Sci. 51*:441–448.

Fonseca, S. M. and Patterson, F. L. (1968). Hybrid vigour in a seven-parent diallel cross of common winter wheat (*Triticum aestivum* L.). *Crop Sci. 8*:85–88.

Hayman, B. I. (1954). Theory and analysis of diallel crosses. I. *Genetics 39*:789–809.

Johnson, V. A., Biever, K. B., Haunold, A., and Schmidt, J. W. (1966). Inheritance of plant height, yield of grain and other plant and seed characteristics in a cross of hard red winter wheat, *Triticum aestivum* L. *Crop Sci. 6*:331–338.

Khadr, F. H. and Morsy, M. S. (1973). Additive and dominance variation, heritability and correlation of quantitative characters in wheat. *Egypt J. Genet. Cytol. 2*:20–30.

Khadr, F. H., Ali, M. A., and Morsy, M. S. (1972). Heritabilities of quantitative traits estimated by different methods in generations of wheat crosses. *Egypt J. Genet. Cytol. 1*:262–269.

Kronstad, W. E. and Foote, W. H. (1964). General and specific combining ability estimates in winter wheat (*Triticum aestivum* L.). *Crop Sci. 4*:616–619.

Liang, G. H. L., Walter, T. L., Mickell, C. D., and Koh, V. O. (1969). Heritability estimates and inter-relationship among agronomic traits in grain sorghum, *Sorghum bicolor* L. Moench. *Can. J. Genet. Cytol. 11*:199–208.

Mather, K. and Jinks, J. L. (1971). *Biometrical Genetics,* 2nd ed., 382 pp. Chapman and Hall, London.

McNeal, F. H. (1960). Yield components in a Lemhi × Thatcher wheat cross. *Agron. J. 52*:348–349.

Paroda, R. S. and Joshi, A. B. (1970a). Genetic architecture of yield and components of yield in wheat. *Ind. J. Genet. Plant Breed. 30*:298–314.

Paroda, R. S. and Joshi, A. B. (1970b). Combining ability in wheat. *Ind. J. Genet. Plant Breed. 30*:630–637.

Soomro, B. A. (1974). A biometrical-genetic analysis of some quantitative characters in a five-parent diallel cross of common wheat (*Triticum aestivum* L.). Ph.D. thesis, Univ. of Alberta, Edmonton.

Soomro, B. A. (1975). Diallel analysis of heading data and plant height in wheat. *Pak. J. Bot. 7*:91–117.

Weibel, D. E. (1956). Inheritance of quantitative characters in wheat. *Iowa State Coll. J. Sci. 30*:450–451.

23

Diallel Analysis of Four Agronomic Traits in Common Wheat

M. B. Yildirim

Department of Agronomy-Genetics
Faculty of Agriculture
Ege University
Bornova, Izmir, Turkey

ABSTRACT

The common wheat cultivars Aköz, Florence, Mentana, Jaral, and Siete Cerros were crossed in 1972 in all possible combinations excluding reciprocals. In 1972–1973 the F_1 hybrids and the five parents were field grown at Bornova in randomized complete blocks. The characters studied were plant height, spike length, 1000-kernel weight, and plant yield. The analysis of data showed that (a) with respect to plant height and 1000-kernel weight all F_1 combinations deviated from the corresponding midparental values, (b) for the same characters the GCA variances were significant and the GCA ÷ SCA ratios high, (c) the characters' plant height, spike length, and 1000-kernel weight were probably controlled by two effective factors each, and (d) plant height had the highest and 1000-kernel weight the lowest heritability ($h^2 = 0.66$ and $h^2 = 0.26$, respectively). It was concluded that a desired response to selection could be expected for plant height and 1000-kernel weight.

INTRODUCTION

The selection of appropriate parents for crossings constitutes one of the important and difficult problems in plant breeding. Various methods of diallel cross analysis have been developed and used in the evaluation of the parental cultivars and their progenies with regard to their potential as breeding materials. The objectives of the present study were (a) investigation of the genetic makeup of some common wheat cultivars by crossing them in a diallel manner, and (b) selection of the most promising hybrid combinations to be used as breeding materials.

MATERIALS AND METHODS

Common wheat cultivars Florence, Mentana, Aköz, Jaral, and Siete Cerros (see Table I) were crossed in all possible combinations excluding reciprocals. The five parents (as selfs) and the F_1 generation of their crosses were sown on November 18, 1972 in the field at Bornova, Izmir. The experimental design used was a randomized blocks design with four replications. The plots were 1-m-long rows with 10-cm spacing between seeds within rows and 30 cm between rows. The plots matured and were harvested plant by plant during the last week of May, 1973. To get rid of border effects, the first and the last plants of each row were discarded. Eight plants per row were used to record data on the following traits.

1. Plant height (cm) measured on the tallest tiller, awns excluded
2. Spike length (cm) measured on up to eight spikes per plant and then averaged
3. Plant yield recorded as the amount of grain (in grams) obtained from individual plants
4. Thousand kernel weight (1000 kwt in grams) determined by averaging the weights of two samples of 200 kernels each and then multiplying by five

Plot means of eight plants for each trait were used in the statistical analyses. The necessary calculations were made by using the computer facilities of the Statistical Laboratory of Ege University. Following the randomized blocks

Table I. The Pedigrees of the Parental Cultivars

Cultivar	Pedigree	Ref.
Aköz	Atlas × Akova-10(A)	Anon. (1962)
Florence	[(White Naple) × (Improved Fife)] × Eden	Gökgöl (1954)
Mentana	[(Rieti) × (Wilhelmine Tarwe)] × Akogomughi	Gökgöl (1954)
Jaral	[(Sonora × T2pp)] × Nai 60-11-18889-101M -IR-3C-4Y	Alcala (personal
Siete Cerros	Penjamo 62 "S" × G655-11-8156-IM -2R-4M	communication, 1974)

analysis of variance (Steel and Torrie, 1960), the effects of heterosis (in %) were calculated by means of procedures used by Matzinger et al. (1959) and Fonseca and Patterson (1968). The general and specific combining abilities (GCA and SCA) were calculated using Griffing's (1956) method of analysis of a diallel cross consisting of parents (selfs) and crosses, excluding reciprocals. The components of variances and covariances and the pertinent ratios reflecting the genetic situation in the diallel cross were calculated following Jinks (1956) and Hayman (1954). The calculations were performed on an IBM 1130 computer using a modified version (Yildirim and Manas, 1974) of a program written by Lee and Kaltsikes (1971) for the IBM 360.

RESULTS OBTAINED

The parental and F_1 cross means for the traits studied are given in Table II. The results of the comparisons for heterosis and heterobeltiosis are summarized in Table III. These results show that (a) on average, heterosis was positive for plant height, spike length, and 1000 kwt, and negative for plant yield; (b) all 10 F_1 crosses were taller and had higher 1000 kwt's than the respective parental means—eight crosses had longer spikes and three crosses had higher yields than the means of the corresponding parents; (c) of the 10 F_1 crosses, six were taller, six had longer spikes, five had higher 1000-kernel weight (1000 kwt), and

Table II. The Trait Measurement-Means of the Parents and Their F_1 Crosses

Parents and F_1 crosses	Plant height (cm)	Spike length (cm)	Plant yield (g)	1000 kwt (g)
P_1 = Aköz	137.7	12.3	17.3	43.8
P_2 = Florence	147.1	10.7	14.7	38.6
P_3 = Mentana	128.4	11.2	15.4	39.1
P_4 = Jaral	91.1	9.4	9.1	31.7
P_5 = Siete Cerros	99.3	11.8	17.5	32.9
$(P_1 \times P_2)F_1$	149.5	13.4	15.8	48.2
$(P_1 \times P_3)F_1$	134.1	12.4	13.8	43.4
$(P_1 \times P_4)F_1$	126.0	11.6	10.4	41.5
$(P_1 \times P_5)F_1$	137.9	13.0	19.2	41.6
$(P_2 \times P_3)F_1$	147.8	13.0	14.5	47.0
$(P_2 \times P_4)F_1$	123.7	11.3	14.2	39.7
$(P_2 \times P_5)F_1$	135.8	12.3	14.0	38.9
$(P_3 \times P_4)F_1$	120.2	11.6	13.8	41.0
$(P_3 \times P_5)F_1$	126.7	11.4	15.9	37.5
$(P_4 \times P_5)F_1$	99.4	10.3	10.8	34.7

Table III. Parental Means, Cross Means, and the Number of Crosses Showing
Heterosis and Heterobeltiosis[a]

Traits	Mean of the parents (P)	Mean of F_1's ($\overline{F}_1$)	Heterosis (%)	$\overline{P}$	Higher $\overline{P}$
				Number of F_1 higher than:	
Plant height (cm)	120.73	130.12	7.78	10	6
Spike length (cm)	11.24	12.05	7.21	8	6
Plant yield (g)	14.81	14.26	−3.71	3	1
1000 kwt (g)	37.23	41.34	11.10	10	5

[a]Total number of F_1 in the diallel table is 10. Heterosis (%) = $(1/\overline{P})(\overline{F}_1 - \overline{P})100$.

only one had higher plant yield than the respective higher parents (heterobeltiosis).

The results of the analysis for combining ability effects of the parental cultivars and the GCA ÷ SCA ratios are given in Table IV. Table V shows that relatively large GCA effects were recorded for the traits, i.e., plant height and 1000 kwt. For the same traits the GCA ÷ SCA ratios were the highest and the GCA variances were significant ($p < 5\%$).

The components of variation of the diallel cross data as estimated using the Jinks–Hayman method of analysis and the pertinent ratios are given in Table V. As shown in this table, component D was significant for all four traits studied, component h^2 was significant for plant height, and component E for plant yield and 1000 kwt. The other components were not significant ($p > 5\%$). The V_r, W_r graphs for plant height, plant yield, and 1000 kwt are shown in Figs. 1, 2, and 3, respectively.

Table IV. General Combining Ability Effects and the GCA ÷ SCA Ratios

Trait	Aköz	Florence	Mentana	Jaral	Siete Cerros	GCA ÷ SCA ratios
	GCA effects of cultivars:					
Plant height	9.04	12.10	2.77	17.06	6.89	11.56[a]
Spike length	0.78	0.62	0.00	−1.11	−0.35	6.86
Plant yield	0.72	0.50	0.36	−2.60	1.00	1.06
1000 kwt	2.59	3.11	1.52	−2.49	−4.73	13.70[a]

[a]GCA variance significant at 5% level.

Table V. The Components of Variation in the Diallel
Cross for the Traits Studied

Parameters and ratios	Plant height	Spike length[a]	Plant yield[b]	1000 kwt
D	570.77*	1.33*	24.45*	22.84*
F	−28.02	−0.14	13.05	−9.83
H_1	90.25	1.18	19.47	19.85
H_2	99.29	1.02	17.65	18.32
h^2	209.30*	1.67	7.30	34.70
E	41.96	0.39	11.92*	8.11*
$(H_1 \div D)^{1/2}$	0.39	0.94	0.89	0.94
$H_2 \div 4H_1$	0.27	0.22	0.22	0.23
$KD \div KR$	0.88	0.89	3.98	0.62
$K = h^2 \div H_2$	2.11	1.64	0.41	1.89
Heritability	0.66	0.31	0.31	0.26
$r_{y_r,(V_r+W_r)}$	−0.80	−0.38	0.89	−0.34

[a]Based on the means of two blocks.
[b]Based on the means of four blocks.

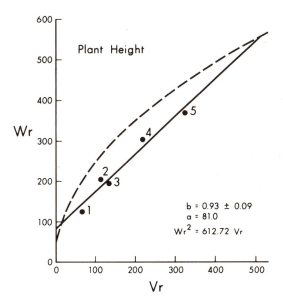

Fig. 1. (V_r, W_r) graph for plant height. The points of (V_r, W_r) intercepts refer to (1) Aköz, (2) Florence, (3) Mentana, (4) Jaral, and (5) Siete Cerros arrays.

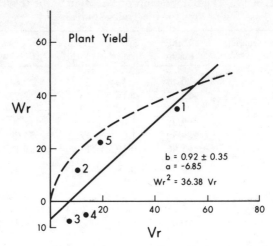

Fig. 2. (V_r, W_r) graph for plant yield. The points of (V_r, W_r) intercepts refer to (1) Aköz, (2) Florence, (3) Mentana, (4) Jaral, and (5) Siete Cerros arrays.

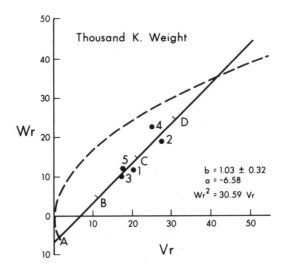

Fig. 3. (V_r, W_r) graph for 1000 kwt. The points of (V_r, W_r) intercepts refer to (1) Aköz, (2) Florence, (3) Mentana, (4) Jaral, and (5) Siete Cerros arrays.

DISCUSSION AND CONCLUSIONS

The possibility of selection of promising crosses in early (F_1 and F_2) generations, especially of those showing potential for transgressive segregation may reduce the amount of work and speed up the process of breeding (Busch et al., 1974). Several investigators (Jinks, 1956; Whitehouse et al., 1958; Crumpacker and Allard, 1962) have proposed appropriate tests to attain this goal. Others (Lupton, 1961; Busch et al., 1974) have advised the use of later (F_4 and F_5) generations in the evaluation of crosses for breeding purposes.

Two crosses in this study seem to be promising, viz. the cross Aköz X Florence for 1000 kwt, and the cross Aköz X Siete Cerros for plant yield. Both crosses showed heterobeltiosis: $\bar{F}$-(higher P) = 4.4 g and 1.7 g, respectively. Associated with the difference between the parents of 5.2 g for 1000 kwt and practically no difference (0.2 g≃ 0) for plant yield, these heterobeltiotic effects show that the Aköz X Florence cross could be used successfully as breeding material for high 1000 kwt, but the value of Aköz X Siete Cerros cross as breeding material for yield performance is rather questionable. However, because Aköz and Siete Cerros appear to be genotypically different (Aköz≃ Siete Cerros < F_1), the occurrence of high-yielding recombinants in the later generations can not be precluded.

Significant GCA variances were found for plant height and 1000 kwt. These results are in agreement with those reported by Busch et al. (1974). The GCA variance is considered to reflect additive genetic variability (Hayman, 1963). The knowledge of additive genetic variability in a hybrid population of a self-pollinating species like wheat, for instance, is important to the plant breeder. In this particular case, the high GCA ÷ SCA ratios for plant height and 1000 kwt (11.56* and 13.70*, respectively) show that the variability with regard to these traits is predominantly of the additive kind, and selection for them could be successful.

Among the genetic components of variation depending on both the additive and the dominance effects (F) or dominance effects (H_1, H_2, and h_2) only h_2 was significant, and that for plant height only. However, considering the relative magnitude of the numerical values of F, H_1, and H_2 and the fact that their nonsignificance at the 5% level of probability does not necessarily imply their absence, the pertinent ratios were calculated and entered in Table V. Assuming them to be valid, the following statements may be made:

1. On the average, dominance $(H_1 \div D)^{1/2}$ was partial (0.39) for plant height and nearly complete (≃ 1.0) for spike length, plant yield, and 1000 kwt.
2. The genes with positive and negative effects were, on the average, in equal proportions ($H_2 \div 4H_1 \simeq 0.25$) in the parents for all four traits studied.

3. More or less equal proportions of dominant and recessive genes in the parents could be assumed for plant height and spike length ($KD \div KR =$ 0.88 $\simeq$ 1 and 0.89 $\simeq$ 1, respectively). For plant yield the genes involved were mostly dominant, and those for 1000 kwt mostly recessive ($KD \div KR$ = 3.98 > 1 and 0.62 < 1, respectively).

4. The traits, namely, plant height, spike length and 1000 kwt were controlled possibly by two groups of genes each ($h^2 \div H_2 \sim 2$). For plant yield the ratio $h^2 \div H_2$ was less than one (0.42 < 1).

5. For spike length, 1000 kwt, and especially plant height, the genes with positive effects were more often dominant than recessive ($r_{y_r} v_r + w_r$ < 0), whereas for plant yield they were predominantly recessive ($r_{y_r}, v_r + w_r$ = 0.89 $\simeq$ 1).

6. The most heritable trait was plant height (heritability = 0.66) and the least heritable was 1000 kwt (heritability = 0.26).

In the present case, the purpose of the investigation was the evaluation of crosses with regard to their potential as materials for breeding new homozygous cultivars of common wheat. Therefore, the most important component of genetical variation is D, which happens to be significant for all four traits studied, and successful selection could be practiced for all four of them.

The study of the (V_r, W_r) graphs (Fig. 1–3) provides information with regard to the overall genetic situation and with regard to individual arrays of crosses and, implicitly, their nonrecurrent parents. Thus, the (V_r, W_r) graph for plant height (Fig. 1) shows that the dominance is partial, that there is no epistasis ($b =$ 0.93 $\simeq$ 1), and that Aköz and Siete Cerros have predominantly dominant and recessive genes, respectively. Because the genes that increase plant height were found to be mostly dominant

$$r_{y_r} v_r + w_r < 0$$

the selection for short straw will be fairly rapid because it is controlled mostly by recessive genes. Selection from the Aköz X Siete Cerros, for instance, would result in a short time in uniform lines as short or shorter than Siete Cerros. For plant yield (Fig. 2) the graph shows a slight overdominance and no epistasis ($b =$ 0.92 $\simeq$ 1). The cultivar Aköz has predominantly recessive genes, whereas Siete Cerros seems to have dominant and recessive genes in more or less equal proportions. Because high plant yield appeared to be controlled predominantly by recessive genes, the selection of high-yielding homozygous lines from the Aköz X Siete Cerros could be fairly rapid. For 1000 kwt (Fig. 3) the graph shows a slight overdominance and there is no indication of epistasis ($b = 1.03 \simeq$ 1). The cultivars Aköz, Siete Cerros, and Mentana appear to have a slight excess of dominant genes. High 1000-kwt was found to be controlled by both dominant and recessive genes with a slight preponderance of dominants

$$r_{y_r, v_r + w_r} = -0.34$$

Consequently, selection for high 1000-kwt in the progeny of Aköz X Siete Cerros, Aköz X Mentana, and Mentana X Siete Cerros would involve the combination of dominant and recessive genes both having positive effects. Thus, the analysis of data shows that from a breeding point of view attention should be given to the Aköz X Siete Cerros progeny. Of course, the other crosses should not be discarded without a fair trial.

REFERENCES

Anonymous (1960–1961). Annual Report, Adapazari Experimental Station, Adapazari, Turkey.

Busch, R. H., Janke, J. C., and Frohberg, R. C. (1974). Evaluation of crosses among high and low yielding parents of spring wheat (*Triticum aestivum* L.) and bulk predictions of line performance. *Crop Sci. 14*:47–50.

Crumpacker, D. W. and Allard, R. W. (1962). A diallel cross analysis of heading date in wheat. *Hilgardia 32*(6):275–318.

Fonseca, S. and Patterson, F. L. (1968). Hybrid vigor in a seven-parent diallel cross in common winter wheat (*Triticum aestivum* L.). *Crop Sci. 8*:85–88.

Gökgöl, M. (1954). General foundations of wheat breeding (in Turkish). Karinca Matb. Ankara.

Griffing, B. (1956). Concept of general and specific combining ability in relation to diallel crossings systems. *Austr. J. Biol. Sci. 9*:463–493.

Hayman, B. I. (1954). The theory and analysis of diallel crosses. *Genetics 39*:235–244.

Hayman, B. I. (1963). Notes on diallel-cross theory. *Stat. Genet. Plant Breed. 982*:571–578.

Jinks, J. L. (1956). The F_2 and backcross generations from a set of diallel crosses. *Heredity 10*:1–30.

Lee, J. and Kaltsikes, P. J. (1971). Letter to the editor. *Crop. Sci. 11*:314.

Lupton, F. G. H. (1961). Studies in the breeding of self-pollinating cereals. 3. Further studies in cross prediction. *Euphytica 10*:209–224.

Matzinger, D. F., Sprague, G. F., and Cockerham, C. C. (1959). Diallel crosses of maize in experiments repeated over locations and years. *Agron. J. 51*:346–350.

Steel, R. G. D. and Torrie, J. H. 1960. *Principles and Procedures of Statistics*. McGraw-Hill, New York.

Whitehouse, R. H. H., Thompson, J. B., and de Valle-Ribeizo, M. A. M. (1958). Studies on the breeding of self-pollinating cereals. 2. The use of diallel cross analysis in yield prediction. *Euphytica 7*:147–169.

Yildirim, M. B. and Manas, O. (1974). A program for the analysis of diallel crosses on an IBM 1130 computer (in Turkish). *Bitki 1*:122–127.

24

The Use of Selection Indices in Maize (*Zea mays* L.)

Mohammad Yousaf
Department of Plant Breeding and Genetics
University of Lyallpur
Lyallpur, Pakistan

ABSTRACT

Estimates of genetic variances for yield and its components—ear number, kernel rows, kernels per row, and kernel weight—and genetic covariances among them were computed for a synthetic population of maize, using 100 S_5 lines randomly chosen out of a lot developed from the population with a minimum of selection. Selection indices for various combinations of yield and its components were then constructed using these estimates of phenotypic and genotypic variances and covariances, and the corresponding estimates of expected genetic advance for yield were compared with that for yield alone. An expected advance of 7% in yield was calculated by considering selection for yield itself. Selection for yield based on the index using all five characters was expected to be 13% more efficient than selection for yield alone. Selection based on the index using kernel rows and kernel weight was almost as efficient as selection for yield itself. However, when the expected genetic advance was computed for one location, this index was 8.3% more efficient. Selection based on any of the components considered alone was much less efficient than that based on yield itself. The actual gain realized for some of the indices involving yield and the various components considered alone was much less efficient than that based on yield itself. The actual gain realized for some of the indices involving yield and the various components compared favorably with the predicted genetic advance.

INTRODUCTION

Improvement of a maize population to be used either directly as a commercial variety or as materials for deriving inbred lines has been the objective of any maize-breeding program. Such an improvement and the choice of means to achieve it are dependent on the extent of genetic variability within a given population with respect to various characters. The improvement of a population is based on selection. Selection indices as objective and theoretically efficient criteria of selection are usually formulated on the basis of several characters.

Robinson et al. (1951) have used different selection indices obtained by Smith's procedure (1936) and have reported that the index for maize based on plant height, number of ears per plant, and yield per plant showed an expected selection response, or genetic advance, in yield 30% higher than that of selection based on yield alone. Subandi et al. (1973) have compared the efficiencies of three types of selection indices in maize crosses and reported them to be more efficient in predicting the genetic advance than the yield itself. They found that simple multiplicative indices were almost as efficient as the ones obtained by means of statistical procedures. Kuhn and Stucker (1973) have evaluated four selection indices for predicting simultaneously the response to selection for yield and the number of ears per plant by using S_1 progeny of two maize populations. They found these indices inefficient and explained this inefficiency in terms of the high heritability of the characters' yield and ear number in their materials.

Selection indices have also been used successfully in soybeans (Johnson et al., 1955) and cotton (Manning, 1955; Miller et al., 1958). Grafius (1956, 1960) suggested that for a desired response to selection the hereditary control of a complex character, such as yield, can be manipulated more efficiently by considering its more simple components. In this study, attempts were made at a test of the potential effectiveness of selection indices obtained from genotypic and phenotypic variance and covariance estimates involving various combinations of yield or its components, or both.

MATERIALS AND METHODS

The population used for the present study was obtained from a synthetic variety developed from five U.S. cornbelt dent-inbred lines and three flint varieties taken from among local land varieties. After being produced in 1966, the synthetic variety was left to sib-pollinate for two generations and was then subjected to selfing. Of the 600 self-pollinated (S_0) plants, 90 were discarded as showing grossly defective agronomic traits, and 510 were used for further inbreeding. The progenies of some of these plants did not survive in the subsequent selfings; therefore, the S_5 generation consisted of 350 inbred lines, which was sufficient for our purpose. Of these 350 lines, 100 were taken at random and partitioned into 10 groups of 10 lines each. Of the 10 lines in each group, five were used as males and five as females in a diallel cross. Sets of 25 F_1 progenies were thus obtained for each of the 10 groups. The synthetic variety was included as a check in each set so that the experiment consisted of a total of 260 entries.

The experiment was grown in 1974 at two locations. The design used consisted of randomized complete blocks with two replications at each location. Each replication consisted of 10 groups of 26 entries (25 F_1 + synthetic) each. The groups within replications and the entries within groups were randomized. Plots were one-row plots of 15 hills each. When possible, 10 plants were harvested from each plot, and on each plant the following data were recorded:

Yield	Grams of grain per plant (at 0% moisture)
Ear index	[(gwt 2) ÷ (gwt 1) + 1] where gwt 2 and gwt 1 are, respectively, the weights of grain in the second and the first ears of a plant
Number of rows of kernels	Average number of rows of kernels in the first ear
Number of kernels per row	Average of three rows in the first ear
100-kernel weight	Weight (grams) of 600 kernels at 0% moisture adjusted to 100 kernels

The genetic design used for this study is generally referred to as design II of Comstock and Robinson (1948, 1952). This design can be used for materials at any level of homozygosity by taking into account the coefficient of inbreeding in computing the genetic expectations of the components of variance.

Analyses of variance were performed for all the characters at each location and for both locations combined, using plant means per plot. The sets of 26 entries each were first analyzed individually followed by pooling the results over all sets. The form of the combined analysis of variance is given in Table I. The estimates of the components of variance were obtained from the mean squares of this combined analysis of variance. The genetic interpretation of the components of variance s_m^2, s_f^2, and s_{mf}^2 were given by Comstock and Robinson (1948, 1952) and by Cockerham (1954). This interpretation assumes regular diploid meiosis, no multiple allelism, no epistasis, no linkage, equal viability of both gametes and zygotes, randomly sampled inbred lines, and random fluctuation of environmental effects. The validity of these assumptions implies that the components of variance s_m^2, s_f^2, and s_{mf}^2 are entirely genetic in nature and that they therefore have the following expectations:

$$s_m^2 = s_f^2 = \tfrac{1}{4}(1 + F)s_g^2 \quad \text{or} \quad (s_m^2 + s_f^2) = \tfrac{1}{2}(1 + F)s_g^2$$

and

$$s_{mf}^2 = \tfrac{1}{4}(1 + F)^2 s_d^2$$

where s_g^2 is the additive genetic variance, s_d^2 is the nonadditive genetic variance (dominance variance), and F is the coefficient of inbreeding of the parent plants

Table I. General Form of the Combined Analysis of Variance

Source of variation	Degrees of freedom (DF)	Expectations of mean squares
Locations (L)	$L-1$	
Replications (r) in L	$(r-1)L$	
Sets (b)	$b-1$	
$b \times L$	$(b-1)(L-1)$	
($b \times r$) in L	$(b-1)(r-1)L$	
Males (m) in b	$(m-1)b$	$s_e^2 + rs_{mfL}^2 + rfs_{mL}^2 + rLs_{mf}^2 + rLs_m^2$
Females (f) in b	$(f-1)b$	$s_e^2 + rs_{mfL}^2 + rms_{fL}^2 + rLs_{mf}^2 + rLs_f^2$
($m \times f$) in b	$(m-1)(f-1)b$	$s_e^2 + rs_{mfL}^2 + rLs_{mf}^2$
($m \times L$) in b	$(m-1)(L-1)b$	$s_e^2 + rs_{mfL}^2 + rfs_{mL}^2$
($f \times L$) in b	$(f-1)(L-1)b$	$s_e^2 + rs_{sfL}^2 + rms_{fL}^2$
($m \times f \times L$) in b	$(m-1)(f-1)(L-1)b$	$s_e^2 + rs_{mfL}^2$
Pooled error	$(m-1)(f-1)(r-1)bl$	s_e^2
Total	$Lbrmf-1$	

involved. In the present case, $F = 0.9375$, and therefore $s_g^2 = 1.03225(s_m^2 + s_f^2)$ and $s_d^2 = 1.06555\, s_{mf}^2$.

The variance among plot means, i.e., the phenotypic variance s_p^2 was calculated for each character as follows:

$$s_p^2 = s_m^2 + s_f^2 + s_{mf}^2 + (1/L)(s_{mL}^2 + s_{fL}^2 + s_{mfL}^2) + (1/rL)s_e^2$$

The estimates of genotypic and phenotypic covariances between any two traits were derived in the same manner as were the corresponding variances.

The selection indices used to determine the expected advance from selection for yield were obtained by means of phenotypic and genotypic variances, as well as by covariances calculated from the data. The procedure followed was that of Robinson et al. (1951). The general form of a selection index is $b_1 X_1 + b_2 X_2 + \cdots + b_n X_n$, where $X_{i=1,2,\ldots n}$ represents the phenotypic value of the ith trait and $b_{i=1,2\ldots n}$ its weight.

The general formulae of the set of simultaneous equations for obtaining the weights b_i required in the calculation of a selection index are

$$b_1 p_{11} + b_2 p_{12} + \cdots + b_n p_{1n} = g_{1y}$$

$$b_1 p_{12} + b_2 p_{22} + \cdots + b_n p_{2n} = g_{2y}$$

$$\cdot \qquad \cdot$$
$$\cdot \qquad \cdot$$
$$\cdot \qquad \cdot$$

$$b_1 p_{1n} + b_2 p_{2n} + \cdots + b_n p_{nn} = g_{ny}$$

where p_{11}, p_{12}, etc., refer to phenotypic variances and covariances, and g_{1y},

g_{2y}, etc., to genotypic covariances among full-sib families with respect to the characters measured and the character to be improved.

The expected genetic advance from the use of a selection index was obtained by means of the formula $k(b_1g_{1y} + b_2g_{2y} + \cdots + b_ng_{ny})^{1/2}$, where k is the selection difference (in standard units), which for a 5% selection pressure in a normally distributed population has a value of 2.06.

RESULTS AND DISCUSSION

Character means of the synthetic variety and of the F_1 progeny of crosses among the inbred lines derived from it are given in Table II. None of the differences between the synthetic variety and the F_1 progeny means in Table II were statistically significant. This shows that the offspring resulting from the mating system used for this study had the same constitution as the original random mating population, and that the partition of the variance among the full-sib and half-sib families was expected to be the same.

The data were analyzed for each location separately, and also for the two locations combined. The results for the combined analyses are given in Table III. As shown in Table III, the variances caused by male and female effects, and to male $\times$ female interaction effects, were significant for all five characters studied. Interactions involving location effects were significant for some, but not all, characters.

The estimates of various components of variance calculated from data in Table III on the basis of the expected mean squares as listed in Table I, are given in Table IV. The estimates of s_m^2, s_f^2, and s_{mf}^2, which are presumably genetical, were significantly different from zero for all the characters studied.

The estimates of genotypic and phenotypic variances and covariances used in obtaining the selection indices, and from them the expected response to selection, are given in Tables V and VI, respectively. The selection responses expected in the present case from the use of various selection indices are given in

Table II. The Means of the Synthetic Variety and the F_1 Progenies

Character	Synthetic variety	F_1 progenies
Yield (g) per plant	164.52	164.45
Ear index	1.04	1.03
Number of rows of kernels per ear	17.74	17.04
Number of kernels per row	41.84	42.46
100-kernel weight (g)	23.31	23.73

Table III. The Results of the Combined Analysis of Variance for Yield and the Four Components of Yield

Sources of variation	DF	Mean squares for characters[a]				
		a	b	c	d	e
Males (m)	40	1956.29^b	0.0145^b	19.07^b	86.21^b	64.70^b
Females (f)	40	1065.27^c	0.0259^b	20.93^b	65.81^b	79.27^b
$m \times f$	160	441.60^b	0.0058^b	0.92^b	11.95^b	4.81^b
$m \times$ locations (L)	40	351.69^b	0.0031	0.29	5.15^c	2.07
$f \times L$	40	379.59^b	0.0060^b	0.50	6.53^b	1.94
$m \times f \times L$	160	191.91	0.0024^b	0.35	3.22^c	1.47
Pooled error	480	157.49	0.0016	0.29	2.40	1.31

[a]Characters: (a) yield, (b) ear index, (c) number of rows of kernels per ear, (d) number of kernels per row, (e) 100-kernel weight.
[b]$p \leqslant 0.01$.
[c]$0.01 < \underline{p} \leqslant 0.05$.

Table VII. In Table VII columns 1–5 show, correspondingly, the number of the order of the selection indices, the characters on which the calculation of the corresponding indices were based, the expected response to selection (increase in yield in grams of grain per plant) from each index, the relative efficiency of the indices in relation to the efficiency of yield alone equated to 100, and the relative (%) selection responses expected from the use of individual indices as criteria of selection for yield. The calculation of these responses was based on the knowledge that the average yield of grain per plant in the synthetic variety (base population) was 164.52 g (see Table II).

Table IV. The Estimates of the Components of Variance

Components of variance	Genetic expectations	Estimates for the characters[a]				
		a	b	c	d	e
s_m^2	$(1 + F)s_g^2 \div 4$	67.75	0.00041	0.910	3.617	2.964
s_f^2	$(1 + F)s_g^2 \div 4$	21.80	0.00082	0.993	2.528	3.699
s_{mf}^2	$(1 + F)^2 s_d^2 \div 4$	62.42	−0.00086	0.143	2.181	0.836
s_{mL}^2	—	15.98	0.00007	0.006	0.193	0.060
s_{fL}^2	—	18.77	0.00036	0.015	0.330	0.948
s_{mfL}^2	—	17.21	0.00039	0.029	0.041	0.079
s_e^2	—	157.49	0.00162	0.292	2.401	1.310

[a]Characters: (a) Yield, (b) ear index, (c) number of rows of kernels per ear, (d) number of kernels per row, (e) 100-kernel weight.

Table V. The Estimates of Additive Genetic Variances and Covariances among Full-Sib Families[a]

Characters	Characters[b]				
	a	b	c	d	e
a	(89.545)	−0.07993	2.3171	−2.1595	11.8300
b	−	(0.00123)	−0.00600	0.00617	−0.00285
c	−	−	(1.903)	−0.15111	1.9278
d	−	−	−	(6.145)	−3.6611
e	−	−	−	−	(6.664)

[a] Estimates of additive genetic variances in parentheses.
[b] Characters: (a) Yields, (b) ear index, (c) number of rows of kernels per ear, (d) number of kernels per row, (e) 100-kernel weight.

The figures in Table VII show that selection for yield based on ear index, number of kernel rows, number of kernels per row, and 100-kernel weight considered individually, are not expected to be as effective as the selection based on plant yield alone. In contrast, the selection index involving all four of them is expected to have an efficiency 9.33% higher than that of yield itself. Generally, indices 2 to 12 are expected to be as efficient as, or more efficient than, the yield alone (index 1) when used as criteria of selection for yield. The figures in columns 4 and 5 (Table VII) show that the highest increase in relative efficiency was 14.44% and that this increase corresponds only to 0.95% increase in response to selection. Furthermore, all selection indices, with the exception of those based on single characters (Nos. 13 to 16), appear to be as good as, or slightly better (0.52−0.95%) than, yield alone when used as predictors of the improvement in yield in relationship to that of the base population.

Table VI. The Estimates of Phenotypic Variances and Covariances among Plot Means

Characters	Characters[b]				
	a	b	c	d	e
a	(217.3179)	0.03092	3.6625	10.9661	16.4771
b	−	(0.00289)	−0.00261	−0.00769	−0.03437
c	−	−	(2.1382)	−0.00520	−2.1072
d	−	−	−	(9.2079)	−3.7044
e	−	−	−	−	(7.9199)

[a] Estimates of phenotypic variances in parentheses.
[b] Characters: (a) Yield, (b) ear index, (c) number of rows of kernels per ear, (d) number of kernels per row, (e) 100-kernel weight.

Table VII. Expected Genetic Advance (Response to Selection in Yield from the Use of Various Selection Indices and Their Relative Efficiency

No. of order of indices	Indices based on characters[a]					Expected increase in yield (advance) (g/plant)	Relative efficiency (%)	Expected relative advance in yield (%)
	a	b	c	d	e			
1	+	−	−	−	−	12.51	100.00	7.60
2	+	+	+	+	+	14.07	112.44	8.55
3	+	+	+	−	+	14.07	112.44	8.55
4	+	−	+	+	+	14.03	112.15	8.53
5	+	+	+	+	−	13.92	111.28	8.46
6	+	+	+	−	+	13.90	111.11	8.45
7	+	+	−	+	−	13.90	111.11	8.45
8	−	−	+	+	+	13.85	110.67	8.42
9	−	+	+	+	+	13.68	109.33	8.31
10	+	−	+	+	−	13.46	107.60	8.18
11	+	−	−	+	−	13.36	106.75	8.12
12	−	−	+	−	+	12.46	99.60	7.57
13	−	+	−	−	−	−2.70	−21.58	−1.64
14	−	−	+	−	−	3.26	26.09	1.98
15	−	−	−	+	−	−1.47	−11.75	−0.89
16	−	−	−	−	+	8.66	69.22	5.26

[a]Characters: (a)Yield, (b) ear index, (c) number of rows of kernels per ear, (d) number of kernels per row, (e) 100-kernel weight.

The estimates of variances and the expected improvements in yield by means of selection presented in this study are, generally, similar to those reported by Horner et al. (1955), Gardner et al. (1953), and Gardner (1961) for different maize populations. Some of the assumptions underlying the calculation of the estimates of genetic variances in the present case may not hold. However, as noted by Comstock and Robinson (1952), Horner (1952), Horner et al. (1955), Robinson et al. (1955), Cockerham (1954), and Kempthorne (1957), the failure of some hypotheses does not seriously affect the estimates of various parameters, and in the presence of considerable additive genetic variation in the population, the improvement by means of selection may not be affected. Selection indices calculated from data on yield and its component appear to be the most efficient ones, a fact noted also by Robinson et al. (1951), and by Subandi et al. (1973). However, some indices based on yield components only, as index 8 in the present case for instance, may be quite satisfactory when used as criteria of selection for yield.

REFERENCES

Cockerham, C. C. (1954). An extension of the concept of partitioning hereditary variance for analysis of covariance when epistasis is present. *Genetics 39*:859–882.

Comstock, R. E. and Robinson, H. F. (1948). The components of genetic variance in populations. *Biometrics 4*:254–266.

Comstock, R. E. and Robinson, H. F. (1952). Estimation of average dominance of genes. Heterosis, pp. 494–516. Iowa State College Press, Ames, Ia.

Gardner, C. O. (1961). An evaluation of effects of mass selection and seed irradiation with thermal neutrons on yield of corn. *Crop Sci. 1*:241–245.

Gardner, C. O., Harvey, P. H., Comstock, R. E., and Robinson, H. F. (1953). Dominance of genes controlling quantitative characters in maize. *Agron. J. 45*:186–191.

Grafius, J. E. (1956). Components of yield in oats: A geometrical interpretation. *Agron. J. 48*:419–423.

Grafius, J. E. (1960). Does overdominance exist for yield in corn? *Agron. J. 52*:361.

Horner, T. W. (1952). Non-allelic gene interactions and the interpretation of quantitative genetic data. Ph.D. dissertation. North Carolina State College Library.

Horner, T. W., Comstock, R. E., and Robinson, H. F. (1955). Non-allelic gene interactions in the interpretation of quantitative genetic data. *NC Agr. Exp. Sta. Tech. Bull.* 118, 117 pp.

Johnson, H. W., Robinson, H. F., and Comstock, R. E. (1955). Genotypic and phenotypic correlations in soybeans and their implications in selection. *Agron. J. 47*:477–483.

Kempthorne, O. (1957). *An Introduction to Genetic Statistics,* 545 pp. Wiley, New York.

Kuhn, W. E. and Stucker, R. E. (1973). Selection indices to improve yield and ears per plant in corn. In *Agronomy Abstracts,* American Society of Agronomy, Madison, Wisconsin.

Manning, A. L. (1955). Response to selection for yield in cotton. *Cold Spring Harbor. Symp. Quant. Biol. 20*:103–110.

Miller, P. R., Williams, Jr., J. C., Robinson, H. F., and Comstock, R. E. (1958). Estimates of genotypic and environmental variances and covariances in upland cotton and their implications in selection. *Agron. J. 50*:126–131.

Robinson, H. F., Comstock, R. E., and Harvey, P. H. (1951). Genotypic and phenotypic correlations in corn and their implications in selection. *Agron J. 43*:283–287.

Robinson, H. F., Comstock, R. E. and Harvey, P. H. (1955). Genetic variances in open pollinated varieties of corn. *Genetics 40*:46–60.

Smith, H. F. (1936). A discriminant function for plant selection. *Ann. Eug. 7*:240–260.

Subandi, Compton, W. A., and Empig, L. T. (1973). Comparison of the efficiencies of selection indices for three traits in two variety crosses of corn. *Crop Sci. 13*:184–186.

25

Quantitative Genetically Nonequivalent Reciprocal Crosses in Cultivated Plants

Rustem Aksel

Department of Genetics
University of Alberta
Edmonton, Alberta, Canada T6G 2E9

ABSTRACT

Quantitative expressions of character difference between reciprocal crosses have been studied by different researchers in a number of plant species, such as *Epilobium, Zea mays, Oryza sativa, Hordeum sativum, Triticum aestivum, Trifolium hybridum, Linum usitatissimum, Nicotiana rustica,* and others. In all cases it was found that the nonequivalence of reciprocal crosses manifested itself beginning with the F_1 generation, with the exception of some flax crosses in which reciprocals differed beginning with the F_2 generation. The nonequivalence of reciprocal crosses usually manifested itself in the inequality of their F_1 and/or F_2 or backcross means; however, there were instances in which their means were the same but the variances were different. Both matroclinous and patroclinous inheritances were reported in plants. Because of the causal complexity of reciprocal differences the experimental results often lack a simple explanation.

INTRODUCTION

As far back as 1901 Correns had expressed the view that in some instances the manifestation of the character in the offspring may depend on both the nuclear and the extranuclear factors; he stated that "A consequence of this view is that the mechanism of development of the offspring will be essentially that of the female parent" (Correns, 1901). Since that time, numerous cases of both qualitative and quantitative expressions of character differences between reciprocal crosses have been investigated. In particular, the qualitative character, cytoplasmic male sterility, most likely because of its actual and prospective importance in the economic exploitation of hybrid vigor in cultivated plants, has been the subject of many studies (see, for example, Edwardson, 1956; Duvick, 1959, 1966; Hadjinov, 1968; Palilova, 1969; Krupnov, 1971). This article gives a short review of cases of quantitative genetic nonequivalence for intraspecific reciprocal crosses in cultivated plants. For a comprehensive study, recourse should be made to pertinent publications.

As stated by Durrant (1965), there is no one universally recognized mechanism which could be considered accountable for character-expression differences between reciprocal crosses. Different methods have been formulated for the analysis of such differences. In the majority of cases, the quantitative genetic nonequivalence of reciprocal crosses manifested itself beginning with the F_1 generation. Instances in which such differences fail to manifest themselves in F_1, but which gain expression in F_2, F_3, and the backcross generations, have been reported for some *Linum* crosses (Durrant and Tyson, 1964; Smith and Fitzsimmons, 1964, 1965; Tyson, 1973). These cases were similar to those of Bateson and Gairdner (1921) and Gairdner (1929) on the inheritance of male sterility in flax. The results of the studies of some quantitative genetically nonequivalent reciprocal crosses in *Zea mays* L. (maize), *Oryza sativa* L. (rice), *Hordeum vulgare* L. (barley), *Triticum aestivum* L. (common wheat), *Linum usitatissimum* L. (flax, linseed), *Trifolium hybridum* L. (Alsike clover), and *Nicotiana rustica* L. are given, in an abridged form, in sequence.

Zea mays L. (Maize)

Richey (1920) reported significant differences in yield between reciprocal crosses of maise. Similar results were also reported by Hoen and Andrew (1957). Fleming et al. (1960) found that the differences between reciprocal crosses of maize occur for many characters and that the degree of expression of these differences depends on the environment. Among the recent studies on reciprocal maize crosses are those of Bhat and Dhavan (1970, 1971) and Garwood et al. (1970). In their 1970 publication, Bhat and Dhavan based their analyses on individual sets, each consisting of two parents, their reciprocal crosses, and backcrosses. The comparisons between the reciprocals in each set were made at three nuclear levels, viz. 75% A as in the backcrosses (A ×B)F_1 × A and (B × A)F_1 × A, 50% A as in the reciprocals (A × B)F_1 and (B × A)F_1, and 25% A as in the backcrosses (A × B)F_1 × B and (B × A)F_1 × B, where A and B refer to the two parents. The characters studied in eight different sets were grain yield (kilograms per hectare), maturity (in days to 75% silking), plant height (centimeters) and ear height (centimeters). In all sets the reciprocal differences for maturity, plant height, and ear height were significant at either one or two nuclear levels. The same was true for yield in all but one set, where the reciprocal differences were significant at all three nuclear levels. From the results obtained, the authors have concluded that in their crosses the cytoplasmic effect expressed itself only when the genes of one parent remained below a certain threshold of concentration in the hybrid nucleus.

For their 1971 study, Bhat and Dhavan reciprocally crossed and backcrossed some of the varieties used for their 1970 work. With the exception of number of ears per plant, the characters considered were the same. The inheritance of number of ears per plant was found to be of the usual nuclear kind. The cause of observed reciprocal differences for grain yield, maturity, plant height, and ear height was explained by the authors as being caused by the sensitivity of nuclear genes to maternal cytoplasm.

Garwood et al. (1970) reciprocally crossed the maize strains Illinois High Oil and Illinois Low Oil and seven inbred lines. The characters studied were plant and ear height as well as oil and fatty acid contents in the kernels. They found that the maternal and paternal effects on oil and fatty acid contents were quite pronounced in the reciprocal crosses, and that these effects were more or less equal. In some of the reciprocal crosses between Illinois High Oil and inbred lines, the oil content, plant height, and ear height showed cytoplasmic effects. However, with the possible exception of ear height, these effects were rather small. It was observed that the cytoplasmic effects were frequently in opposition to what would have been expected from maternal differences.

Oryza sativa L. (Rice)

Chandraratna and Sakai (1960) studied the inheritance of seed weight (grams per 100 seeds) in F_1, F_2, and F_3 generations of reciprocal crosses between two rice varieties that differed significantly for this character ($\bar{P}_1$ = 1.78 g and $\bar{P}_2$ = 3.02 g/100 seeds). The analyses of family (generation) means and of second-degree statistics were based on biometrical models formulated by the authors on the assumption that a system of extranuclear determinants interacting with the genotype was transmitted to the progeny through the maternal cytoplasm, thereby affecting the character expression in the progeny. As far as their data were concerned, the authors found that the maternal effect in seed-weight inheritance was 32%. Narrow- and broad-sense heritabilities were estimated to be 40% and 77%, respectively. On theoretical grounds it was concluded that heritability must be inversely correlated with the maternal effect and that the difference between reciprocals would be expected to diminish with each subsequent generation of selfing, a fact that appears to apply to their data. In the opinion of Sakai et al. (1961), cytoplasmic inheritance of polygenic characters is important from the points of view of evolution and breeding work, because it decreases the amount of genetic variation and covariation between two consecutive generations of the hybrid population, and thereby lowers the efficiency of selection.

Hordeum vulgare L. (Barley)

The inheritance of several metrical traits in reciprocal crosses of barley were studied by Nečas (1961–1963, 1966). For his 1966 study Nečas used as parents two two-rowed varieties (*Hordeum vulgare* L. ssp. *distichum* Thell) and three six-rowed varieties (*Hordeum vulgare* L. ssp. *polystichum* Schnitz *et* Keller). The characters studied were plant shape (habitus), tillering, development of lateral spikelets, spike length, seed weight, germination velocity (energy of germination) of seeds, and β-amylase activity. The evaluation of data obtained involved testing the significance of differences between reciprocal crosses, as well as plotting the frequency distribution of data for the parents and their reciprocal crosses. With respect to plant shape, the reciprocals were definitely different in F_1. These differences appeared to persist as well in F_2 and F_3 generations, but were blurred by segregation. Data on tillering were available for the F_1 generation of two crosses only, and only in one cross were the reciprocals significantly different. As the average tiller numbers of the reciprocals were practically the same as those of their female parent, the inheritance appeared to be completely maternal. The trends of the inheritance of development of lateral spikelets in reciprocal crosses, recorded on a five-grade scale, were mainly of maternal type, and persisted in F_2, F_3, and the backcross generations. But most of the reciprocal differences were not significant at the 5% level of probability. With regard to spike length, the differences between reciprocals were not significant in either F_1 or F_2 generations, but they did figure significantly in most of the backcrosses, where the general and consistent trend was toward the female parent. The inheritance of seed weight in reciprocal crosses and backcrosses was preponderantly matroclinous, and this trend persisted in the F_2 and the F_3 generations; however, in most, if not in all cases, the reciprocal differences were not significant at the $P = 5\%$ level. Strong maternal effects in the F_1 generation of reciprocal crosses were recorded for the character-germination velocity of the seeds. The segregating generations were not studied, and it is therefore not known if the observed differences between the reciprocal crosses were persistent. The β-amylase activity was studied in only the parents and the F_1 generation of their reciprocal crosses. Of the eight differences between the reciprocals, seven were statistically significant, of which five showed matroclinous and two patroclinous mode of inheritance. Because the segregating generations were not studied, it is unknown whether these differences were persistent.

Triticum aestivum L. (Common Wheat)

It appears that intraspecific reciprocal cross differences in *Triticum* have a rather low frequency of occurrence. Reciprocal differences in common wheat

· crosses have been observed for some qualitative and quantitative characters. Thus, Lyashchenko (1971) reported that of the 17 reciprocal crosses between spring (alternative) and winter common wheat varieties, four showed maternal inheritance of habit of growth (development). Soomro (1974), in a study of the genetics of quantitative traits in a five-parent diallel cross of common wheat, found that the differences in plant height between reciprocal crosses of varieties INIA and Chinook and especially of INIA and Marquis were persistently significant over environments (two locations) and generations (F_1, F_2, and back-crosses).

A current project in progress at the Department of Genetics, University of Alberta (Canada) is centered on the study of inheritance of quantitative traits in reciprocal crosses and backcrosses between winter and spring varieties of common wheat. The results obtained from a preliminary yield trial on the F_2 generation of reciprocal crosses are given in Table I (Aksel, unpublished). The F_1 generation of all three crosses headed when spring-sown, thus showing that the spring habit of growth was inherited as a dominant trait. The seed-producing plant density in the V-belt-sown F_2 plots appeared to be the same for all three pairs of reciprocals (roughly 75% of the emerged plants). Therefore, as far as this trial was concerned, the comparisons between reciprocals were valid and reliable. Of the three reciprocal pairs, two have produced a higher grain yield when the female parent was the spring variety, and one when the female parent was the winter variety. In this last case 1000-kernel weight was positively associated with the yield of grain. For one pair of reciprocals, total yield and grain yield were positively associated.

Table I. Winter by Spring Common Wheat Reciprocal Cross Differences for Total Yield (Straw + Grain), Grain Yield, and 1000-Kernel Weight in F_2 Generation[a]

Reciprocal crosses[b]	Total yield (kg/100 m²)	Grain yield (kg/100 m²)	Kernel weight (g/1000 kernels)
(J × K)F_2	158.33 ± 5.00	14.77 ± 1.13	24.29 ± 0.77
(K × J)F_2	202.00 ± 9.67	25.57 ± 1.37	24.21 ± 0.32
Difference	−43.67 ± 11.00[c]	−10.80 ± 1.73[c]	ns
(S × K)F_2	195.00 ± 5.00	34.47 ± 1.13	25.00 ± 0.77
(K × S)F_2	201.33 ± 9.67	39.87 ± 1.37	26.07 ± 0.32
Difference	ns[d]	−5.40 ± 1.73[c]	ns
(L × G)F_2	171.00 ± 5.00	21.60 ± 1.13	25.35 ± 0.77
(G × L)F_2	158.00 ± 9.67	13.33 ± 1.37	23.29 ± 0.32
Difference	ns	+8.27 ± 1.73[c]	2.06 ± 0.83[c]

[a]Seeding date: May 14, 1974. Plot size: 3 m². Replications: 4.
[b]Winter parents: Jones Fife (J), Sakhalin (S), and Leda (L). Spring parents: Khush-ha1 (K), and Gabo (G).
[c]$0.01 < p < 0.05$.
[d]ns, $p > 0.05$.

Linum usitatissimum L. (Flax, Linseed)

Durrant and Tyson (1964) studied the inheritance of plant, side-shoot, and center-shoot weights in a six-parent diallel cross of *Linum usitatissimum* L. The parental set of the diallel cross consisted of two flax varieties, two linseed varieties, and the genotrophs Large (L) and Small (S) produced by Durrant (1962*a,b*) from a plastic flax variety Stormont Cirrus by means of environmental induction. The analysis of the F_1 and F_2 diallel cross data showed that, with regard to generation means, the reciprocal crosses were the same. But the variances within the F_2 reciprocals were significantly different. The variances within $(L \times S)F_2$ and $(S \times L)F_2$, for instance, were found to be 357 and 671, respectively. These differences in variation were not reflected in the effectual reduction of the dominance in the respective F_2 reciprocals. According to Durrant and Tyson, this suggests that the change in dominance might have been caused by processes other than segregation. The variances of log plant weights of F_2 families were further analyzed by Durrant (1965). This analysis showed that the male parents were largely determining the character of the offspring when crossed to genotroph S, and female parents were largely determining the character of the offspring when crossed to genotroph L. The nonequivalence of reciprocal crosses has not expressed itself in an overall trend toward either a matro- or a patroclinous inheritance. Both types of inheritance were present in the diallel cross.

In another study, Tyson (1973) used a four-parent diallel cross. The parental set consisted of genotrophs L and S and the varieties Mandarin and Dakota. The character studied was plant weight. No differences between the mean measurements of the reciprocal crosses were observed in the F_1 generation. The complete data obtained from the reciprocal crosses and backcrosses, selfs included, were arranged into five 4×4 diallel tables of the $(P_1, F_{1(12)}, F_{1(21)}, P_2)^2$ type. Detailed analyses made on the logarithmic (ln) values of progeny means in these five tables showed that in most cases the reciprocals were different. Cytoplasmic action and interaction effects were detected in the segregating generations, and it was found that a depressant cytoplasmic effect was transmitted through the female gametes of L.

The inheritance of plasticity was studied by Durrant and Timmis (1973) in reciprocal crosses and backcrosses between the plastic (Pl) and nonplastic (R) flax varieties Stormont Cirrus and Royal, respectively. The materials were tested for plasticity by determining the changes in the amount of DNA when grown in specific change-inducing environments of nitrogen (N) and phosphorus (P). The nuclear DNA contents of 4-week-old shoot apices were measured by Feulgen photometry according to the procedure described by Evans (1968). The DNA measurements in the two parents and the F_1 generation of their reciprocal crosses grown in N and P environments showed that the changes in DNA contents were induced in Pl and $(Pl \times R)F_1$, but not in $(R \times Pl)F_1$ and R. The amount of nuclear DNA was much higher in $(Pl \times R)F_1$ than in its reciprocal. The difference in plasticity between the reciprocals manifested itself also in their F_2 generation grown in a noninducing environment, showing thus the change to be heritable. However, because the difference between the reciprocals in F_2 was diminished, these workers have expressed the view that the induced change may eventually disappear.

A second group of materials consisting of the same two parents, their reciprocal crosses, and the first and repeated backcrosses were grown by the authors in the change-inducing N and P environments, where they were tested for nuclear DNA content. The statistical analysis of experimental data showed that the components of variation attributable to environmental and genotypic differences, and to genotype $\times$ environment interaction effects, were all significant at the 5% level of probability. Similar results were obtained for a third group involving the same parents, Pl and R, and their first backcrosses, and grown in the same change-inducing condition but at a lower pH. The induced (N − P) differences between the plastic and nonplastic parents in this third group were slightly higher than those in the second group. If the (N − P) differences obtained by the authors for the second group are adjusted to a level comparable to that given by them for the third group, the results of the two groups can then be shown jointly, as in Table II. The interpretation of the results in this table is that given by the authors themselves, but restated in a slightly different form, viz.

1. In plasmatypically Pl families, the change from a plastic to a nonplastic type appears to be gradual and follows the reduction of the plastic (Pl) content

Table II. Induced (N−P) Differences in *Linum*
Varieties Stormont Cirrus (Pl) and Royal (R) and in
Their Reciprocal Crosses and Backcrosses

Group	Family	Pl in the nucleus (%)	N − P (%)
I	Pl	100.000	18.1
	Pl⁵ × R	96.875	21.3
	Pl² × R	75.000	19.1
	Pl × R	50.000	17.9
	Pl × R²	25.000	15.0
	Pl × R⁵	3.125	2.7
II	R	0.000	2.5
	R⁵ × Pl	3.125	−2.0
	R² × Pl	25.000	—
	R × Pl	50.000	0.6
	R × Pl²	75.000	—
	R × Pl⁵	96.875	2.0

in the nucleus. When repeated backcrossing to the nonplastic parent R reduces the Pl content of the nucleus to 3.125%, the plasticity is lost (the N − P differences for Pl × R^5 and R are 2.7% and 2.5%, respectively, i.e., practically the same).

2. In plasmatypically R families, the change of the nuclear content from 0% Pl to 96.875% Pl has not conferred plasticity to the plants (the N − P difference for R and R × Pl^5 are, respectively, 2.5% and 2%, i.e., not significantly different).

These results led the authors to the conclusion that the plastic parent Stormont Cirrus must contain nuclear and cytoplasmic factors, both of which have to be present for the plastic character to manifest itself, but at the same time the other parent, viz. the nonplastic parent Royal, although deprived of these factors, must possess sites at which changes in the amount of nuclear DNA could occur when the necessary factors were provided by a plastic parent such as Stormont Cirrus. In these experiments, the authors have found that the induced change in nuclear DNA was always associated with a corresponding change in plant weight. Their view was that the two characters were probably controlled by the same regulatory system.

The inheritance of seed weight in *Linum* was studied by Smith and Fitzsimmons (1964, 1965). Reciprocal crosses and backcrosses of linseed varieties Redwing and Beta-210 plus Redwing and Humpata were used as materials. Beta-210 and Humpata have considerably higher 1000-seed weights than Redwing. A detailed account of the results obtained from Redwing (*R*) and Beta-210 (*B*) reciprocal crosses and backcrosses was given by Smith and Aksel (1974). The generalized expression, or model, for the expected mean measurement of a family was formulated as follows (Aksel, 1974):

$$E_{\bar{x}}(XY)F_n = m + (p-r)[d] + q([h] + \Delta_{[h]}) + \Delta_{[d]}$$

where X and Y are the female and the male parents, respectively, ($X = R,B,(RB)F,(BR)F_1$ and $Y = R,B(RB)F_1$, $(BR)F_1$ in this particular case); p, q, and r are the cross- and generation-specific coefficients ($p + q + r = 1$); $\Delta_{[h]}$ and $\Delta_{[d]}$ represent the amounts of change in genotypic values $[h]$ and $[d]$ owing to plasma sensitivity of paternal genes in heterozygous and homozygous states, respectively. The system of linear equations deriving from the model may or may not have a solution, depending on particular assumptions, a fact not stated explicitly at the time (Aksel, 1974). For Smith-Fitzsimmons's data, the system of equations had a solution.

The difference $\bar{x}(RB)F_n - x(BR)F_n$ was practically zero for $n = 1$, but was significant for $n = 2$ and $n = 3$ (−1.60 ± 0.29** and −1.11 ± 0.15**, respectively). It was therefore obvious that reciprocal crosses were not equivalent with respect to the character seed weight, but this nonequivalence manifested itself beginning with the F$_2$ generation and persisted in the F$_3$ generation. Appropriate tests on backcrosses and their first selfed generation led to the same conclusion. Moreover, there were indications that the nuclear genes of Beta-210 were sensitive to Redwing cytoplasm, whereas those of Redwing were not affected by the cytoplasm of Beta-210. Subsequently, the 22 hybrid family means were partitioned equally into two supposedly genotypically similar, but plasmatypically different, groups. The family means in either group, and those of the two parents, were expressed in terms of appropriate parameters, and the resulting two systems of linear equations were solved in the manner of a joint scaling test (see, for example, Mather and Jinks, 1971). The analysis of the results obtained led to the conclusion that the nonequivalence of reciprocal crosses resulted in this particular case from the joint action of nuclear and cytoplasmic factors. It was estimated that the nuclear genes of Beta-210, when acting in Redwing cytoplasm, have lost $\simeq 75\%$ of their expressivity, about 20% of this loss being caused by the suppressive action of nuclear factors, and the rest by that of cytoplasmic factors carried by Redwing. Some gene–dosis effects were detected in the plasmatypically Beta-210 backcrosses.

Trifolium hybridum L. (Alsike Clover)

In 1947, Yates published his method of analysis of data from all possible reciprocal crosses between a set of parental lines (Yates, 1947). Basically, the method assesses the breeding values of the parents and tests for the presence and reliability of differences between reciprocal crosses. The experimental data used by Yates were on fertility in a 12-parent F_1 diallel cross of Alsike clover, the fertility being expressed as the number of seeds obtained per 100 fertilized florets. Out of 12 parents, five were found to exceed the rest for fertility in their crosses. The observed differences between the reciprocal crosses were, on the average, neither large nor quite significant. Nevertheless, at least for some reciprocal crosses in the set, there were strong indications as to the direction of crossing which could secure the better fertility in their offspring.

Nicotiana rustica L.

A study of reciprocal-cross differences for metrical traits in *Nicotiana rustica* L. was conducted by Jinks et al. (1972). Two varieties, #2 = P_1 and #12 = P_2, were reciprocally crossed and backcrossed. The parents and their F_1 reciprocal crosses were tried in 18 environments. The F_2, F_3, B_1, B_2, $F_2 \times P_1$, $F_2 \times P_2$, $F_2 \times F_1$, and F_2 biparental generations of reciprocals were included in some or most of these trials. The characters studied were flowering time (days after an arbitrary date) and final plant height (centimeters). The analysis of data on F_1 generation showed significant reciprocal differences for both characters. These differences were of a matroclinous type for final height and mostly of a patroclinous type for flowering time. A detailed biometrical analysis of complete data by means of appropriately devised tests showed that the reciprocal effects have persisted up to at least two further generations, that there was interaction between the maternal lines and paternal contributions, and that the two characters studied were interdependent.

CONCLUSION

The phenotypic variation within a plant species is usually attributed to nuclear genetic differences among the individuals and to the action of environmental agencies. Cytoplasmic differences are seldom, if ever, associated with the question of variability. The main reasons for this exclusion, or neglect, possibly are the relatively low frequency of the occurrence of cytoplasmic differences, their causal complexity, and the absence of a clear-cut and generally valid pattern of their inheritance. The present review of some cases of quantitative genetically nonequivalent reciprocal crosses shows that such crosses may have different means beginning with the F_1 or a subsequent generation, that they may have the same means but different variances within the same segregating generation, or, possibly, both different means and variances. Ignoring the transient physiologic—maternal effects, it appears that the cause of persistent differences between some reciprocal crosses is either cytoplasmic, manifesting itself as matroclinous inheritance, or both cytoplasmic and nuclear, in which case the inheritance is either matroclinous or patroclinous, depending on the mode of action of, or interaction between, the cytoplasmic and nuclear factors. There is no question that cytoplasmic factors, like the nuclear factors, contribute to heritable variation of both the qualitative and quantitative characters in a plant species, and, as such, should not be ignored or neglected in the study of variability in plants.

REFERENCES

Aksel, R. (1974). Analysis of means in the case of non-equivalent reciprocal crosses in autogamous plants. *Theoret. Appl. Genet. 45*:96–103.

Bateson, W. and Gairdner, A. E. (1921). Male sterility in flax, subject to two types of segregation. *J. Genet. 11*:269–275.

Bhat, B. K. and Dhavan, N. L. (1970). Threshold concentration of plasmonsensitive polygenes in the expression of quantitative characters of maize. *Theoret. Appl. Genet. 40*:347–350.

Bhat, B. K. and Dhavan, N. L. (1971). The role of cytoplasm in the manifestation of quantitative characters of maize. *Genetica 42*:165–174.

Chandraratna, M. F. and Sakai, K.-I. (1960). A biometrical analysis of matroclinous inheritance of grain weight in rice. *Heredity 14*:365–373.

Correns, I. C. (1901). Die Ergebnisse der neuesten Bastardforschungen für die Vererbungslehre. *Ber. Deut. Bot. Ges. XIX*:71–94.

Durrant, A. 1962*a*. The environmental induction of heritable change in *Linum. Heredity 17*:27–61.

Durrant, A. 1962b. Induction, reversion and epitrophism of flax genotrophs. *Nature* *196*:1302–1304.

Durrant, A. (1965). Analysis of reciprocal differences in diallel crosses. *Heredity 20*: 573–607.

Durrant, A. and Timmis, J. N. (1973). Genetic control of environmentally induced changes in *Linum*. *Heredity 30*:369–379.

Durrant, A. and Tyson, H. (1964). A diallel cross of genotypes and genotrophs of *Linum*. *Heredity 19*:207–227.

Duvick, D. N (1959). The use of cytoplasmic male sterility in hybrid production. *Econ. Bot. 13*:167–195.

Duvick, D. N. (1966). Influence of morphology and sterility on breeding methodology. In *Plant Breeding*. Univ. of Iowa Press, Ames, Ia.

Edwardson, J. R. (1956). Cytoplasmic male sterility. *Bot. Rev. 22*:696–738.

Evans, G. M. (1968). Nuclear changes in flax. *Heredity 23*:25–28.

Fleming, A. A., Kozelnicky, G. M. and Brown, E. B. (1960). Cytoplasmic effects on agronomic characters in a double-cross maize hybrid. *Agron. J. 52*:112–115.

Gairdner, A. E. (1929). Male sterility in flax. II. A case of reciprocal crosses differing in F_2. *J. Genet. 21*:117–127.

Garwood, D. L., Weber, E. J., Lambert, R. J. and Alexander, D. E. (1970. Effect of different cytoplasms on oil, fatty acids, plant height and ear height in maize (*Zea mays* L.). *Crop Sci. 10*:39–41.

Hadjinov, M. I. (1968). Genetic foundations of cytoplasmic male sterility (in Russian). In *Heterosis: Theory and practice*. L., "Kolos" (cited after Krupnov, 1971). *Genetika* *7*:159–174.

Hoen, K. and Andrew, R. H. (1959). Performance of corn hybrids with various ratios of flint-dent germ plasm. *Agron. J. 51*:451–454.

Jinks, J. L. (1956). The F_2 and backcross generations from a set of diallel crosses. *Heredity 10*:1–30.

Jinks, J. L., Perkins, J. M. and Gregory, S. R. (1972). The analysis and interpretation of differences between reciprocal crosses of *Nicotiana rustica* varieties. *Heredity 28*: 363–377.

Krupnov, V. A (1971). Sources of cytoplasmic male sterility in plants (in Russian with English summary). *Genetika 7*:159–174.

Lyashchenko, I. F. (1971). Genetic peculiarities of alternative wheats (in Russian). *Genetika* *7*:20–29.

Mather, K. and Jinks, J. L. (1971). *Biometrical Genetics*. Cornell Univ. Press, Ithaca, N.Y.

Nečas, J. (1961). Inheritance of kernel size in barley (Czechoslovakian, with summary in Russian and German). *Sbor. CSAZV, Rostl. Vyroba 7*:1607–1634.

Nečas, J. (1962). Inheritance of spike length in barley (Czechoslovakian, with summary in Russian and English). *Biologia 17*:401–414.

Nečas, J. (1963). Inheritance of spike length in barley (Czechoslovakian, with summary in Russian and English). *Biologia 18*:195–209.

Nečas, J. (1966). Unequality of reciprocal crosses of barley (English, with summary in German). *Z. Planz. 55*:260–275.

Palilova, A. N. (1969). Cytoplasmic male sterility in plants. Minsk, "Nauka i tekhnika" (cited after Krupnov, 1971). *Genetika 7*:159–174).

Richey, F. D. (1920). The inequality in reciprocal corn crosses. *J. Amer. Soc. Agron. 12*:185–196.

Sakai, K.-I., Iyama, S.-Y. and Narise, T. (1961). Biometrical approach to cytoplasmic inheritance in autogamous plants. *Bull. Int. Stat. Inst. 38*:249–257.

Smith, W. E. and Aksel, R. (1974). Genetic analysis of seed-weight in reciprocal crosses of flax (*Linum usitatissimum* L.). *Theoret. Appl. Genet. 45*:117–121.

Smith, W. E. and Fitzsimmons, J. E. (1964). Maternal inheritance of seed weight in flax. *Can. J. Genet. Cytol. 6*:244.

Smith, W. E. and Fitzsimmons, J. E. (1965). Maternal inheritance of seed weight in flax. *Can. J. Genet. Cytol. 7*:658–662.

Soomro, B. A. (1974). A biometrical-genetic analysis of some quantitative characters in a five-parent diallel cross of common wheat (*Triticum aestivum* L.). Ph.D. thesis, Faculty of Graduate Studies and Research, Univ. of Alberta, Edmonton.

Tyson, H. (1973). Cytoplasmic effect on plant weight in crosses between flax genotypes and genotrophs. *Heredity 30*:327–340.

Yates, F. (1947). Analysis of data from all possible reciprocal crosses between a set of parental lines. *Heredity 1*:287–301.

V

Prospects of Breeding
for Physiological·Characters

26

Physiological Basis
of Salt Tolerance in Plants

Leon Bernstein

1795 New Hampshire Drive
Costa Mesa, California 92626

ABSTRACT

For most plants, and under most field conditions, osmotic effects of salinity greatly predominate in restricting growth and yields. In certain cases, however, specific ion effects may be decisive. These may involve either nutrition, as in calcium deficiency in some lettuce varieties, tomato, and bell peppers, or direct toxicity (chloride or sodium toxicity, or both) in tree and vine crops. Rootstocks, or varieties that restrict the uptake of toxic ions, increase the salt tolerance of some susceptible fruit crops. Salinity-induced nutritional imbalance can, in some cases, be corrected by selecting better adapted varieties and in others by the use of foliar nutrient sprays. Recent evidence indicates simple single-gene control over uptakes of chloride and sodium, but the more general osmotic effects appear to be complex and under multigenic control.

INTRODUCTION

Saline soils contain excessive concentrations of soluble salts that depress the growth and yield of most crop plants. For decades, opposing schools of thought have debated whether growth depression is caused primarily by osmotic or by specific ion effects. Some of the arguments for specific ion effects are flawed by failure to distinguish between salts in solution and undissolved salts and by failure to take into account the different water-retentive capacities of different soils (Bernstein, 1975). Yet it is apparent that specific ion effects as well as osmotic effects do occur. Although the evidence indicates that under field conditions the osmotic effect predominates for most crops, specific ions—either by affecting nutrition or by direct toxicity—can be important (and in some cases, even decisive).

Before discussing salinity, the related problem of soil sodicity should be briefly considered. In Pakistan, as in many areas in which salinity is a problem, sodicity frequently occurs along with salinity. In sodic soils, the exchangeable sodium percentage (ESP) exceeds 15%, i.e., exchangeable sodium occupies 15% or more of the exchangeable cation sites in the soil with concomitant reduction in exchangeable calcium and magnesium. Sodic soils may affect plant growth adversely in three distinct ways: (1) exchangeable sodium tends to disperse soils, impairing permeability to air and water; (2) the decrease in exchangeable Ca and Mg may, under nonsaline conditions, cause deficiencies of these elements; and (3) Na may be directly toxic to species susceptible to Na toxicity. When sodic soils are nonsaline, all soluble cation concentrations are low, and Ca^{2+} and Mg^{2+} may be deficient nutritionally. In saline sodic soils, ionic concentrations are higher, and Ca^{2+} and Mg^{2+} concentrations may be nutritionally adequate. To illustrate, consider two soils, both with a sodium adsorption ratio (SAR) of 36 (equivalent to an ESP of 34), one nonsaline (total soluble salts in the saturation extract 8 meq/liter), the other saline (total salt concentration of 80 meq/liter). The nonsaline soil will have a soluble Ca + Mg concentration of only 0.1 meq/liter, which is deficient for most crops, whereas the saline soil will have 8 meq/liter of Ca + Mg, which is usually nutritionally adequate. Although SAR determines ESP and, by difference, exchangeable Ca and Mg percentages, it does not indicate the nutritional adequacy of sodic soils, which depends on the absolute concentrations of these ions in the soil solution. Also, adverse soil physical conditions caused by exchangeable sodium tend to be less severe under saline conditions because high salt concentrations tend to flocculate soils and counteract the dispersive effects of exchangeable sodium. In saline soils, therefore, the effects of salinity predominate and the effects of sodicity are minimal, unless the salts are leached, leaving the soil nonsaline—sodic. Of course, plants specifically sensitive to Na toxicity, as detailed below, will be severely injured by sodicity in any case.

SALT-TOLERANCE RANGE AND EFFECTS OF SALINITY ON PLANTS

Salt-sensitive species, such as garden peas, are affected by salinity as low as −1 bar, equivalent to an electrical conductivity of the saturation extract (EC_e) of about 1.5 mmho/cm. Even low salinities cause obvious symptoms of salt damage, such as dieback of shoots, in such species. Moderately tolerant species (e.g., bell peppers) exhibit only progressive reduction in growth and yield with salinities ranging up to −5 bar (EC_e 7.5 mmho/cm). Tolerant species such as garden beets may show only a small decline in growth over this salinity range. Among all crop plants, there is about a 10-fold range in salt tolerance. The highly sensitive strawberry plant is severely affected at an EC_e of 2 mmho/cm, whereas the most tolerant Bermuda grass varieties are comparably affected at EC_e of 20 mmho/cm (Bernstein, 1964a, 1965).

The absence of specific injury symptoms poses a problem in selecting salt-tolerant individuals from a segregating population. Biochemical properties as well as visible signs of salt injury have been studied with the aim of determining plant characters that would indicate the salt tolerance of an individual. Because enzymes in halophytic bacteria are more resistant to salts in the assay medium than are those of glycophytic bacteria (Ingram, 1957), a similar effect was sought by comparing the enzymes of seed plant halophytes (the salt bush *Atriplex spongiosa*) with those of glycophytes. The enzymes of Atriplex were, however, found to be as salt sensitive as those of maize or beans (Greenway and Osmond, 1972; Osmond and Greenway, 1972). Moreover, the activities of the enzymes studied (see also Weimberg, 1970) were found to be unaffected by salinity in the growth medium. Although results to date have been negative, the search to identify biochemical properties associated with salt tolerance continues, because it is argued that slower growth rates must be caused by some enzyme(s) that limit growth under saline conditions.

Growth regulators are agents that could obviously be involved in decreasing growth under saline conditions (for references and discussion see Bernstein, 1975). An early report by Marth and Frank (1961) indicated that growth retardants increase resistance to lethal doses of salinity. Later studies by Bernstein (unpublished) showed that the inhibitory effects of continuous salinity and growth retardants are simply additive in reducing the growth of soybeans. More recent studies by Mizrahi et al. (1971) indicate that salinity, like water stress, reduces the cytokinin and increases the abscissic acid contents of leaves. Both changes reduce stomatal aperture and, therefore, according to Mizrahi and co-workers, promote adjustment to salinity. Bernstein (1975), however, suggests that these effects of salinity on growth substance levels may be transitory and may not persist under continuous saline treatments.

OSMOTIC EFFECTS OF SALINITY

When single salts (e.g., chlorides or sulfates of Na, Ca, and Mg) are added to a nutrient solution, the predominant influence of the osmotic factor is clearly evident. Although one salt may be more inhibitory than the others in individual experiments, the added inhibition is evidently caused by nutrient imbalance. Thus, bean plants are inhibited more by $CaCl_2$ than by NaCl, whereas the reverse is true for maize (Bernstein, 1964b). Beans are avid Ca accumulators and high concentrations of Ca impair the uptake of K and Mg causing nutritional deficiencies or imbalance. In contrast, maize cannot absorb enough Ca from a saline medium unless the Ca concentration is increased above the usual nutrient level. For both beans and maize, mixed salt solutions (e.g., Ca + Na salts) correct the nutritional balance and improve growth and yield to the best level attainable at a given osmotic potential. Furthermore, the plants tolerate large variations in the proportions of salts that contribute to salinity. In saline fields a mixture of salts rather than a single salt gives rise to salinity; therefore, the osmotic effects of salinity generally predominate, and a measure of osmotic potential (or some related measure, such as EC) provides a good index of the effective salinity.

Another line of evidence that indicates the relative unimportance of specific ion effects in salt tolerance is the lack of correlation between salt uptake and salt tolerance. Data for truck crops show a general similarity of leaf chloride levels among plants that differ markedly in salt tolerance (Bernstein, 1964b). Similarly, there is no correlation between leaf Na levels and salt tolerance. Some crops that restrict Na transport to the leaves ("Na excluders," such as beans, potatoes, and maize) are more salt-sensitive than others that accumulate Na (broccoli, tomato). Ecologists recognize that halophytes employ two distinct strategies under saline conditions. Euhalophytes take up salts to offset the osmotic effects of salinity whereas glycohalophytes restrict salt uptake and increase their internal concentration of organic substances to effect osmotic adjustment. Crop plants also utilize both methods for increasing their internal solute concentrations. Some take up salts, others exclude them.

As already noted, internal tolerance to absorbed salts does not seem to be a differentiating factor between salt-tolerant and salt-sensitive species, even when halophytes and glycophytes are compared. Unlike bacterial cells in which salts appear to be freely diffusible (100% free space), the cells of higher plants by compartmentation apparently restrict intracellular salt distribution so that enzyme sites are protected from injurious salt concentrations.

OSMOTIC ADJUSTMENT AND GROWTH

The osmotic gradient for water entry into plants would be drastically reduced and even lost were it not for the osmotic adjustment of plants to saline media. The osmotic potential of all plant parts, roots, stems, and leaves, decreases to match the decrease in osmotic potential caused by salination of the root media, thus maintaining the osmotic gradient for water entry (for references, see Bernstein, 1975). Despite this osmotic adjustment, growth is less. I have proposed that the growth reduction is the mechanism for osmotic adjustment. All cells of a plant must, under saline conditions, achieve and maintain higher solute concentrations to maintain osmotic gradients. The initial effect of an increase in salinity is a check in growth; growth is subsequently resumed, albeit at a slower rate than before salination.

During the check in growth, osmotic adjustment occurs, initially by an increase in K salts of organic acids. After a day or two, other ions, such as Cl^-, and Ca^{2+}, or Na^+, replace the K salts in maintaining the higher salt concentrations. In some species, as in carrots, increased sugar concentrations may effect much of the osmotic adjustment. Whatever the mechanism, the required increased solute concentration can be maintained in a cell population that increases more slowly than is possible under nonsaline conditions for which lower internal solute concentrations are adequate.

SPECIFIC ION EFFECTS THROUGH NUTRITION

Although mixed salt solutions are nutritionally balanced for most species, exceptions do occur (for literature references see Bernstein, 1964b). Sulfate salinity generally reduces the uptake of Ca^{2+} and increases the uptake of monovalent ions (Na^+ and K^+). This effect does not usually cause any nutritional problem, but some lettuce varieties were shown by Doneen and Grogan (1954) to become Ca deficient as a result of sulfate salinity. Tomatoes and bell peppers develop blossom-end rot under saline conditions unless the proportion of soluble Ca is markedly increased in the saline soil solution. Blackheart of celery is a similar Ca-deficiency disorder that may be aggravated by salinity. Geraldson (1956, 1957) showed that these disorders can be prevented by properly timed foliar sprays of dilute $CaCl_2$ or $Ca(NO_3)_2$.

Carrot varieties exhibit marked differences in Ca and K nutrition under nonsaline conditions. The varieties that take up more K and less Ca are more salt tolerant than are those that take up more Ca and less K, as salinity increases the uptake of Ca and decreases the uptake of K in carrots (Bernstein and Ayers, 1953).

For the vast majority of crops studied, nutritional effects of salinity like those described for lettuce, tomato, and carrots, do not occur. When a crop is affected nutritionally, varieties resistant to the effect may be available, or simple remedial treatments, such as foliar sprays, may be quite effective in correcting the disorder. Specific ion-uptake mechanisms, such as the high-affinity mechanism for K uptake (mechanism 1), appear to ensure an adequate uptake by most crops of ions present in low concentrations despite a preponderance of other ions in the root medium.

SPECIFIC ION EFFECTS VIA TOXICITY

Although nonwoody crop plants, including field, forage, and vegetable crops, show no specific sensitivity to Cl^- or Na^+, woody crop plants, such as trees, vines, and most ornamentals, do (Bernstein, 1965). The accumulation of about 0.5–1.0% Cl^- on a dry-leaf basis in woody crop plants generally causes characteristic marginal or leaf-tip necrosis. Woody species that transport Na^+ to the leaves develop leaf necrosis when Na^+ content reaches 0.25–0.5% of the leaf dry weight. Differences among species in tolerance to Cl concentration of the root medium are caused primarily by differences in rate of uptake and transport of Cl^- to the leaves. Among rootstocks for each crop group—citrus, stone-fruit trees, and avocados—there is a two- to threefold difference in rate of transport of Cl^- to the leaves, hence tolerance to external Cl concentration. Among grape rootstocks, a difference as large as 15-fold in chloride transport has been shown (Bernstein et al., 1969).

The relative importance of specific ion toxicity and osmotic effects in susceptible fruit crops depends on the sensitivity of the crop to the osmotic effect of salinity. Strawberry plants, which are extremely salt-sensitive, exhibit characteristic leaf necrosis on chloride treatments, but not on sulfate treatments. Yet, growth is so limited by the osmotic effect that it is the same with both types of salinity at a given osmotic potential. For more tolerant species, such as the stone-fruit trees, about half the total growth depression may be caused by Cl^-, the other half by osmotic effects. When specific ion toxicity is an important factor, as it is for most woody crop plants, the use of rootstocks or varieties that restrict the transport of the toxic ion can markedly increase the salt tolerance of the crop.

CONCLUSIONS

The evidence strongly indicates that salinity affects most crops by means of an osmotic mechanism and that specific ion effects are rare, except among woody species for which rootstocks that restrict the transport of the toxic ions (primarily Cl^-) are available. The predominance of osmotic effects is in one sense unfortunate because genetic control over ion transport appears to be much simpler than that over osmotic effects. In an exceptional case that requires more critical examination, Abel and MacKenzie (1964) reported the tolerance of soybean varieties to be inversely related to chloride accumulation. Moreover, chloride accumulation in soybeans is regulated by a single gene, with chloride "exclusion" dominant over chloride accumulation (Abel, 1969). The greater tolerance of tideland grass ecotypes compared to upland ecotypes has also been attributed to decreased transport of chloride and sodium in the former (Hannon and Barber, 1972). In contrast, responses related to the osmotic properties of saline media appear to be complex and controlled by the many genes that influence plant–water relations and the osmotic properties of plants. This inference received striking support from the finding that tissue cultures of halophytes are no more salt tolerant than those of glycophytes (Strogonov et al., 1970). Salt tolerance thus appears to be a property of the whole plant, rather than of isolated parts or organs, which further complicates not only the transfer of salt tolerance to a sensitive crop, but also the recognition of individuals possessing the multifaceted attributes of salt tolerance.

REFERENCES

Abel, G. H. (1969). Inheritance of the capacity for chloride inclusion and chloride exclusion by soybeans. *Crop Sci. 9*:697–698.

Abel, G. H. and MacKenzie, A. J. (1964). Salt tolerance of soybean varieties (*Glycine max* L. Merrill) during germination and later growth. *Crop Sci. 4*:157–161.

Bernstein, L. (1964*a*). Salt tolerance of plants. *U.S. Dept. Agri., Agri. Inf. Bull. 283*:23 pp.

Bernstein, L. (1964*b*). Effects of salinity on mineral composition and growth of plants. *Plant Anal. Fert. Probl. 4*:25–45.

Bernstein, L. (1965). Salt tolerance of fruit crops. *U.S. Dept. Agri., Agri. Inf. Bull. 292*:8 pp.

Bernstein, L. (1975). Effects of salinity and sodicity on plant growth. *Annu. Rev. Phytopathol. 13*:295–312.

Bernstein, L. and Ayers, A. D. (1953). Salt tolerance of five varieties of carrots. *Proc. Amer. Soc. Hort. Sci. 61*:360–366.

Bernstein, L., Ehlig, C. F., and Clark, R. A. (1969). Effect of grape rootstocks on chloride accumulation in leaves. *J. Amer. Soc. Hort. Sci. 94*:584–590.

Doneen, L. D., and Grogan, R. G. (1954). Lettuce tolerance to the sulfate ion. *Amer. Soc. Hort. Sci.* (oral communication, Western Section).

Geraldson, C. M. (1956). Watch nutrient intensity and balance; by checking soil solution soluble salts, we can prevent blossom-end rot of tomatoes and peppers and blackheart of celery. *Sunshine State Fla. Agri. Exp. Sta. Res. Rep. 1*(3):10–11.

Geraldson, C. M. (1957). Control of blossom-end rot of tomatoes. *Proc. Amer. Soc. Hort. Sci. 69*:309–317.

Greenway, H. and Osmond, C. B. (1972). Salt responses of enzymes from species differing in salt tolerance. *Plant Physiol. 49*:256–259.

Hannon, N. J., and Barber, H. N. (1972). The mechanism of salt tolerance in naturally selected populations of grasses. *Search Sydney 3*:259–260.

Ingram, M. (1957). Micro-organisms resisting high concentrations of sugars or salts. In *7th Symp. Soc. Gen. Microbiol.*, pp. 90–133. Cambridge Univ. Press, Oxford.

Marth, P. C. and Frank, J. R. (1961). Increasing tolerance of soybean plants to some soluble salts through application of plant growth-retardant chemicals. *J. Agri. Food Chem. 9*:359–361.

Mizrahi, Y., Blumenfeld, A., Bittner, S., and Richmond, A. E. (1971). Abscisic acid and cytokinin contents of leaves in relation to salinity and relative humidity. *Plant Physiol. 48*:752–755.

Osmond, C.B. and Greenway, H. (1972). Salt responses of carboxylation enzymes from species differing in salt tolerance. *Plant Physiol. 49*:260–263.

Strogonov, B. P., Kabanov, V. V., Shevjakova, N. I., Lapina, L. P., Komizerko, E. I., Popov,

B. A., Dostanova, R. Kh. and Prykhod'ko, L. S. (1970). *Structure and Function of Plant Cells in Saline Habitats.* (Translated from Russian by A. Mercado, Wiley, New York, 1974.)

Weimberg, R. (1970). Enzyme levels in pea seedlings grown on highly salinized media. *Plant Physiol. 46*:466–470.

27

Prospects of Breeding
for Salt Tolerance in Rice

M. Akbar, A. Shakoor, and M. S. Sajjad

Nuclear Institute for Agriculture and Biology
Lyallpur, Pakistan

ABSTRACT

Variations with regard to salt tolerance were observed in rice varieties, Blue bonnet, IR-8, Jhona-349, and Magnolia. Crosses (F_1) between relatively salt-resistant (Jhona-349) and salt-sensitive (Magnolia) varieties were highly resistant to salinity. The F_2 population resulted in some salt-resistant combinations. In the F_3 and F_4 populations, some desirable salt-resistant progenies were selected. Results obtained suggest that selection for salt tolerance may be possible within hybrid populations.

INTRODUCTION

Soil salinity is one of the most important problems of crop production in arid and semiarid zones in which canal irrigation is practiced. In Pakistan, out of 37.4 million acres of irrigated land about 10.1 million acres are affected by salinity. With the increase in population, effective utilization of these soils has become necessary, either by reclamation or by growing some salt-resistant agricultural crops on marginal saline soils. Breeders have utilized the genetic variability to develop varieties that can tolerate cold, drought, and floods, and show resistance to diseases and insects. However, exploitation of genetic variability for salt tolerance in a breeding program has seldom been considered. It is true that most of the cultivated crops have been bred for growing on normal soils. However, marked differences with regard to salt tolerance do exist among genera, species, and varieties of various field crops (Hayward and Wadleigh, 1949; Bernstein and Hayward, 1958; Dewey, 1960; Yoshida, 1967; Akbar et al., 1972). In nature, salinity, like other stresses, often results in the evolution of races or ecotypes through natural selection adapted to this condition (Dewey, 1960, 1962; Tanimoto, 1969). Some species of the genus Agropyron are highly resistant to salinity. Other alien species may also be screened for salt tolerance, and attempts should be made to test the possibilities of transferring this trait into cultivated forms. There appears to be no antagonism between resistance and productivity. Increased tolerance with increased yield has been reported (Strogonov, 1964). If natural genetic variation for salt tolerance could be combined with both the right type of plant and the resistance to pests, it may be possible to evolve improved varieties suited to saline conditions.

Unfortunately, no species has been studied adequately for the genetic basis of salt tolerance (Dewey, 1960), and no systematic efforts have been made to collect and maintain germ plasm which is salt tolerant. Most of the research work on salt tolerance deals with the ecology, physiology, and anatomic changes that take place in cultivated plants grown under saline conditions, but little has been done to breed varieties adapted to adverse soil conditions such as salinity, alkalinity, and acidity.

Salt tolerance is a complex character and is highly influenced by environmental factors, such as soil, temperature, light, and type of salinity. Combined efforts in such diverse fields as plant breeding, plant physiology, and soil chemistry may lead to some success. From the viewpoint of plant breeding, quick and reliable methods are needed to screen varieties for their reaction to salt tolerance during early stages of development. Information on the relationship between salt tolerance and any morphologic character can provide some marker genes for salt tolerance.

In previous studies, rice varieties Jhona-349 and Magnolia were found to be relatively salt resistant and salt sensitive, respectively (Akbar et al., 1972). In the F_2 population, a few salt-resistant plants, namely, P-15, P-21, P-57, and P-129, were selected (Table I). The selection of these plants was based mainly on their seed-setting performance, for it was observed that this character was affected drastically by salinity when compared with other morphological characters. The present chapter deals with the study concerning the performance of F_3 and F_4 generations grown under saline conditions.

MATERIALS AND METHODS

The salt-resistant F_2 single-plant selections, P-15, P-21, P-57, and P-129, along with the parents Jhona-349 and Magnolia, were grown in artificially salinized field basins (20 ft × 20 ft × 3 ft) during the summer of 1974 at the

Table I. Morphologic Characterics of Some Promising Salt-Resistant Plants in the F_2 Population

Plant No.	Height (cm)	Productive tillers/plant	Heading date (days)	Panicle length (cm)	Number of primary branches/panicle	Number of spikelets/panicle	Seed setting (%)
P-15	212.2	18	98	31.5	11.9	164.2	84.8
P-21	185.0	18	93	28.2	10.7	146.8	85.0
P-57	170.0	17	111	26.1	11.5	126.6	90.8
P-129	141.0	16	97	27.4	10.0	138.8	82.2
				Parents			
Jhona-349	142.9	19	100.0	23.3	9.6	139.1	70.8
Magnolia	156.4	14	99.4	27.9	12.5	147.4	32.1

Nuclear Institute for Agriculture and Biology at Lyallpur. The characteristics of the saline soil in the basins were pH 8.4, EC_e (electrical conductivity) 7.5 mmhos/cm at 25°C, and 27 ESP (exchangeable sodium percentage). The desired salinity level was achieved by adding tubewell water, which contained TSS (total soluble salts) 35, HCO_3^- 17.5, $Ca^{2+} + Mg^{2+}$4.8 and Na^+30.2 meq/liter with a value of 19.5 SAR (sodium adsorption ratio). The nursery was sown in normal soil and 5-week-old seedlings were transplanted in saline field basins. Selection in the F_3 was based mainly on panicle fertility. The performance of the relatively salt-resistant progenies, selected in the F_3, was again studied in the salinized field basins in the summer of 1975. The salinity parameters were pH 8.5, EC_e 5.0, and ESP 35. The data on various morphologic characters were taken in both years of study.

RESULTS AND DISCUSSION

Data on various morphologic characters of F_3 progenies are given in Table II. In spite of normal vegetative growth, the progenies, P-15-74, P-21-74, P-57-74, and P-129-74, and the parents, Jhona-349 and Magnolia, generally produced little grain. Seed setting was markedly affected as compared to other morphological characters studied. This demonstrates that the rice plant is highly sensitive to salinity after the boot stage (Ota et al., 1955; Iwaki, 1956; Bernstein and Hayward, 1958; Pearson and Ayers, 1960; Yoshida, 1967; Akbar et al., 1972). Therefore, the character seed setting may be given more emphasis in breeding programs for salt tolerance in rice. Progenies P-15-74, P-21-74, and P-129-74 reacted like the sensitive parent Magnolia with respect to this character and failed to produce any desirable segregants. However, progeny P-57-74 performed better than did other progenies and both the parents under saline conditions (Table II); seven salt-resistant plants were selected. These salt-resistant plants had more than 82% seed setting, compared with the parents, Jhona-349 (31.5%) and Magnolia (12.0%) (Table III). However, some of these plants were late in heading. In the previous studies (F_2), when the desired salinity level (4000 ppm) was achieved by adding equal amounts of NaCl and $CaCl_2$, plants P-15, P-21, P-129 and Jhona-349 behaved as though they were salt resistant (Akbar, 1973), but in the present studies Jhona-349, P-15, P-21, and P-129 progenies were indeed salt sensitive. This discrepancy may be the result of a high percentage of sodium, high pH, and other environmental factors. The type of salinity, temperature, pH, soil, and other environmental factors play an important role in the response of plants to salinity (Richards, 1969). The seven single-plant selections obtained from the relatively salt-resistant P-57-74 family show that some sort of interaction of genes may be present. These single-plant selections might have general resistance for salt stress as compared to the salt-sensitive progenies that may have specific resistance. The studies for general

Table II. Behavior of Various F_3 Progenies under Saline Conditions

Progeny	Plant height (cm)	Number of productive tillers/plant	Heading date (days)	Panicle length (cm)	Number of primary branches/panicle	Number of spikelets/panicle	Seed setting (%)
P-15-74	116.2 ± 2.53	8.4 ± 2.83	106	19.2 ± 1.56	6.2 ± 1.07	56.2 ± 11.88	14.3 ± 9.59
P-21-74	103.0 ± 2.41	8.5 ± 2.22	105	21.7 ± 3.50	7.4 ± 1.60	77.8 ± 20.64	10.6 ± 9.67
P-57-74	111.4 ± 3.40	6.4 ± 1.99	112	21.9 ± 2.87	8.9 ± 1.60	86.1 ± 24.59	55.4 ± 4.48
P-129-74	80.5 ± 2.52	5.5 ± 1.90	102	18.7 ± 2.21	5.5 ± 1.34	63.8 ± 20.88	10.4 ± 8.55
Parents							
Jhona-349	91.3 ± 2.33	5.0 ± 2.33	113	20.6 ± 1.76	8.0 ± 1.20	74.0 ± 10.46	31.5 ± 11.70
Magnolia	96.3 ± 3.46	4.0 ± 1.90	102	20.3 ± 3.28	7.9 ± 1.42	84.2 ± 20.07	12.0 ± 11.84

Table III. Morphologic Characteristics of Single-Plant Selections Obtained from Relatively Salt-Resistant Family P-57-74 in F_3 Generation

Progeny	Plant height (cm)	Number of productive tillers/plant	Heading date (days)	Panicle length (cm)	Number of primary branches/panicle	Number of spikelets/panicle	Seed setting (%)
P-57-74-79	109	5	120	23.0 ± 1.43	8.2 ± 0.83	70.2 ± 23.78	85.1 ± 8.79
P-57-74-92	119	7	110	23.1 ± 2.56	9.0 ± 2.38	88.6 ± 27.98	85.3 ± 11.41
P-57-74-93	88	4	107	23.9 ± 4.27	9.5 ± 1.73	88.8 ± 23.62	87.9 ± 9.02
P-57-74-96	97	10	120	21.8 ± 1.89	8.9 ± 1.37	82.4 ± 20.60	82.2 ± 6.79
P-57-74-97	97	6	110	20.7 ± 1.86	8.2 ± 1.71	72.3 ± 22.67	94.5 ± 1.37
P-57-74-106	119	8	120	22.8 ± 2.37	10.8 ± 2.05	107.9 ± 32.42	95.0 ± 2.45
P-57-74-108	124	5	116	27.5 ± 5.31	9.4 ± 1.14	106.0 ± 21.88	94.7 ± 1.45
Parents							
Jhona-349	91.3 ± 2.52	5.0 ± 2.33	113	20.6 ± 1.76	8.0 ± 1.20	74.0 ± 10.46	31.5 ± 11.70
Magnolia	96.3 ± 3.46	4.0 ± 1.90	102	20.3 ± 3.28	7.9 ± 1.42	84.2 ± 20.07	12.0 ± 11.84

Table IV. Morphologic Characteristics of Seven Strains under Saline Conditions (in F_4 Generation)

Strains	Plant height (cm)	Number of productive tillers/plant	Heading date (days)	Panicle length (cm)	Number of primary branches/panicle	Number of spikelets/panicle	Seed setting (%)
P-57-74-79	125.7 ± 2.64	9.7 ± 0.43	108	22.6 ± 0.87	8.9 ± 0.54	79.1 ± 8.20	89.4 ± 4.89
P-57-74-92	120.8 ± 2.96	6.4 ± 0.52	100	24.2 ± 0.77	12.8 ± 0.94	147.4 ± 13.96	77.2 ± 8.26
P-57-74-93	125.6 ± 2.49	10.7 ± 0.57	108	25.0 ± 0.67	10.0 ± 0.42	102.4 ± 7.46	92.0 ± 2.27
P-57-74-96	132.2 ± 3.29	10.0 ± 0.58	108	23.1 ± 0.66	12.1 ± 0.54	101.1 ± 7.04	93.7 ± 1.70
P-57-74-97	121.1 ± 2.85	9.9 ± 0.97	102	21.2 ± 0.74	11.5 ± 0.67	113.5 ± 9.63	84.0 ± 2.47
P-57-74-106	136.6 ± 2.81	10.6 ± 0.74	105	24.7 ± 0.97	11.0 ± 0.70	112.3 ± 9.22	86.9 ± 4.43
P-57-74-108	118.7 ± 2.99	7.9 ± 0.79	99	23.8 ± 0.78	10.5 ± 0.56	106.6 ± 9.33	89.9 ± 4.19
Jhona-349	96.5 ± 3.24	6.2 ± 0.46	101	20.8 ± 0.51	9.2 ± 0.43	79.7 ± 9.56	36.4 ± 3.27

and specific tolerance need thorough investigations under field conditions. In the F_4 generation, strains P-57-74-79, P-57-74-92, P-57-74-93, P-57-74-96, P-57-74-97, P-57-74-106, and P-57-74-108 exhibited a higher degree of tolerance than did the better parent Jhona-349 (Table IV). Their seed setting ranged from 84.0 to 93.7%, except for strain P-57-74-92 (77.2%). Similarly, other yield components showed better resistance to salinity than did the Jhona-349. However, some strains were late in heading.

In general, these results indicate that selection for salt tolerance within a hybrid population resulting from appropriate crossings may produce salt-resistant lines. The possibility of increasing the salt tolerance of most of the legumes and of crested wheat grass by selection was reported by Hutton (1971) and Dewey (1962), respectively. However, under field conditions, many factors are involved which may also influence the extent of tolerance. Therefore, it seems advisable that the breeding objectives preferably be based on the general tolerance, rather than on the specific tolerance. The new variety evolved for saline areas must have the ability to cope with all the adverse conditions of the habitat. Earlier investigations have shown that there is no relationship between any morphologic character studied and resistance to salinity in rice varieties (Akbar et al., 1972). Similarly, no relationship could be established between apiculus pigmentation and resistance to salinity (Akbar et al., 1975). However, in a separate study conducted by Akbar et al. (1976), it was found that Jhona-349 (relatively salt resistant) was also radioresistant, whereas Magnolia was found to be relatively radiosensitive as well as susceptible to salinity. These studies need confirmation. A definite relationship, if established, may help the breeder to screen plant-breeding material on a larger scale in early developmental stages. Efforts must also be made to discover some relationship between an easily recognizable character and salt tolerance.

REFERENCES

Akbar, M. (1973). Breeding for salt-resistant varieties of rice. Ph.D. thesis, Univ. of Osaka Prefecture, Osaka, Japan.

Akbar, M., Yabuno, T., and Nakao, S. (1972). Breeding for saline-resistant varieties of rice. I. Variability for salt tolerance among some rice varieties. *Jap. J. Breed.* 22:272–284.

Akbar, M., Yabuno, T., and Chaudhry, A. S. (1975). Inheritance of apiculus pigmentation in some rice varieties and its possible relation to salinity. *Nucleus 12* (1–2):31–33.

Akbar, M., Inoue, M., and Hasegawa, H. (1976). Comparative radiosensitivity in Indica and Japonica rice. *Nucleus 13*:25–29.

Bernstein, L., and Hayward, H. E. (1958). Physiology of salt-tolerance. *Annu. Rev. Plant Physiol. 9*:25–46.

Dewey, D. R. (1960). Salt tolerance of twenty-five strains of Agropyron. *Agron. J. 52*:631–635.

Dewey, D. R. (1962). Breeding crested wheat grass for salt tolerance. *Crop Sci. 2*:403–407.

Hayward, H. E., and Wadleigh, C. H. (1949). Plant growth on saline and alkali soils. *Advan. Agron. 1*:1–38.

Hutton, E. M. (1971). Variation in salt response between tropical pasture legumes. *SABRAO Newsl 3*(2):75–81.

Iwaki, S. (1956). Studies on salt injury in the rice plant. (In Japanese with English summary.) *Mem. Ehime Univ. Sect. 6 (Agr.) 2*:1–156.

Ota, K., Ogo, T., and Sasai, K. (1955). Studies on salt injury to crops. IX. (In Japanese with English summary.) *Okayama Agri. Exp. Sta. Bull. 51*.

Pearson, G. A., and Ayers, A. D. (1960). Rice as a crop for salt-affected soil in process of reclamation. *U.S. Dept. Agri. Prod. Res. Rep. 43*:13 pp.

Richards, L. A. (1969). Diagnosis and improvement of saline and alkali soils. *U.S. Dept. Agri. Hbk 60*.

Strogonov, B. P. (1964). *Physiological Basis of Salt Tolerance of Plants.* (Translated from Russian.) I.P.S.T., Jerusalem.

Tanimoto, T. T. (1969). Differential physiological response of sugarcane varieties to osmotic pressures of saline media. *Crop Sci. 9*:683–688.

Yoshida, S. (1967). Salt tolerance of rice plant. *Annual Report IRRI*, pp. 32–36.

28

Plant Responses to High Temperatures

C. Y. Sullivan, N. V. Norcio, and J. D. Eastin

Agricultural Research Service, USDA
The University of Nebraska
Lincoln, Nebraska

ABSTRACT

Research has shown that there are wide diversities in heat tolerance among crops, and that differences occur not only between crop species, but also among genotypes within the species. Sufficient variability occurs to select for genotypes with high heat tolerance. Under field conditions, drought stress often accompanies heat stress, and there are usually interactions of plant response to these two stresses. Consequently, heat and drought resistance are usually considered together in field response, but each mechanism must be considered separately in order fully to understand the response. An example is given in which sorghum is regarded as having greater stress resistance than corn from field performance. However, results showed that cellular tolerance to high temperatures was higher in corn than in sorghum and higher in pearl millet than in corn. This was true not only of cellular membrane stability, but also of isolated chloroplast activity and photosynthesis of intact leaves under controlled conditions. Results also showed that the drought-avoidance mechanisms were inadequate in corn as compared to sorghum; therefore, corn-leaf tissue may be more frequently exposed to high temperatures owing to decreased evaporative cooling, and the critical limits of high temperature and desiccation tolerance exceeded, resulting in leaf "firing," even though cellular tolerance is greater than that of sorghum. In pearl millet, both heat tolerance and drought-avoidance mechanisms appear well developed. Tests have shown that heat tolerance frequently correlates positively with desiccation tolerance, but because they do not always correlate, different mechanisms must be involved in each kind of tolerance. Heat hardening occurs under natural conditions and may contribute significantly to total plant performance. Once plants are heat hardened there may be long-lasting effects. The age or stage of development of the plants at which high-temperature exposure occurs may also have a marked influence on the response. The relative resistance to high-temperature injury may change among genotypes as they age. Leaf temperatures in the range of 43°–45°C may have marked effects on photosynthesis of sorghum, with distinct differences shown in genotype response. The response of hybrids to high temperatures may be determined by one or both parents. Photosynthesis by plants selected for high heat tolerance by a leaf-disc technique was shown to be more stable at high temperatures than that of plants with low heat tolerance. The leaf-disc technique may be used for rapid field screening.

INTRODUCTION

Plants have adapted to many environmental extremes because of genetic diversity and natural selection pressures. Under cultivated conditions, plant breeders select and manipulate plants according to the traits they desire. The breeder may empirically select for what appears to be high-temperature resistance, but if the component physiological mechanisms that contribute to the overall response were understood, it should at least shorten selection and breeding procedures and likely result in the development of plants tolerant of greater heat.

There are many aspects to high-temperature responses of plants, but much of this chapter is concerned with our own cooperative research between the U.S. Department of Agriculture, Agricultural Research Service, and the University of Nebraska, Lincoln, Nebraska.

Under field conditions it is usually unknown to what extent plants are directly affected by high temperatures. This is mainly because drought stress often accompanies high temperatures, and a distinction is seldom made between responses to these two concomitant stresses. In fact, heat resistance and drought resistance are frequently referred to as a single stress resistance. Hunter et al. (1936), Heyne and Laude (1940), and Heyne and Brunson (1940), for example, classified corn seedlings as to their drought resistance based on resistance to high temperatures at low relative humidities. Similarly, Tatum (1954) concluded that the major effect of heat was increased evaporation and transpiration, rather than its direct effect. Kaloyereas (1958) related the thermal stability of chlorophyll to drought resistance of pine trees. Kilen and Andrews (1969) positively correlated field firing of corn with heat tolerance as evaluated by the chlorophyll stability index of Kaloyereas, and by heating seedlings in a forced air dryer at 54.5°C with 15–20% relative humidity for 5 h and visually estimating recovery. Julander (1945) heated range and pasture grasses in glass tubes in a water bath and also concluded from recovery counts that heat resistance was a measure of drought resistance. Williams et al. (1969) positively correlated results of heat-chamber tests with field drought resistance of sweet corn.

Yet it is well known that plants have optimum temperatures for growth and development, and at higher temperatures various forms of injury or alterations in growth and metabolism may occur in the absence of drought stress. It is evident that direct heat injury occurs.

HEAT EFFECTS ON DEVELOPING PANICLES

Pasternak and Wilson (1969) showed that sorghum exposed to heat waves at the boot stage, or soon after, had reduced seed set if the flower parts were still enclosed in the leaf sheaths, but was shown to have little effect on florets fully emerged from the boot. This agreed with our recent results with developing sorghum panicles treated with hot water. Field-grown plants were severed near the ground, and the shoot was brought to the laboratory where the leaves and sheaths were stripped from the stalks to expose the panicles. The panicles were then submerged in hot water for 15 min at $52°C$. Heat injury was evaluated visually and by electrical conductivity measurements 24 h after treatment (Sullivan, 1972). Visual estimates of injury agreed with the conductivity method. Table I shows that heat tolerance increased as the panicles matured, based both on length and dry weight. Panicles emerging from the boot were much more heat tolerant than were young developing panicles.

Downes (1972) showed that high temperatures during floral initiation reduced the number of florets that developed and adversely affected both grain and stover yields in sorghum, even if the temperatures were reduced to more favorable conditions after the treatment.

Working with the Nebraska sorghum physiology group, Dickinson (1976) placed plastic bags over sorghum heads to induce heat stress at several different growth stages and left them on for different lengths of time. He found for short-term heat stresses that the most significant period for reducing grain yield was about 7 to 9 days after bloom began at the tip of the panicle. He surmised from review of the literature that this was the time at which starch formation started, and that starch granular size and number were limited by the heat stress (Hoshikawa, 1962; Nagato and Ebata, 1966; Wardlaw, 1970).

HEAT HARDENING

It was believed for some years that heat hardening analogous to drought and cold hardening did not occur (Levitt, 1956). However, it is now well docu-

Table I. Heat Tolerance of Developing Sorghum
Panicles

Sorghum	Panicle length or fresh weight	% Injury[a] (at 52°C)
	Length (cm)	
8568	15.8	13.3
	44.9	5.9
8573	12.5	15.0
	45.6	6.5
8619	5.6	12.7
	57.3	3.2
Tx-414	2.7	52.3
	5.6	39.8
	9.8	12.1
	Fresh weight (g)	
8614	2.91	22.2
	0.52	56.6
8617	5.10	36.0
	0.55	56.1
8622	2.36	12.3
	.75	43.6
8573	4.69	6.3
	2.58	26.5
	0.49	61.7
Martin	1.86	29.4
	0.55	45.7

[a] Values are averages of three plants.

mented that heat hardening occurs when plants are exposed to subinjurious high temperatures (Levitt, 1972).

Sullivan and Kinbacher (1967) found that bean plants exposed to 44°C for 2–4 h per day reached their maximum hardiness in about 4 days (Table II). Unhardened plants were 50% injured at about 47°C, and the hardened plants at about 50°C, as determined by the electrical conductivity method.

Coffman (1957) used temperatures of 48.5°–51°C for 45 min to heat-harden winter oats; he found that heat tolerance was higher after exposure to bright sunlight than when shaded. Similarly, Heyne and Laude (1940) found heat tolerance higher in corn in the afternoon after exposure to sunlight. Coffman (1957) concluded that heat resistance is an inherited characteristic in oats, and susceptibility is dominant over resistance.

Table II. Heat Tolerance of Hardened (H) and
Unhardened (UH) Bean Leaves[a]

Days hardened	Temperature causing 50% injury	
	H	UH
3	50.4	46.0
4	49.2	47.4
4	50.8	47.8
4	50.1	46.4
6	51.8	47.2
9	50.8	47.9
10	50.1	45.9
Average	50.5[b]	46.9[b]
S.D.	± 0.75	± 0.81

[a]From Sullivan and Kinsbacher (1967).
[b]Significant at the 1% level.

Alexandrov (1964) showed that very short heat shocks of even one or a few seconds increased heat hardiness of certain plants. Yarwood (1967) found optimum hardening of a number of plants at elevated temperatures for no more than 20 s at 50°C.

Once heat hardened, whether by shock or longer high-temperature exposures, the heat-hardened condition may persist (Schroeder, 1963; Alexandrov, 1964), although Alexandrov (1964) showed that dehardening occurred after 24 h. Our results with cabbage, shown in Table III, did not indicate a noticeable

Table III. Dehardening of Two Heat-Hardened
Cabbage Varieties[a]

Days after hardening	Golden acre (% injury)		Bonanza (% injury)	
	Hardened	Unhardened	Hardened	Unhardened
1	48.7[b]	95.6[b]	28.0[b]	94.2[b]
2	46.5	–	31.4	–
3	71.9	91.7	56.6	92.8
8	69.6	97.6	59.5	95.9
15	66.7	97.9	57.1	88.4

[a]Potted plants were heat hardened for 4 h/day at 45°–46°C for four consecutive days in a heat chamber.
[b]Percent injury as evaluated by electrical conductivity with leaf discs after treatment at 48°C for 1 h. Values are means of four determinations.

decline in hardening until more than 2 days after hardening, and then an appreciable level of hardiness remained for at least 15 days.

There is some evidence that heat hardening may have a lifelong influence on some plants. Smith (1973) heat-hardened four sorghum hybrids at approximately 2 weeks of age in growth chambers at 46°C for 3.5–5 h per day for four consecutive days. Controls were treated equally except the temperature was held at 29.4°C during the heat-treatment period. The plants were grown together during the time between heat treatments. Two days after the treatment, the plants were transplanted in the field and grown normally with irrigation to maturity. At harvest, grain yield of the heat-hardened plants was significantly 7% greater on the average than that of unhardened controls. There were no significant differences in bloom date. This short period of stress acclimation in the early life of these plants in some way made them perform better under the existing climatic conditions, perhaps by increased tolerance to heat stress during a critical stage of floral development.

Even heat treatment of seeds may increase the heat tolerance of plants grown from seeds (Kydrev and Kolev, 1962).

In contrast, when Jones (1947) heat-treated maize seedlings at 40°, 50°, and 60°C for 1 h and transplanted them in the field, the treated plants were less vigorous throughout the season, flowered later than untreated, and were subject to pollen sterility in all treated lots.

Differences in the ability of genotypes to heat harden naturally may also account for differences in field stress resistance. Table IV shows the heat tolerance of four sorghums before and after heat hardening in growth chambers at about 3 weeks of age. Heat tolerance was evaluated by the electrical conductivity method with leaf discs. The relative ranking of heat tolerance changed when they were exposed to high temperatures. Some genotypes may fail to harden appreciably, while others harden very noticeably. In this experiment, sorghum CK-60 did not heat-harden to the extent of the others, and its relative tolerance was lower than the other sorghums after the high-temperature treat-

Table IV. Effect of Heat Hardening on the
Relative Heat Tolerance of Four Sorghum
Genotypes[a]

Day/night temp. (°C)	
31/27	42/27
CK-60	9084
9084	RS-610
RS-610	C-7078
C-7078	CK-60

[a]The sorghums are ranked from highest to lowest in heat tolerance.

ment. It was later found with field-grown plants, however, that as the plants aged and neared the boot and bloom stage there were no evident differences in heat-tolerance levels of RS-610, CK-60, and Combine-7078 (see Table XII). The yellow endosperm sorghum 9084, however, remained high in heat tolerance (see Table VII).

MEASURING HEAT TOLERANCE

Alexandrov (1964) reviewed several methods of measuring heat resistance. Among the methods evaluated were vital staining, depression of protoplasmic streaming, exit of electrolytes, changes in protoplasmic viscosity, luminescence of chloroplasts, infiltrated fluorochromes, retardation or cessation of respiration, and photosynthesis. He concluded that photosynthesis and protoplasmic streaming were among the most sensitive to high temperatures.

In our laboratory electrolyte leakage from leaf discs bathed in deionized water and measured by electrical conductivity has been used extensively to evaluate heat tolerance. This method is a modification of a method used for freezing resistance (Dexter et al., 1932). The most recent procedure for our method is given by Sullivan (1972).

A number of crop species have been tested for heat tolerance by this method. Some of the results are shown in Table V. The grain crops millet, corn and sorghum were among the highest in heat tolerance. It was interesting that cabbage developed fairly high heat tolerance when tested during hotter summer months. Results of selection for heat tolerance among some cabbage varieties are shown in Table VI. The variety Bonanza was significantly higher in heat tolerance than the other varieties during testing in July and August. There was a

Table V. Heat Tolerance of Some Field-Grown Crops

Plant	Temp. (°C)[a]
Pearl millet	47.7 – 54.6
Dent corn	46.6 – 54.1
Grain sorghum	45.0 – 52.8
Cabbage	45.4 – 52.0
Sweet corn	43.8 – 48.6
Tomato	44.2 – 48.4
Dry bean	43.9 – 47.4
Beet	43.6 – 47.2
Spinach	44.0 – 46.1

[a]Temperature causing 50% injury after 1-h exposure using fully grown plants.

Table VI. Heat Tolerance of Cabbage During July
and August

| | Temp. (°C) causing 50% injury | |
Variety	July	August
Golden acre	45.0 a[a]	46.3 a[a]
Bonanza	46.5 b	47.2 b
Ferry's hollander	45.7 a	46.1 a
Red acre	45.5 a	46.1 a

[a]Values not followed by the same letter in a column are significantly different at the 5% level of probability.

noticeable increase in heat tolerance during August, but there was relatively no change from July in the varietal ranking.

In another experiment heat injury, as evaluated by the electrical conductivity method, was compared to visual observations of leaf injury to shoots of potted bean plants after they were submerged in hot water at the same temperature and for the same length of time as the leaf discs were treated. The results of evaluated heat injury were nearly the same by the two methods (Sullivan et al., 1968).

We have used the conductivity test extensively in screening for heat tolerance of sorghum genotypes. Table 7 shows the variability found in one group tested. Temperatures causing 50% injury ranged from 45 to 52°C, a difference of 7°C. The averages for several dates tested ranged from 46.6 to 51.1, or a difference of 3.5°C. Table VIII shows differences found by the conductivity

Table VII. Heat Tolerance of Sorghums as Determined by the Conductivity
Method with Leaf Discs[a, b]

| | Sorghum | | | | | | | | |
Date	9084	2140	9024	9103	RS-610	RS-501	Martin	Caprock	9039
7/11–20	51.4	–	51.6	–	50.9	50.7	–	–	45.0
7/21–23	–	52.0	–	–	50.0	50.4	51.2	46.2	49.5
8/1–10	47.6	46.7	48.5	50.8	–	49.6	46.2	48.3	46.0
8/11–20	50.7	49.8	47.9	47.8	49.2	–	46.3	46.0	46.0
8/21–31	50.5	–	–	50.4	47.4	45.0	49.2	–	–
Mean	50.1	49.5	49.3	49.7	49.4	48.9	48.2	46.8	46.6

[a]Each value is the mean of duplicate samples of 20 plants each. Values are the temperature (°C) at 50% injury.
[b]From Sullivan (1972).

Table VIII. Heat Tolerance of Grain Sorghum, Corn and Pearl Millet

	% Injury (48°C, 1 h)	
	Late bloom to early grain filling	Late grain filling
	Sorghum	
M.35-1	21.6 b[a]	29.3 cd[a]
CK-60	−	53.1 e
C-7078	−	45.9 e
RS-610	70.2 c	46.3 e
2140	−	38.5 d
C42y	84.0 c	
	Millet	
Tift 23A	4.6 a	18.2 b
BIL 3B	−	16.5 ab
H.B.-1	−	12.6 a
	Corn	
Conico	33.0 b	21.7 bc
Hays Golden	30.5 b	−

[a]Values not followed by the same letter in a column are significantly different at the 5% level.

method among sorghums, pearl millet, and corn. The sorghum M.35-1, which was found to have high heat tolerance, is a heat- and drought-resistant sorghum from India (Rao and Murty, 1963). It was interesting and surprising to find that corn had higher cellular heat tolerance than was found for most of the sorghums. The pearl millets had the highest heat tolerance. In another experiment the chlorophyll stability index (Kaloyereas, 1958, as modified by Murty and Majumder, 1962) was compared to heat tolerance measured by the electrical conductivity method with leaf discs (Table IX). There was good agreement between the two methods, and again, M.35-1 had high heat tolerance as evaluated by both methods. Corn was more tolerant than the sorghums by the CSI method and using the leaf-disc method corn had greater tolerance than did sorghum RS-610. Pearl millet had greater heat tolerance than either corn or sorghum by both methods.

INTERACTION OF HEAT AND DROUGHT STRESS

The results in which corn was found to be more heat tolerant than sorghum were initially very perplexing to us, as it is generally accepted that corn is more

Table IX. A Comparison of the Chlorophyll Stability
Index (CSI) and Heat Tolerance of Leaf
Discs of Sorghum, Corn, and Millet[a, b]

	Sorghum		Corn	Millet
Method	(M.35-1)	(RS-610)	(N-705)	(Tift-23B)
CSI	0.061 c[c]	0.101 d	0.047 b	0.021 a
Heat tol.	31.1 b[c]	50.3 c	27.0 b	12.8 a

[a]Expressed as percent injury after treatment for 1h at 48°C.
[b]From Sullivan (1972).
[c]Values not followed by the same letter across a line are
significantly different at the 5% level of probability.

stress susceptible and usually "fires" sooner than sorghum. However, when we
examined the data further, and the interactions between drought and heat
responses of these crops were considered, the high-temperature tolerance of corn
became more meaningful.

Sullivan and Eastin (1973) grew corn and a tall sorghum with sand-nutrient
cultures in large tanks in a greenhouse. At about 4 weeks plant-age, droughting
began by withholding water. Several parameters were measured during the
drought period, including soil- and leaf-water potential, diffusive resistance,
stomatal width, and green leaf area. The plants droughted slowly for a period of
35 days, as the large tanks had some reserve water in the bottoms at the
beginning of the drought. Table X summarizes some of the results during and at

Table X. A Comparison of the Response of M.35-1
Sorghum and Hays Golden Corn to an Extended
Drought[a]

Measurement	Sorghum	Corn
Water potential of root media (day 35 of drought)[b]	−16.3 bar	−14.8 bar
Leaf-water potentials (day 35 of drought)	−16.8 bar	−26.9 bar
Leaf-water potentials at which lower stomata closed[c]	−14 bar	−12 bar
Green leaf area		
before drought	799 dm²	995 dm²
after drought	633 dm²	239 dm²
% reduction	21	76

[a]Adapted from Sullivan and Eastin (1973).
[b]Average of 15 and 45 cm depth, measured with soil psy-
chrometers.
[c]Considered closed with diffusive resistance greater than 75
sec·cm^{-1}

the end of the drought period. Corn stomata closed at higher leaf-water potentials (less stress) than did those of the sorghum, as others have reported (Pallas and Bertrand, 1966; Sanchez-Diaz and Kramer, 1971), but corn leaf-water potentials dropped about 10 bars lower than that of the sorghum, that is, the mechanisms for avoidance of leaf desiccation were more effective in sorghum than in corn.

Early stomatal closure and reduced leaf-water potentials usually result in higher leaf temperatures because of less evaporative cooling. It is therefore believed that corn has been inadvertently selected, naturally or artificially, to tolerate higher leaf temperatures, but drought mechanisms are still inadequate, and the limits of desiccation tolerance are exceeded; thus, leaf "firing" occurs when corn is drought and heat stressed. This occurred in our experiment, and green leaf area was reduced considerably more in the corn than in the sorghum, even though drought stress to the roots was slightly less for the corn than for sorghum. This is a case in which high cellular heat tolerance of a crop does not necessarily imply overall greater resistance to combined heat and drought stress.

HEAT EFFECTS ON PHOTOSYNTHESIS

Alexandrov (1964) concluded that photosynthesis was a plant process that is quite sensitive to high temperatures. We measured the thermal stability of the Hill reaction by isolated chloroplasts (Sullivan and Eastin, 1969). Table XI

Table XI. Thermal Stability of the Hill Reaction in Chloroplasts Isolated from Sorghum, Corn, and Pearl Millet.[a]

	July				
	Sorghum				Pearl millet
Parameter	RS-610	CK-60A	C-7078	M.35-1	H.B.-1
Mean (4 rep.)	0.66 a	0.52 a	0.53 a	0.18 b	0.98 c
S.D.	0.17	0.17	0.03	0.11	0.03
	August				
	Sorghum		Corn		Pearl millet
Parameter	RS-610	M.35-1	Conico	Hays G.	Tift 23B
Mean (4 rep.)	0.31 a	0.15 a	0.68 c	0.60	0.96 d
S.D.	0.06	0.08	0.18	0.21	0.06

[a]Measured in μmoles O_2 evolved per milligram chlorophyll per hour at $25°C$ after 15-min exposure to $25°$ or $43°C$. Expressed as the ratio of the activities at $43°/25°C$. Field-grown plants.
[b]Means not followed by the same letter are significantly different at the 5% level.

Table XII.   Electroconductivity Test for Percent Injury to Leaf Discs after 1 hr at 48°C, Relative to Controls at 25°C[a]

	July				
	Sorghum				Pearl millet
Parameter	RS-610	CK-60A	C-7078	M.35-1	H.B.-1
Mean (4 rep.)	60.9 c[b]	60.1 c	59.2 c	29.0 b	7.8 a
S.D.	5.5	0.6	11.8	12.9	2.7
	August				
	Sorghum			Corn		Pearl millet
Parameter	RS-160	C-42y	M.35-1	Conico	Hays G.	Tift 23B
Mean (4 rep.)	70.2 c	84.0 c	21.6 b	33.0 b	30.5 b	4.6 a
S.D.	7.2	4.8	3.2	6.1	9.5	3.0

[a] The second fully expanded leaf from the top of 20 plants sampled for each test. Field-grown plants.
[b] Means not followed by the same letter are significantly different at the 5% level.

shows the results of two experiments, one conducted in July at bloom or early grain filling, and the other in August or during late grain filling. When the ratios of oxygen evolution at 43°C to that at 25°C were compared, pearl millet had very high thermal stability and corn again had greater thermal stability than sorghum, as was also found by the leaf disc method (Table XII). The exception to agreement with the leaf-disc method was that the thermal stability of the Hill reaction by chloroplasts of sorghum M.35-1 was less than that of the other sorghums, whereas it was higher with the leaf-disc method. The suggestion was made that under natural conditions this damage is repaired by resynthesis, although this was not confirmed. Response of this variety in high-temperature growth-chamber experiments tends to support this view (Sullivan, unpublished data).

Norcio (1976) measured photosynthesis of sorghum leaf sections under controlled temperature conditions in the laboratory and found that in some cases an increase of 1.5°C, when approaching the high-temperature limit, may mean the difference between near-optimum rate and complete cessation of photosynthesis (Table XIII). Marked differences in genotype response to high temperatures causing sharp reduction in photosynthesis were also found, as shown in Fig. 1. The sorghum 4104 was selected from M.35-1 conversion lines for high heat tolerance by the electrical conductivity method with leaf discs (Sullivan, 1972). Some differences in temperature optimum for photosynthesis

Table XIII. Effects of Temperature on
Photosynthesis of RS 626 Sorghum[a]

Temperature (°C)	Photosynthesis (μmoles O_2/dm² /h)
40.0	51.9
41.5	49.5
43.0	−39.5

[a]From Norcio (1976).

were also found among genotypes, as measured by oxygen evolution with temperature-controlled leaf sections, an example of which is shown in Fig. 2. The sorghum 9040 also had high heat tolerance when tested by the electrical conductivity method with leaf discs.

In another experiment, photosynthesis was measured at high temperatures in two sorghum hybrids, the parent lines of one of the hybrids, and two corn lines. Figure 3 shows Redlan (the female parent of hybrid RS-691) unrelated and the unrelated hybrid RS-626, which we found to be heat susceptible by the leaf-disc test, were more susceptible to high-temperature inactivation of photosynthesis than were RS-691 and 9040 and corn lines N7A and N142. The hybrid RS-691 and its male parent 9040 maintained photosynthesis at a high level at 43°C, as

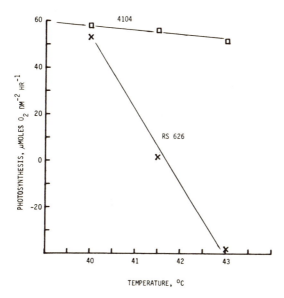

Figure 1. Effects of high temperatures on photosynthesis of two sorghum genotypes (from Norcio, 1976).

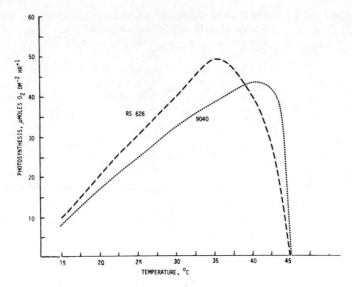

Fig. 2. Differences in temperature optimum for photosynthesis of two sorghum genotypes (from Norcio, 1976).

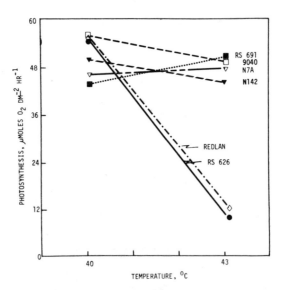

Fig. 3. High-temperature effects on photosynthesis of sorghums RS-626, RS-691, 9040, and Redlan, and corn N7A and N142 (from Norcio, 1976).

compared to markedly reduced rates by Redlan and RS-626. The two corn lines also maintained photosynthesis at the high temperature in agreement with our previous results, which showed that corn had high cellular and chloroplast heat tolerance.

Norcio (1976) also found a positive correlation between the ability to maintain photosynthesis at high temperatures and cellular heat tolerance of sorghums, as determined by the leaf-disc method.

When transpiration and evaporative cooling decrease as a result of water deficits, leaf temperatures may increase considerably above ambient (Ansari and Loomis, 1959; Tanner, 1963; Gates, 1968). We have recorded leaf temperatures of dry land-grown sorghum hybrids very near that reported by Norcio to sharply decrease photosynthesis in some genotypes, and as expected, a significant positive correlation was found between leaf temperatures, measured with an infrared noncontact thermometer, and leaf diffusive resistance to water-vapor transfer. This same group of 15 hybrids was tested for heat tolerance near the maximum stress period of 1974, a high heat-stress year, and there was a significant positive correlation between heat tolerance and yield that same year (Sullivan et al., 1975). These hybrids were made from selected M.35-1 conversion males (shortened height) crossed with Martin, Wheatland, and Redlan females.

The results and discussion we have presented show that genetic differences in heat tolerance occur. We have further shown that plants can be selected for high-temperature tolerance.

CONCLUSION

These differences in cellular heat tolerance and ability to photosynthesize and carry on metabolic functions at high temperatures may markedly affect plant productivity in hot environments. Although our knowledge is increasing, much is still unknown about the effects and interactions of high-temperature stress. This is certainly an area in which additional research should be fruitful.

REFERENCES

Alexandrov. V. Ya. (1964). Cytophysiological and cytoecological investigations of heat resistance of plant cells toward the action of high and low temperatures. *Quart. Rev. Biol. 39*:35–77.

Ansari, A. Q. and Loomis, W. E. (1959). Leaf temperatures. *Amer. J. Bot. 46*:713–717.

Coffman, F. A. (1957). Factors influencing heat resistance in oats. *Agron. J. 49*:368–373.

Dexter. S. T., Tottingham, W. E., and Graber, L. F. (1932). Investigations of the hardiness of plants by measurement of electrical conductivity. *Plant Physiol. 7*:63–78.

Dickinson, T. E. (1976). Caryopsis development and the effect of induced high temperatures in *Sorghum bicolor* (L.) Moench. M.S. thesis. Univ. of Nebraska, Lincoln.

Downes, R. W. (1972). Effect of temperature on the phenology and grain yield of *Sorghum bicolor. Aust. J. Agri. Res. 23*:584–594.

Gates, D. M. (1968). Transpiration and leaf temperatures. *Annu. Rev. Plant Physiol. 19*:211–238.

Heyne, E. G. and Brunson, A. M. (1940). Genetic studies of heat and drought tolerance in maize. *J. Amer. Soc. Agron. 32*:803–814.

Heyne, E. G. and Laude, H. H. (1940). Resistance of corn seedlings to high temperatures in laboratory tests. *J. Amer. Soc. Agron. 32*:116–126.

Hoshikawa, K. (1962). Studies on the ripening of wheat grain. 4. Influence of temperature upon the development of the endosperm. *Proc. Crop Sci. Soc. Jap. 30*:228–231.

Hunter, J. W., Laude, H. H., and Brunson, A. M. (1936). A method for studying resistance to drought injury in inbred lines of maize. *J. Amer. Soc. Agron. 28*:694–698.

Jones, D. F. (1947). Effect of temperature on the growth and sterility of maize. *Science 105*:390–391.

Julander, O. (1945). Drought resistance in range and posture grasses. *Plant Physiol. 20*: 573–599.

Kaloyereas, S. A. (1958). A new method of determining drought resistance. *Plant Physiol. 33*:232–233.

Kilen, T. C. and Andrews, R. H. (1969). Measurement of drought resistance in corn. *Agron. J. 61*:669–672.

Kydrev, T. G. and Kolev, V. M. (1962). Thermal treatment of dry wheat seeds and its effect on the plants. *Fiziol. Rast.* (AIBS Transl., *Sov. Plant Physiol.*)*8*:460–463.

Levitt, J. (1956). *The Hardiness of Plants,* 278 pp. Academic Press, New York and London.

Levitt, J. (1972). *Responses of Plants to Environmental Stresses,* 697 pp. Academic Press, New York and London.

Murty, K. S. and Majumder, S. K. (1962). Modifications of the technique for determination of chlorophyll stability index in relation to studies of drought resistance in rice. *Curr. Sci. 31*:470–471.

Nagato, K. and Ebata, M. (1966). Effects of high temperature during ripening period of the development and quality of rice kernels. *Proc. Crop Sci. Soc. Jap. 34*:59–66.

Norcio, N. (1976). Effect of high temperature and water stress on photosynthesis and respiration rates of grain sorghum. Ph.D. thesis. The Univ. of Nebraska, Lincoln.

Pallas, J. E. and Bertrand, A. R. (1966). Research in plant transpiration: 1963. *Prod. Res. Rept. No. 89,* ARS, USDA, Georgia Agr. Expt. Sta. and Meteor. Dept. U.S. Army Elect. Res. Dev. Activ.

Pasternak, D. and Wilson, G. L. (1969). Effects of heat waves on grain sorghum at the stage of head emergence. *Aust. J. Exp. Agr. Animal Husb. 9*:636–638.

Rao, G. N. and Murty, B. R. (1963). Growth analysis in grain sorghums of deccan. *Indian J. Agri. Sci. 33*:155–162.

Sanchez-Diaz, M. F. and Kramer, P. J. (1971). Behavior of corn and sorghum during water stress and during recovery. *Plant Physiol. 48*:613–616.

Schroeder, C. A. (1963). Induced temperature tolerance of plant tissue in vitro. *Nature (London) 200*:1301–1302.

Smith, D. H. (1973). Selected studies of heat tolerance in grain sorghum (*Sorghum bicolor* (L.) Moench). M. S. thesis. The Univ. of Nebraska, Lincoln.

Sullivan, C. Y. (1972). Mechanisms of heat and drought resistance in grain sorghum and methods of measurement. In *Sorghum in Seventies* (Rao, N. G. P. and House, L. R. eds.), pp. 247–264.

Sullivan, C. Y. and Eastin, J. D. (1969). Effects of heat and drought on the photosynthetic activity of isolated chloroplasts from sorghum, corn and pearl millet. *Agron. Abst. Amer. Soc. Agron.,* p. 30.

Sullivan, C. Y. and Eastin, J. D. (1973). Stomatal control of water loss in sorghum and corn and relation to desiccation tolerance. In *The Physiology of Yield and Management of Sorghum in Relation to Genetic Improvement. (Annu. Rept. 7, Univ. of Nebr., USDA, ARS, NCR)* pp. 58–64. The Rockefeller Foundation, Lincoln, Nebr.

Sullivan, C. Y. and Kinbacher, E. J. (1967). Thermal stability of fraction I protein from heat hardened *Phaseolus acutifolius* Gray 'Tepary Buff.' *Crop Sci.* 7:241–244.

Sullivan, C. Y., Eastin, J. D., and Kinbacher, E. J. (1968. Finding the key to heat and drought resistance in grain sorghum. University of Nebraska, *Farm, Ranch and Home Quarterly 15*:7–9.

Sullivan, C. Y., Ogunlela, V. B., Ross, W. M., and Eastin, J. D. (1975). Selecting for heat and desiccation tolerance in field grown sorghum. In *The Physiology of Yield and Management of Sorghum in Relation to Genetic Improvement (Annu. Rept. 8., Univ. of Nebr., USDA, ARS, NCR)* pp. 118–125. The Rockefeller Foundation, Lincoln, Nebr.

Tanner, C. B. (1963). Plant temperatures. *Agron. J. 55*:210–211.

Tatum, L. A. (1954). Breeding for drought and heat tolerance. *Rep. 9th Hybrid Corn Ind. Res. Conf. 9*:22–28.

Wardlaw, I. F. (1970). The early stage of grain development in wheat: Response to light and temperature in a single variety. *Aust. J. Biol. Sci. 23*:765–774.

Williams, T. V., Snell, R. S., and Cress, C. E. (1969). Inheritance of drought tolerance in sweet corn. *Crop Sci. 9*:19–23.

Yarwood, C. E. (1967). Adaptation of plants and plant pathogens to heat. In *Molecular Mechanisms of Temperature Adaptation* (Prosser, C. L., ed.) pp. 75–89. Am. Assoc. Adv. Sci., Washington, D.C.

29

Effect of High-Temperature Stress on the Growth and Seed Characteristics of Barley and Cotton

Riaz A. Khan
Department of Agronomy
University of Agriculture
Lyallpur, Pakistan

ABSTRACT

The existence of a sensitivity gradient to a uniform high-temperature stress applied at stages during seed maturation can be demonstrated in barley. The germination of freshly harvested seed is depressed following heat stress at 7–10 days after awn emergence, but is enhanced by the same stress applied 3 weeks after awn emergence. The depression is attributed to reduced viability associated with thermal injury. The stimulation following stress at more mature stages of seed development is related to a thinner seed coat, increased permeability as evidenced by faster imbibition rate, and decreased content of water-soluble inhibitors in the seed. These effects of environmental stress during seed maturation aid in explaining differences noted in the germinability at harvest of seed produced in successive years or produced in the same year at different locations.

Seed of American Cotton, var. AC 134, was stressed at 50°, 60°, 70°, 80°, and 90°C for 24 or 48 h before seeding. Stresses at 50° to 70°C increased seedling emergence and subsequent performance of the cotton plants, but higher temperatures caused thermal injury or killed the seed.

INTRODUCTION

During the normal progress of growth, a plant in the field experiences continually changing conditions of the environment. When these environmental conditions lie outside the "optimal range," a stress is exerted on the plant. The effects of a given stress vary with the stage of development of the organism at the time of exposure.

Temperature stress at a critical period of development has been shown to affect subsequent growth in several crop species. Jennings and de Jesus (1964) demonstrated that direct exposure of freshly harvested rice seed in envelopes to 50°C for 4–5 days broke dormancy in many varieties. Kydrev and Kolev (1962) reported that wheat seedlings emerging from seeds stressed at 50°–80°C for 1 h showed, subsequently, a greater resistance to dry and hot environments. Jones (1947) found corn seedlings exposed to 1 h of heat just after emergence developed into shorter plants, flowered later, and had considerable pollen sterility. Dotzenko (1967) stressed White Wonder millet plants at 2° or 35°C during anther emergence. The seed produced after 2°C exposure required prechilling before germination, whereas that stressed at 35°C did not. Laude (1967), studying Atlas barley, suggested the existence, during seed maturation, of a sensitivity gradient to high-temperature stress. Thus, it appears that critical periods of high sensitivity prevail at seed, early seedling, near-flowering, and seed maturation stages. Stress during one of these periods of growth may alter subsequent growth and development of the plant.

It is reasonable to assume that supraoptimal but sublethal stress applied during a period of high sensitivity may trigger subsequent responses as yet not well appreciated but of significant physiological and agricultural importance. Consequently, the objective of the present study was to explore these possibilities in cotton and barley using high temperature as the stress factor. In barley, the effect of brief exposures during seed maturation to supraoptimal but sublethal temperatures on the germinability of freshly harvested seeds was studied. Particular attention was directed to the influence of heat stress applied at successive stages of seed maturation as well as to the resultant changes in the seed characteristics. In cotton, after high-temperature treatments of the seeds, a study was made of seedling emergence and subsequent performance of the plants.

MATERIALS AND METHODS

Barley

Potted plants of Atlas barley grown under greenhouse as well as outdoor conditions were subjected to heat stress at different stages during seed maturation. The plants were introduced into the stress chamber when the air temperature in the chamber reached 38°C. Thereafter, the temperature was raised gradually to the desired maximum and held at that temperature for the intended duration. Subsequently the plants were cooled for 30 min to near greenhouse temperature before returning them to the prestress conditions. Seed was harvested when all green coloration had left the spike, and germination tests commenced immediately in a controlled environment growth chamber at constant 20°C with a daily photoperiod of 8 h. Daily emergence was recorded for 21 days. Duncan's Multiple Range test was used to establish statistical significance among treatment means.

Cotton

Air-dried seeds of cotton var. A.C.134 were stressed at 50°, 60°, 70°, 80°, and 90°C for 24 or 48 h in a temperature controlled cabinet. Germination tests, commenced 1 day after the temperature stress, were measured in terms of seedling emergence. The emergence rate index was calculated by the method of Kappleman and Buchanan (1968).

Stressed and nonstressed seeds also were grown simultaneously in 24-cm-diameter pots filled with 30 lb sandy clay loam soil fertilized with 80 lb urea nitrogen per 2×10^6 lb soil. One plant per pot was grown to maturity to observe subsequent effects of heat stress on flowering, fruiting, and yield of seed cotton. A further three rows each of stressed and nonstressed seeds were planted in replicated plots of 7.5- × 28-ft plots in the field, using a completely randomized block design. Fifty seeds were sown in each row. When the seedlings were 15 cm (6 in.) high, they were thinned to 23 plants per row, and nitrogen was added at 60 lb per acre at the preflowering stage.

RESULTS AND CONCLUSIONS

Effects of Heat Stress during Seed Maturation on Seed Characteristics and Seedling Growth in Barley

The existence of a sensitivity gradient to a uniform high temperature applied at stages during seed maturation was demonstrated when the stressed seed was planted immediately after harvest. The stress temperature used was 1–2 h at 54°C after 90 min of heating from 38° to 54°C. Maximum germinability was obtained more quickly from the seed stressed about 3 weeks after awn emergence. This germination rate remained more or less constant with the age of the seed up to 3 months. Seed of greater age was not tested. Germinability was lowered considerably when seed was stressed in earlier stages as well as when stressed at 29 days after awn emergence. However, the germinability obtained from the seed stressed in earlier stages remained poor when germinated 1–90 days after harvesting, whereas that of the seed stressed at 29 days after awn emergence increased like the control seed with the passage of time. The existence of a sensitivity gradient was revealed also by plants grown outdoors. Increased germinability at harvest was shown by barley varieties other than Atlas when stressed at $40°$ and $54°C$ during seed maturation, suggesting that the observed response is general in barley.

Stimulation in germinability at harvest of the seed stressed some 3 weeks after awn emergence was associated with a thinner seed coat, increased seed coat permeability and faster imbibition rate, and decreased content of a water-soluble inhibitor in the seed.

The dormancy and germinability of seed stressed at the earlier stages of development differed from that of seed stressed later. A comparison was made of seed removed from the parent plant at 10 days or at 21 days after awn emergence. Seed removed from the parent plants 10 days after awn emergence showed no seed dormancy, while that removed at the 21-day stage showed characteristic fresh seed dormancy as in control seed harvested at seed maturity. These observations indicate that at 10 days after awn emergence the factor or factors causing seed dormancy, possibly an inhibitor, had not accumulated in sufficient concentration to give seed dormancy. A level of inhibitor potency causing seed dormancy developed later, but before the seed was 21 days from awn emergence. Heat stress at 21 days destroyed or inactivated, or at least reduced, this dormancy factor, and the result was the stimulation in germination noted in these studies. Inhibitor potency assayed by excised embryo and lettuce seed bioassays showed less inhibitor is present in seed stressed at the 21-day stage than in unstressed seed of the same age. Heat stress at 10 days after awn emergence, if intense enough to arrest further seed development and to cause injury to the seed (detectable by excised embryo germination and tetrazolium tests), resulted in reduced germinability, but if less severe, seed development continued and this seed, if harvested at maturity, exhibited typical fresh seed dormancy like the controls.

Seedlings from seed stressed at relatively mature stages were like those from control seed. These seedlings were also more vigorous than those obtained from plants at 10 days after awn emergence; they produced uniformly normal seedlings compared with controls, despite the fact the seed was only one-third as heavy as the control seed. This suggests that the depression noted in growth of the seedlings raised from seed stressed at earlier stages was associated with deleterious thermal effects. This contention was further confirmed when seed at the earlier stage was less severely stressed, to prevent heat injury to the seed, and it produced normal seedlings as compared with the controls. However, higher temperature or longer exposure for any one stage of seed maturation resulted in reduced seed viability and stunted seedlings with narrow leaves. Seed size and weight did not appear to be associated with measurable differences in germinability of seedling growth in this study.

Effects of Heat Stress to Cotton Seed on Subsequent Plant Growth

Seedling emergence 7 days after planting was significantly higher with a matching emergence rate index for seeds stressed at $50°–70°C$ for 24 or 48 h, as compared with nonstressed seeds. However, this difference in germinability of the nonstressed (control) and the stressed seeds disappeared by the fourteenth day after planting, by which time all the viable control seeds had emerged. Emergence from the seeds stressed at 80°C was very poor, the seedlings were abnormal, stunted and discolored, and most of them died shortly after emergence, while a temperature of 90°C killed the seeds. These observations suggest that whereas 50°–70°C may have a stimulatory effect on germinability, a stress at a higher temperature may cause thermal injury or heat killing of the seed.

The imbibition rate was significantly greater for the heat-stressed seed than for the controls. The increased permeability of stressed seed, as evidenced by the faster imbibition rate, may be one of the factors causing faster emergence.

The faster emergence from stressed seeds enabled seedlings to become better established before the soil dried, as compared with the more slowly emerging seedlings from nonstressed seed. This initial difference in establishment of seedlings was manifest also in their subsequent growth and yields. The flowering, fruiting, and yield of seed cotton was generally higher in plants from stressed seeds grown outdoors in pots. These observations were further confirmed in the field, where a presowing temperature stress of 70°C for 24 or 48 h, 1 day after harvest or after 3 months' dry storage, resulted in a significant increase in yield of seed cotton. This increase in yield was more consistent when the stress was applied to freshly harvested seed.

Average summer temperatures during growth of the crop were 3.5°C higher than normal (37°C), rainfall was 13.7 cm (5.4 in.) less than normal (28.2 cm, 11.5 in.), and supply of irrigation water was reduced considerably because of low water levels in the rivers. Under these conditions of higher summer temperature and severe drought, plants from the stressed seed showed relatively greater resistance. The heat stress probably hardened the embryo within the seed, so that plants developing from such embroys had greater resistance to the extremes of weather and performed better than the control plants, as was indicated from the significant differences in their yield. This observation is supported by the work of Schroeder (1963), who showed that plant tissue can acquire hardiness to high temperature by a brief exposure to heat treatment at 50°C. Such hardening of plants to high temperature has also been claimed to be associated with hardening to drought (Levitt, 1951). Similarly, induction of resistance to high temperature and drought in wheat seedlings emerging from seeds stressed at 50°–80°C for 1 h was reported by Kydrev and Kolev (1962).

REFERENCES

Dotzenko, A. D. (1967). Temperature stress during anther extrusion. *Western Regional Research Publ. Tech. Bull. 97, Colo. Exp. Sta., Fort Collins,* pp. 12–17.

Jennings, P. R. and de Jesus, J., Jr. (1964). Effect of heat on breaking seed dormancy in rice. *Crop Sci. 4*:530–533.

Jones, D. F. (1947). Effect of temperature on the growth and sterility of maize. *Science* *105*:390–391.

Kappleman, A. J., Jr. and Buchanan, G. A. (1968). Influence of fungicides, herbicides and combinations on emergence and seedling growth of cotton. *Agron. J. 60*:660–662.

Kydrev, T. G. and Kolev, V. M. (1962). Thermal treatment of dry wheat seeds and its effect on the plant. *Fiziol. Rast. 8*:460–463.

Laude, H. M. (1967). Temperature stress during seed maturation. *Western Regional Research Publ. Tech. Bull. 97, Colo. Exp. Sta., Fort Collins,* pp. 17–19.

Levitt, J. (1951). Frost, drought and heat resistance. *Annu. Rev. Plant Physiol. 2*:245–268.

Schroeder, C. A. (1963). Induced temperature tolerance in plant tissue *in vitro. Nature, (London) 200*:1301–1302.

30

Plant Genotype Effects
on Nitrogen Fixation in Grasses

Johanna Döbereiner

Empresa Brasileira de Pesquisa Agropecuaria
UEPAE Itaguai via Campo Grande
Rio de Janeiro, Brazil

ABSTRACT

Potentials for nitrogen fixation of economic importance have been shown now for a number of tropical forage grasses, sorghum, maize, rice, and perhaps even wheat. The exploitation of this potential, however, will be dependent on the identification of the limiting factors and agronomically feasible practices to eliminate them. Environmental effects are pronounced but rather difficult to manipulate. Whenever possible, preference should be given to plant-breeding practices.

Differences between cultivars and even ecotypes of *Paspalum notatum* in relation to the occurrence of *Azotobacter paspali* were shown several years ago. Differences in nitrogenase activity were then confirmed in this species, in *Pennisetum purpureum,* and in *Digitaria decumbens.* Among S_1 lines of maize, several could be selected with nitrogenase activity many times higher than that of the original cultivar.

Considerable nitrogenase activity has now been shown in wheat. Estimates from 24-h intact soil core assays indicate up to 400 g N/h/day being fixed at flowering stage. Extracted root assays correlated well with the intact system (correlation coefficient $r = 0.87$), but gave values less than one-third of those obtained with intact soil–plant systems. Differences between cultivars were at the limit of significance.

INTRODUCTION

Potentials for nitrogen fixation of economic importance have been shown now for a number of tropical forage grasses (Balandreau and Villemin, 1973; Day et al., 1975), sorghum, maize (Balandreau and Dommergues, 1972; Bülow and Döbereiner, 1975), and rice (Yoshida and Ancajas, 1971). Although most results have been obtained by the indirect C_2H_2 reduction method, confirmation by $^{15}N_2$ incorporation has been reported for *Paspalum* and *Digitaria* (De-Polli et al., 1977). The association of these species with nitrogen-fixing bacteria seems to be much less perfect than the nodule symbioses of legumes with *Rhizobium* or those of nonleguminous species with *Actinomyces* sp., and are therefore more vulnerable to environmental effects, which often are difficult to control. Much research is necessary to understand the mechanism of the grass associations. The exploitation of this novel nitrogen source will be dependent on the identification of the limiting factors and agronomically feasible practices to eliminate them. Plant-breeding practices with the objective of obtaining more stable and more efficient grass—bacteria associations rank among the most promising possibilities. The present chapter reviews the available information related to plant genotype effects on N_2 fixation in grass.

Forage Grasses

A number of years ago differences were shown between cultivars and ecotypes of *Palpalum notatum* in their rhizosphere effects on the occurrence of *Azotobacter paspali* (Döbereiner, 1970); plant genotype effects on nitrogenase activity on roots extracted from the soil are presented in Table I. The broad-leaved tetraploid types are much more propitious for *A. paspali* growth than the fine-leaved Pensacola types from Florida and the hybrid seems to be intermediate. Nitrogenase activity and forage yield were similar, except for the hybrid, which seemed to be able to obtain more nitrogen from the soil. These data indicate that selection for high forage yield and for high nitrogen fixation seems possible. Significant differences between nitrogenase activity in intact soil—plant cores of variou• *Digitaria* genotypes can be observed in Table II. Several such observations during the entire growth cycle would be necessary to evaluate nitrogen-fixing capacities for selection. The high amount of nitrogen taken out by the forage from the extremely poor soil is additional evidence that nitrogen fixation should be substantial. Tentative balance accounts indicate yearly mean gains of more than 0.5 kg N/ha/day, which would be still more than the amounts estimated by the nitrogenase activity in cores measured in summer.

Maize and Sorghum

Extremely high nitrogenase activities have been reported on selected S_1 lines of maize and also some sorghum plants (Table III). As can be seen from the high

Table I. Differences between Cultivars and Ecotypes of P. notatum in Their Capacity to Support A. paspali and Fix Nitrogen and Their forage Production and Nitrogen Assimilation[a,b]

Cultivar or ecotype	Type of leaf	N$_2$-ase activity (nmoles C$_2$H$_4$/g roots/ha)				Forage production (g dry matter/m^2 after 4 months)	Nitrogen assimilation in leaves (g N/m^2 after 4 months)
		11/72[c]	1/73	3/73	11/73		
T7 Batatais Km 47	Broad	1.02	78.1[d]	79.6[d]	6.7	829[d]	17.11[d]
61 Batatais Matão	Broad	1.15	63.2	42.0	5.9	592	11.41
53 Typhen hybrid	Intermediate	3.43	18.2	22.8	6.8	1010	21.60
48 Pensacola Florida	Fine	1.36	13.8	20.6	4.9	620	12.78
50 Pensacola Argentina	Fine	2.02	29.0	24.4	4.2	303	6.57
55 Pensacola hybrid	Fine	1.42	5.6	13.4	4.8	402	7.37

	Number of microcolonies A. paspali/g dry root-surface soil			
	11/72[c]	1/73	3/73	11/73
T7 Batatais Km 47	7,700	2,325[e]	9,950[e]	14,300[e]
61 Batatais Matão	4,665	3,272	13,050	8,450
53 Typhen hybrid	1,167	1,170	1,350	8,350
48 Pensacola Florida	16	37	2,900	5,400
50 Pensacola Argentina	0	12	320	150
55 Pensacola hybrid	0	50	37	250

[a] Means of 4 replicate plots, 2 samples each.
[b] From Day et al. (1975).
[c] At transplant.
[d] Difference significant at $p = 0.01$.
[e] Difference significant at $p = 0.05$.

328   Johanna Döbereiner

Table II. Nitrogenase Activity and Nitrogen Yield of Three Commercial Cultivars of *Digitaria decumbens* and Three *Digitaria* Hybrids[a,b]

| Genotype | g N/ha/day | | |
	N$_2$ fixed estimated from C$_2$H$_2$ assays[c]	N in forage[d]	N gain not accounted for[e]
Pangola	881	1501	405
Transvala	485	1482	216
Slenderstem	970	1400	468
Hybrid 46-2	234	2022	1090
Hybrid 97-2	265	2101	1279
Hybrid 159-4	446	1789	967

[a] From Schank and Day (1975).
[b] All data are means of four replicate plots.
[c] Estimates from 24-h assays with 10-cm-wide intact soil–plant cores taken in March 1975, based on the theoretical 3 : 1 C$_2$H$_2$: N$_2$ conversion rate.
[d] Mean daily nitrogen increase in forage as determined by Kjeldahl analysis taken between Nov., 1973, and May, 1975.
[e] Calculated from total N in forage after 18 months minus difference in soil nitrogen content (0–20 cm) minus 200 kg N added as fertilizer. Mean N% in soil at beginning of experiment was 0.080 and at the end 0.072.

variability, although there were differences at the 5% level between lines and the original cultivar, the variation between individual plants was very high, so that these lines can not be considered uniformly higher; rather, a few S$_1$ plants with extremely high activity were found in these lines. Seeds of these plants were pooled for one generation of cross-pollination and are under test at the time of writing this chapter. Furthermore, the extent to which the differences among S$_1$ plants and lines were caused by the pronounced differences in the growth cycle is not known (Döbereiner et al., 1975).

Rice

Although it has been suggested that N$_2$ fixation in grass associations might be limited to C$_4$ grasses that should have more photosynthetic products available for this purpose, Yoshida and Ancajas (1971) showed substantial rhizosphere nitrogen fixation in rice, which was attributable to the presence of heterotrophic bacteria. More recent data also indicate differences between cultivars in rice (Table IV).

Table III. Nitrogenase Activity on Roots of Field-Grown Maize,
Sorghum, and Teosinte in Summer (January) and after Cool Nights (April)[a]

	January			April		
	Number of samples	Mean	Maximum observed	Number of samples	Mean	Maximum observed
Maize						
Cv. Piranão	24	646[b]	1870	7	1098	2104
Cv. UR-1	30	234	1650	–	–	–
S$_1$ line 122[c]	10	7124	13700	10	706	3013
61	10	2026	6846	10	606	2372
130	10	1870	4612	10	364	2125
102	10	1793	6121	10	920	3303
115	10	418	1533	10	486	1103
Sorghum						
Redlan A × B	4	1364	2973	16	1053	9833
Teosinte[d]						
Jutiapa	3	0		4	75	303
Bolsas	3	0		5	244	717

[a]From Bülow and Döbereiner (1975).
[b]Values represent nmoles C_2H_4/ha/g dry roots. All results are from field experiments at UFRRJ, in gray hydromorphic soil fertilized with PK and sprayed with 1 kg/ha of ammonium molybdate 1 or 2 months after planting. All plants were near flowering stage when the samples were taken. Mean maximal and minimal temperatures in January were 30.8° and 21.5°C and in April 28.7° and 17.9°C, respectively.
[c]Seed kindly provided by Dr. W. C. Galinat, Univ. of Massachusetts.
[d]These S$_1$ lines from Cv. UR-1 were selected among 276 lines in two 12 × 12 simple lattice field experiment, after prescreening of one plant per line. Difference between selected lines in January were significant at $p = 0.05$, although variations within lines were very high.

Wheat

Some preliminary data on nitrogenase activity in wheat have been discussed previously (Döbereiner et al., 1975). Table V shows that in spite of a large sample variation there is a 5% level of significance for varietal differences in both locations. Because of the difference in climatic conditions between Rio de Janeiro and Brasilia all the cultivars were different. In both locations the plants were sampled on the same day for all cultivars, and it is therefore impossible to eliminate growth stage effects. Intact soil–plant cores of wheat showed pronounced day–night fluctuations which, in contrast to *Paspalum* cores, responded more slowly to changes from day to night and had no night peak (Fig. 1). Although these cores were all collected at the flowering stage, there were large differences between individual cores taken in the same field. Extrapolation from the C_2H_2 reduction rates to nitrogen fixation, calculated on an area basis and from the 24-h rates, indicates the possibility of N_2 fixation in the range of 40 and 500 g N/ha/day at the flowering stage (Table VI).

Table IV. Nitrogenase Activity ($C_2 H_2$) in Rice
Cultivars in Intact Soil–Plant Systems
(nmoles $C_2 H_4$/ha/g roots)[a]

Rice cultivar	Seedlings in test tubes[b]	Plants at heading stage in pots with rice paddy soil[c]
Soil	0	0
IR 5	9900	87
IR 8	5000	78
IR 26		67
GBS 236		110
Bali Kamhong 37		98
Arlesienne	5500	
Cigalon	6400	
Delta	9800	
Cesariat	11400	
Cristal	11700	

[a]Differences between cultivars in both experiments highly significant. The pot experiment (Lee et al., 1975) contained 42 cultivars, but only the most active ones are computed here.
[b]Rinaudo et al. (1975).
[c]Lee et al. (1975).

Table V. Nitrogenase Activity on Extracted Wheat Roots Collected from Cultivar Trials at Flowering Stage in the Field

Rio de Janeiro[a]		Brasilia[b]	
Cultivar	nmoles $C_2 H_4$/ha/g roots	Cultivar	nmoles $C_2 H_4$/ha/g roots
Noroeste-66	210	IRN 152	74
St. Helena	175	S-61	73
BH-1146	138	Tanori	72
IRN-52663	138	IAC-5	49
LAI-434	130	S-42	39
IAS-20	118	Sonora-64	34
Reg. 260	80	BH-46	16
Sonora-63	73	S-60	20
IAS-49	64	S-79	11
L.s.d. 5%	92	Jacuí	11
CV	86%	D. Feliciano	5
		L.s.d. 5%	53
		CV	96%

[a]Data from Rio de Janeiro are means of two plants 10 replicates (5 inoculated, 5 not). There was no effect of seed inoculation and *Spirillum lipoferum* occurred abundantly on the roots of both (Nery et al., 1975).
[b]Data from Brasilia are means of 4 plants from 4 replicates each. There was no inoculation, and all collected roots showed abundant *S. lipoferum* occurrence (Peres and Silva, 1975)

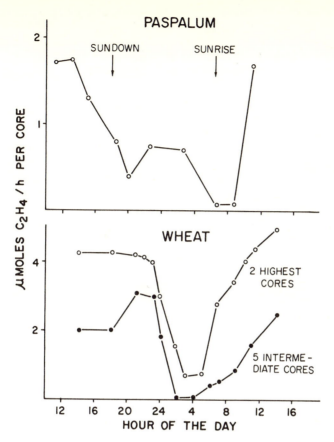

Fig. 1. Day–night cycle in N_2-ase activity in intact soil–plant cores of Paspalum notatum (Döbereiner and Day, 1973) and wheat (cv. Sonora) at flowering stage (Nery and Peres, 1975). Paspalum data are from three groups of three cores used alternatively for measuring 1-h C_2H_2 reduction rates after 1-h preincubation for gas equilibration. In these cores the leaves were inside the assay vessel during the assay. Wheat cores in plastic bags with aerial parts outside the bags were assayed for 24-h period under C_2H_2. The numbers of replicate cores are stated in the figure.

Table VI. Nitrogenase Activity in Ten Intact Wheat Cores (cv. Sonora) Collected at Random in the Field at Flowering Stage

	nmoles C_2H_4/h/core	Fixed N_2/day (μg/10 cm^3 core)	g N_2/day/ha[a]
Mean 2 most active cores	2641	597	506
Mean 5 intermediate cores	1137	276	238
Mean 3 least active cores	180	44	38
Mean all cores	—	—	229

[a]Estimate by the theoretical C_2H_2 : N_2 3 : 1 ratio from 24-h rates based on the $\emptyset$ of 10-cm area of the cores corrected for 15-cm distance between rows.

DISCUSSION

One of the major difficulties for plant-breeding work, where the purpose is that of increasing nitrogen fixation, is still the inadequacy of the methods of estimation of nitrogenase activity in large numbers of plants. Intact soil–plant cores are inadequate because of the amount of labor and material required. The meaningfulness of extracted root assays as a quantitative measure of the ability to fix nitrogen has been questioned (Hardy et al., 1975; Rinaudo et al., 1975) because these assays have to be done after 10–16-h preincubation treatments under low pO_2 which overcome a lag in C_2H_2 reduction onset. The activity of extracted *Paspalum notatum* roots and the soil in the cores came close to that of the intact systems (Döbereiner et al., 1972). In wheat and *Digitaria* a highly significant correlation of extracted root activity with that of intact cores was found (Fig. 2), although the intact activity was about three

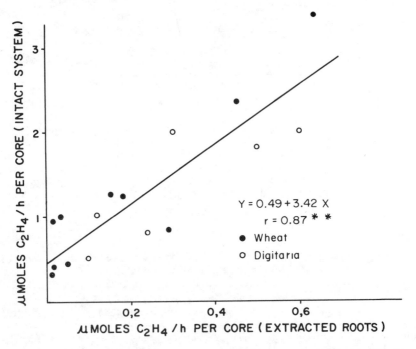

Fig. 2. Correlation of intact core N_2-ase activity in wheat cores (same as in Fig. 1) and Digitaria cores (assayed as stated for Paspalum in Fig. 1) with the N_2-ase activity of extracted roots obtained from the same cores, preincubated overnight at pO_2 0.02 atm, and assayed at pO_2 0.01 atm with 12% C_2H_2 (2-h rates).

times higher. This seems not to be the case in maize and sorghum where roots extracted from almost inactive intact cores showed activities of up to 400 and 1800 nmoles C_2H_4/ha/g roots, respectively (Tjepkema and van Berkum, 1976). In contrast, reproducible seasonal variations (Döbereiner et al., 1975), molybdenum effects, and varietal differences obtained also in maize and sorghum indicate that extracted root assays seem at least to provide relative values for comparison.

But once the assay problems have been overcome then the possibilities for plant breeding work seem attractive. Comparisons may be considered of physiological differences between genotypes with high and low activities for root anatomy, root physiology, translocation, and photosynthetic efficiency. Furthermore, the extension of seasonal and day peak activities seems possible. Studies of the interaction of nitrate assimilation with nitrogenase activity should represent the key elements for eventual success in attaining the goal of grain cultivars that obtain part of their nitrogen from biological fixation, and thereby can be maintained with low nitrogen fertilizer supplements.

ACKNOWLEDGMENTS

This contribution is from the Program for International Cooperation in Training and Basic Research on Nitrogen Fixation in the Tropics sponsored by the National Research Council, the Empresa Brasileira de Pesquisa Agropecuaria, and the Universidade Federal Rural do Rio de Janeiro.

REFERENCES

Balandreau, J. and Dommergues, Y. (1972). Assaying nitrogenase (C_2H_2) activity in the field. *Bull. Ecol. Res. Comm. (Stockh.)* 17:247–254.

Balandreau, J. and Villemin, G. (1973). Fixation biologique de l'azote moleculaire en savanne de Lampto (Basse Côté d'Ivoire). Résultat préliminaires. *Rev. Ecol. Biol. Sol.* 10:25–33.

von Bülow, J. F. W. and J. Döbereiner, (1975). Potential for nitrogen fixation in maize genotypes in Brazil. *Proc. Natl. Acad. Sci. USA* 72:2389–2393.

Day, J. M., Neves, M. C. P., and Döbereiner, J. (1975). Nitrogenase activity on the roots of tropical forage grasses. *Soil Biol. Biochem.* 7:107–112.

De Polli, H., Matsui, E., Döbereiner, J., and Salati, E. (1977). Confirmation of nitrogen fixation in two tropical grasses by $^{15}N_2$ incorporation. *Soil Biol. Biochem.* 9:119–123.

Döbereiner, J. (1970). Further research on *Azotobacter paspali* and its variety specific occurrence in the rhizosphere of *Paspalum notatum* Flugge. *Centralbl. Bakt. Parasitenkunde II.* 124:224–230.

Döbereiner, J. and Day, J. M. (1975). Dinitrogen fixation in the rhizosphere of tropical grasses. In *IBP Synthesis Meeting: Nitrogen in the Biosphere* (Stewart, W. D. P., ed.), Vol. 1, Chap. 3, pp. 39–52. Cambridge Univ. Press, Oxford.

Döbereiner, J., Day, J. M., and Dart, P. J. (1972). Nitrogenase activity and oxygen sensitivity of the *Paspalum–notatum–Azotabacter paspali* association. *J. Gen. Microbiol.* *71*:103–116.

Döbereiner, J., Day, J. M., and von Bülow, J. F. W. (1975). Associations of nitrogen fixing bacteria with roots of forage grass and grain species. II. *Int. Winter Wheat Conf. Proc.* pp. 221–237. Zagreb, Yugoslavia.

Hardy, R. W. F., Filner, P. and Hageman, R. H. (1975). Nitrogen Input. In *Crop Productivity–Research Imperatives, International Conference, Tennessee,* p. 160. Michigan State University and Kettering Foundation, East Lansing.

Lee, Kuk-ki, Bonifácio, V., and Watanabe, I. (1975). Non-symbiotic nitrogen fixation in paddy soils. *IRRI Saturday Seminar.*

Nery, M., Peres, J. R. R., and Döbereiner, J. (1975). Unpublished data.

Peres, J. R. R. and da Silva, A. R. (1975). (*Unpublished data from our laboratory and Centro Nacional de Pesquisa de Cerrado, Brasilia.*)

Rinaudo, G., Hames-Farad, I., Mouraret, M., and Dommergues, Y. (1975). N_2-fixation in the rice rhizosphere: Methods of measurement; practices suggested to enhance the process. *Biological Nitrogen Fixation in Farming Systems of the Humid Tropics, Conference Ibadan, Nigeria.*

Schank, S. and Day, J. M. (1975). (*Unpublished data from our laboratory.*)

Tjepkema, J. D. and van Berkum, P. (1976). (*Unpublished data from our laboratory.*)

Yoshida, T. and Ancajas, R. R. (1971). Nitrogen fixation by bacteria in the root zone of rice. *Proc. Soil Sci. Amer. 35*:156–157.

VI

Seed Storage Proteins

31

Storage Proteins in Cereals

Hans Doll
Agricultural Research Department
Research Establishment Risø
DK-4000 Roskilde, Denmark

ABSTRACT

The seed protein of cereals comprises many different proteins that are synthesized and accumulated in the endosperm during seed development. The total amount of protein produced depends heavily on the availability of nitrogen. High-yielding cereals are generally very effective in their utilization of the available nitrogen for protein production, and the prospect of genetic improvements in this respect seems limited. Traditionally, the protein of the cereal endosperm is classified into albumin, globulin, prolamin, and glutelin. The most typical and best-known storage protein is found in the prolamin fraction, which is present in high or medium amounts in maize, sorghum, wheat, and barley, whereas the prolamin content is low in rice and oats. Prolamin is deposited in protein bodies in the starchy endosperm, and it has a low content of the amino acids that are essential for man and nonruminant animals. It has been shown in maize, sorghum, and barley that prolamin synthesis is controlled by a limited number of genes and that an inactivation of these genes is not lethal for the plant. Genotypes with reduced prolamin synthesis have a substantially increased concentration of lysine and other essential amino acids in the seed protein, because these amino acids are much more abundant in the other endosperm proteins. The low-prolamin genotypes, normally termed high-lysine types, offer great possibilities for improving the nutritional value of cereal protein. However, the somewhat reduced grain yield of most high-lysine types indicates that an inactivation of the prolamin synthesis impairs the accumulation of carbohydrates in the endosperm.

337

INTRODUCTION

Considering the origin of our food, it is true that most of the protein consumed by humans derives from grain cereals directly or through animal production. This great contribution of cereals to our protein supply is merely a consequence of the even more central role played by grain cereals in our supply of metabolizable energy. The low content of protein in cereal grains, and especially the poor nutritional quality of most cereal protein, have led to great efforts to improve this protein genetically both in quantity and quality. Even though such improvements are very important, it should always be kept in mind that the production of starch, for example, in cereals is probably just as important as the protein production. Therefore, protein should not be improved at the expense of other important properties of the cereals.

This chapter gives a brief introduction to the classification, formation, and deposition of storage protein in cereals, as well as an evaluation of the possibilities of improving the storage protein genetically. Barley is the principal example in this chapter. This does not imply that storage protein is best known in barley—it simply reflects the author's field of work. No attempt is made to give a thorough review of the topic, as this was done by Altschul et al. (1966) and more recently by Sylvester-Bradley and Folkes (1976). Also, the reviews by Nelson (1969), Millerd (1975), and Dure, III (1975) contain much information on this subject.

FORMATION AND DEPOSITION OF STORAGE PROTEIN

The cereal grains are characterized by their large, highly developed endosperm, a typical storage organ, which contains all the components necessary for the initial growth of the embryo at germination. All the protein present in the mature endosperm may be considered as storage protein from the point of view that it can be utilized by the embryo at germination. However, the endosperm contains many different proteins that are very different with respect to formation, composition, and function, only some of which have typical storage properties. These differences are of greatest importance for an understanding of the possibilities for obtaining a better nutritional value of the endosperm protein.

Seed proteins are traditionally classified into albumin, globulin, prolamin, and glutelin according to their solubility in water, salt solution, alcohol, and basic or acid solutions, respectively. This protein fractionation, proposed by Osborne (1895), has proved very convenient in a broad characterization of the seed protein. However, since the Osborne fractionation is based on the physicochemical properties of the proteins, it tells us little about their physiological properties. Furthermore, because fractionation is not performed in exactly the same way in different cereals and different laboratories, comparisons are difficult.

The diversity of the endosperm protein is best illustrated by following its formation during endosperm development. The results of one such study are presented in Fig. 1, which shows the results obtained by Brandt (1976), who observed the formation of protein and dry matter in the barley endosperm. The dry weight of the endosperm can be used as a measure of the total accumulation of storage products in the endosperm. The gain in dry weight started about 8 days after flowering and leveled out around 20 days later. Albumin was very different from the other Osborne protein fractions with respect to formation pattern. The albumin, in which the enzymes and free amino acids are found, was present in considerable amounts very early in the development of the endosperm, and it preceded both the gain in dry weight and the other protein fractions (Fig. 1). The globulin, prolamin, and glutelin fractions were formed relatively late compared with the main increase in endosperm dry weight (Fig. 1), which indicates that the synthesis of storage protein is delayed compared with the starch synthesis.

Although the globulin, prolamin, and glutelin are synthesized at about the same time (Fig. 1), they contain proteins that are very different in function and amino acid composition. The globulin and some part of the glutelin have almost the same amino acid composition as the albumin fraction (Brandt, 1976). These

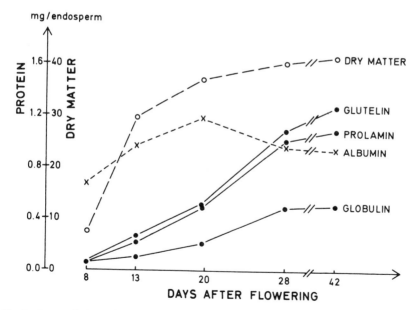

Fig. 1. Accumulation of protein and dry matter in the barley endosperm during development (Brandt, 1976).

fractions probably consist mainly of proteins related to membranes and cell walls, and only the latter fraction, the glutelin, is generally considered a storage protein. The most typical storage protein is present in the prolamin fraction, which is entirely different from the other endosperm protein fractions in amino acid composition. Generally, prolamin has a low content of the amino acids essential for humans and nonruminant animals (e.g., lysine), whereas the content of glutamic acid and proline is extremely high (Brandt, 1976).

Prolamin is also different from the other protein fractions because of the way in which it is deposited in the endosperm. Special protein stores have been detected and termed protein bodies in maize (Khoo and Wolf, 1970), wheat (Buttrose, 1963), sorghum (Adams and Novellie, 1975), and barley (Ory and Henningsen, 1969). Most of the protein in the protein bodies is prolamin (Tronier et al., 1971; Christianson et al., 1974; Ingversen, 1975). Therefore, the storage nature of the prolamin is further emphasized by its deposition in special bodies. It should be noted that the protein bodies in the starchy endosperm differ from the protein-containing aleuron grains found in the aleuron cells (Jacobsen et al., 1971).

AMOUNT OF STORAGE PROTEIN FORMED

All the protein produced in a cereal crop derives from inorganic nitrogen taken up from the soil. Hence, the amount of nitrogen available limits the ultimate protein production, and this production may strongly depend on environmental factors. In these respects cereals differ from legumes, which have the ability to utilize photosynthetically stored energy to reduce atmospheric nitrogen to ammonia.

The dependence of protein formation on nitrogen availability is illustrated in Figs. 2 and 3, which show how the protein production per seed and per unit area, respectively, is related to the supply of nitrogen fertilizer. The figures were made from the results of an experiment with barley grown outdoors in pots (Andersen and Køie, 1975, and personal communication). On a per-seed basis, the amount of albumin plus globulin, which were extracted together, was independent of nitrogen fertilization, whereas the glutelin, and especially the prolamin fractions, increased substantially with increasing nitrogen supply (Fig. 2). This means that the prolamin and the glutelin fractions contain the typical storage proteins, i.e., particularly those accumulated in the seeds when more nitrogen is available.

Figure 3 shows the relationship between nitrogen application and amount of nitrogen (protein) harvested per unit area in the entire plants (straw plus seeds) as well as in the seeds. Both the total and the seed nitrogen increased drastically when more nitrogen was available. The increase in the amount of nitrogen in the seeds was partly attributable to the increase in protein per seed (Fig. 2) and

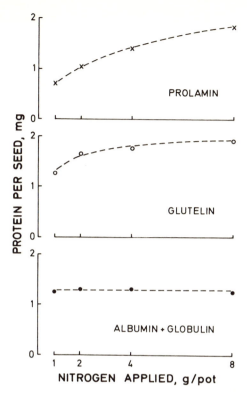

Fig. 2. Formation of different protein fractions in barley seeds as influenced by nitrogen fertilization (Andersen and Køie, 1975).

partly to an increased number of seeds per pot. The slopes of the two curves in Fig. 3 reflect, respectively, the ability of the barley to absorb nitrogen from the soil and to translocate it into the seeds. At the lowest nitrogen application, 87% of the supplied nitrogen was taken up by the plants and 83% of the absorbed nitrogen was accumulated in the seeds. Both the uptake and the translocation efficiency declined at higher nitrogen supply, and it is seen that the barley crop was able to take up considerably more nitrogen than it could translocate into the seeds. In the present experiment the maximum grain yield was obtained with 3 g nitrogen per pot. Hence, the barley was also able to absorb much more nitrogen than it could utilize for grain production.

Concerning the possibilities of improving the production of seed protein in cereals genetically, this can be achieved by improving either the ability to absorb nitrogen or the ability to accumulate the absorbed nitrogen in storage protein in the seeds. A comparison of old and new barley varieties (Sandfaer and Haahr, 1975) demonstrated only little genetic variation in nitrogen uptake, but the new, high-grain-yielding varieties had a higher production of seed protein than did the

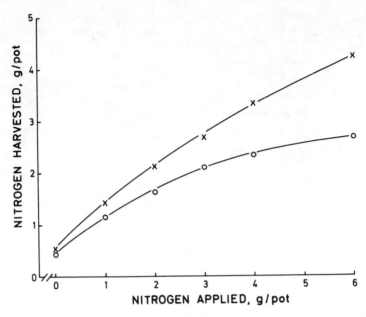

Fig. 3. *Relationship between nitrogen supply and amount of nitrogen harvested in straw plus seeds, upper curve, and in the seeds, lower curve (from Andersen and Køie, 1975).*

old varieties with a low grain yield. Because neither the translocation ability nor the seed protein was considered in the breeding of these new varieties, breeding for high grain yield seems to cause an increased protein accumulation in the seeds. The low genetic variation in nitrogen uptake, as well as the abundant absorption of nitrogen demonstrated in Fig. 3, may be the effect of a substantial selection for this trait in barley and other cereals. Nitrogen has probably long been a major limiting nutrient in most agricultural areas. Therefore, genotypes that can take up more nitrogen from the soil have had a higher yield such that they have been favoured both by natural selection and by the intensive selection for higher production.

GENETIC CONTROL OF STORAGE-PROTEIN FORMATION

Although the description of cereal storage protein was initiated many years ago (Osborne, 1895), many details of the synthesis, composition, and function of this protein are still unknown. However, the intensive efforts to improve the nutritive value of cereal protein have provided further information and stimulated research on this subject.

The protein in the glutelin fraction has not been studied in great detail, mainly because it is difficult to dissolve and handle in chromatographic and electrophoretic studies. Most of this protein is probably related to cell walls and membranes and is therefore of vital importance for the development of the endosperm.

The best-known protein is prolamin, which is found in considerable amounts in all the important cereals apart from rice and oats. The prolamin fraction contains several different proteins (Altschul et al., 1966; Mesrob et al., 1970). Køie et al. (1976) classified the barley prolamin into three subfractions, A, B, and C, on the basis of electrophoretic mobility, staining behavior, and response to nitrogen fertilization. It was shown that the B and especially the C prolamin are produced in response to nitrogen fertilization.

All three barley prolamin subfractions contain several electrophoretic bands (Køie et al., 1976). A difference between two varieties with respect to the electrophoretic banding pattern of the B fraction was found to arise from two codominant alleles (Oram et al., 1975). The composition of the C fraction also varies genetically. These genetic variations in electrophoretic mobility within the prolamin subfractions are probably without nutritive significance.

All information indicates that prolamin is perhaps the only real storage protein fraction in cereals, that is, it is a fraction synthesized mainly for the purpose of supplying the embryo with nitrogen compounds at germination. It has been emphasized that a reduction or blocking of the synthesis of such proteins would probably not be lethal for the plant, and that a reduced prolamin content is expected to cause a much better nutritional value of the seed protein. The validity of this hypothesis was proved by the detection of the opaque-2 and floury-2 genes in maize (Mertz et al., 1964; Nelson et al., 1965). Both of these so-called high-lysine types have a drastically decreased prolamin content and a much higher concentration of essential amino acids, especially lysine, in the seed protein than ordinary maize. Similar types have now been found in sorghum (Singh and Axtell, 1973) and barley (Munck et al., 1970; Doll et al., 1974). The latter study in barley shows that high-lysine types are induced relatively frequently by mutagenic treatments.

Barley mutant 1508 contains only about one-third of the normal prolamin content (Ingversen et al., 1973), and the lysine content of the protein in this mutant is therefore increased nearly 50% compared with the parent variety. This change is the result of a single recessive gene (Doll, 1973) that blocks the synthesis of several protein bands with high molecular weight in the prolamin fraction (Brandt, 1976; Køie et al., 1976). However, several other genes are involved in the synthesis of the prolamin in barley. A number of different high-lysine mutants, in which the increase in lysine is attributable to single-gene action (Doll, 1976), have a reduced prolamin synthesis, although the reduction is less than in mutant 1508. Preliminary studies indicate that the mutants have their high-lysine genes in at least six different loci.

Studies of high-lysine types of maize, sorghum, and barley have indicated no principal difference between these cereals with respect to the genetic control of the prolamin synthesis. Apparently, the selected genes are mutations in a common storage protein synthesis present not only in these three cereals but also in wheat. An intensive search for high-lysine wheat (Johnson et al., 1970; Siddiqui and Doll, 1973) indicated no varieties or mutants with a drastically reduced prolamin synthesis. However, this may be because of the hexaploidy of bread wheat, which renders the detection of recessive mutants much more difficult.

To the author's knowledge, the exact step blocked in the storage protein synthesis is not yet known for any low-prolamin/high-lysine cereal. Apparently the genes involved act solely in the endosperm. This may be seen from the fact that a heterozygote for the high-lysine gene in mutant 1508 produces both high-lysine seeds and normal seeds on the same plant. However, the endosperm seems even further independent of the mother plant concerning the composition of the storage protein. Studies of the amino acid metabolism in maize (Sodek and Wilson, 1970) and barley (Brandt, 1975) demonstrated a considerable conversion of lysine to glutamic acid and proline in the normal genotype. This lysine conversion was much reduced in the respective high-lysine types, opaque-2 and mutant 1508. Hence, the cereal endosperm is apparently able to convert the amino acids received from the mother plant according to the requirements of the actual protein synthesis.

The last topic to be dealt with concerns the utilization of the genetic variation in storage protein composition in the breeding of varieties with a better nutritional value of the seed protein. The main difficulty in this breeding is the reduced grain yield of nearly all high-lysine cereals. Even though the productivity of, for example, opaque-2 maize has been considerably improved compared with normal maize, many reports and unpublished studies strongly indicate that high-lysine genes in general reduce the grain yield, and that a considerable breeding effort is needed to overcome this negative effect.

The effect of the high-lysine gene in mutant 1508 on the two main yield components, single seed weight and number of seeds per unit area, is illustrated in Fig. 4. Mutant 1508 was crossed with a normal lysine variety, Sultan, and the offspring lines that were homozygous for either the high-lysine or the corresponding normal gene were selected and propagated. In this material the high-lysine gene is distributed at random in a common, segregating genetic background. Therefore, an evaluation of the effects of the high-lysine gene based on a comparison of the segregated high-lysine and normal lines is not likely to be invalidated by unknown mutations or the genetic background.

A field test of 21 high-lysine and 17 normal lines showed that the two groups of lines had the same number of seeds per unit area, but the single seed weight, and thereby the grain yield, of the high-lysine lines was on average reduced by 15% (Fig. 4). The two groups of lines had the same yield of seed protein ($N \times 6.25$) per unit area, but the protein concentration of the high-lysine seeds was increased as much as the single seed weight was reduced. These results show that the high-lysine gene in mutant 1508 not only changes the storage protein composition but also impairs the grain filling considerably. The

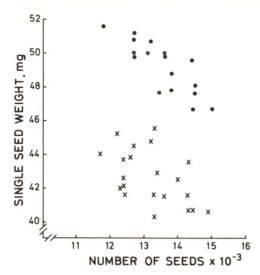

Fig. 4. The effect of a high-lysine gene on seed size and number of seeds per unit area. (X) Lines homozygous for the high-lysine gene, (●) corresponding normal lines.

gene has no significant effect on the number of seeds formed or on the amount of protein accumulated in the seeds.

The reduced seed size of mutant 1508 is visible as seed shriveling, and all the segregated high-lysine lines mentioned above have shrunken seeds. In a genetic study of five other high-lysine mutants having shrunken seeds, grain shriveling was completely linked with the high-lysine character (Doll, 1976). Therefore, reduced grain filling appears to be a pleiotropic effect of these high-lysine genes. So far, we have only found two mutants with an increased lysine content, nos. 7 and 56 (Doll et al., 1974), which apparently have nonshriveled seeds.

Altogether, it seems justified to conclude that most barley high-lysine genes interfere with the accumulation of carbohydrates, which is the main storage compound in the endosperm. We hope that this relationship between the accumulation of storage protein and carbohydrates is indirect, so that it will be possible to obtain a satisfactory nutritive quality of the seed protein in cereals without affecting the carbohydrate production, which is an equally important character of the cereals.

REFERENCES

Adams, C. A. and Novellie, L. (1975). Composition and structure of protein bodies and spherosomes isolated from ungerminated seeds at Sorghum bicolor (Linn.) *Moench. Plant Physiol. 55*:1–6.

Altschul, A. M., Yatsu, L. Y., Ory, R. L., and Engleman, E. M. (1966). Seed proteins. *Annu. Rev. Plant Physiol. 17*:113–136.

Andersen, A. J. and Køie, B. (1975). N fertilization and yield response of high lysine and normal barley. *Agron. J. 67*:695–698.

Brandt, A. B. (1975). *In vivo* incorporation of ^{14}C lysine into the endosperm proteins of wild type and high-lysine barley. *FEBS Lett. 52*:288–291.

Brandt, A. B. (1976). Endosperm protein formation during kernel development of wild type and a high-lysine barley mutant. *Cereal Chem. 53*:890–901.

Buttrose, M. S. (1963). Ultrastructure of the developing wheat endosperm. *Aust. J. Biol. Sci. 16*:305–317.

Christianson, D. D., Khoo, U., Nielsen, H. C., and Wall, J. S. (1974). Influence of opaque-2 and floury-2 genes on formation of proteins in particulates of corn endosperm. *Plant Physiol. 53*:851–855.

Doll, H. (1973). Inheritance of the high-lysine character of a barley mutant. *Hereditas 74*:293–294.

Doll, H. (1976). Genetic studies of high lysine barley mutants. In *Barley Genetics III*, pp. 542–546. Thiemig, Munich.

Doll, H., Køie, B. and Eggum, B. O. (1974). Induced high lysine mutants in barley. *Radiat. Bot. 14*:73–80.

Dure III, L. S. (1975). Seed formation *Annu. Rev. Plant Physiol. 26*:259–278.

Ingversen, J. (1975). Structure and composition of protein bodies from wild-type and high-lysine barley endosperm. *Hereditas 81*:69–76.

Ingversen, J., Køie, B., and Doll, H. (1973). Induced seed protein mutant of barley. *Experientia 29*:1151–1152.

Jacobsen, J. F., Knox, R. B., and Pyliotis, N. A. (1971). The structure and composition of aleuron grains in the barley aleurone layer. *Planta 101*:189–209.

Johnson, V. A., Mattern, P. J., and Schmidt, J. W. (1970). The breeding of wheat and maize with improved nutritional value. *Proc. Nutr. Soc. 29*:20–31.

Khoo, U. and Wolf, M. J. (1970). Origin and development of protein granules in maize endosperm. *Amer. J. Bot. 57*:1042–1050.

Køie, B., Ingversen, J., Andersen, A. J., Doll, H., and Eggum, B. O. (1976). Composition and nutritional quality of barley protein. In *Evaluation of Seed Protein Alterations by Mutation Breeding*, pp. 55–61. IAEA, Vienna.

Mertz, E. T., Bates, L. S. and Nelson, O. E. (1964). Mutant gene that changes protein composition and increases lysine content of maize endosperm. *Science 145*:279–280.

Mesrob, B., Petrova, M., and Ivanov, Ch. P. (1970). A comparative study of hordein fractions. *Biochim. Biophys. Acta 200*:459–465.

Millerd, A. (1975). Biochemistry of legume seed proteins. *Annu. Rev. Plant Physiol. 26*:53–72.

Munck, L., Karlsson, K. E., Hagberg, A., and Eggum, B. O. (1970). Gene for improved nutritional value in barley seed protein. *Science 168*:985–987.

Nelson, O. E. (1969). Genetic modification of protein quality in plants. *Advan. Agron. 21*:171–194.

Nelson, O. E., Mertz, E. T., and Bates, L. S. (1965). Second mutant gene affecting the amino acid pattern of maize endosperm proteins. *Science 150*:1469–1470.

Oram, R. N., Doll, H., and Køie, B. (1975). Genetics of two storage protein variants in barley. *Hereditas 80*:53–58.

Ory, R. L. and Henningsen, K. W. (1969). Enzymes associated with protein bodies isolated from ungerminated barley seeds. *Plant Physiol. 44*:1488–1498.

Osborne, T. B. (1895). The proteids of barley. *J. Amer. Chem. Soc. 17*:539–567.

Sandfaer, J. and Haahr, V. (1975). Barley stripe mosaic virus and the yield of old and new barley varieties. *Z. Pflanz. 74*:211–222.

Siddiqui, K. A. and Doll, H. (1973). Screening for improved protein quality mutants in wheat. *Z. Pflanz. 70*:143–147.

Singh, R. and Axtell, J. D. (1973). High lysine mutant gene (hl) that improves protein quality and biological value of grain sorghum. *Crop Sci. 13*:535–539.

Sodek, L. and Wilson, C. M. (1970). Incorporation of leucine-[14] C and lysine-[14] C into protein in the developing endosperm of normal and opaque-2 corn. *Arch. Biochem. Biophys. 140*:29–38.

Sylvester-Bradley, R. and Folkes, B. F. (1976). Cereal grains: Their protein components and nutritional quality. *Sci. Prog. 63*:241–263.

Tronier, B., Ory, R. L., and Henningsen, K. W. (1971). Characterization of the fine structure and proteins from barley protein bodies. *Phytochemistry 10*:1207–1211.

32

Nutritional Aspects of Cereal Proteins

Bjørn O. Eggum

Institute of Animal Science
Rolighedsvej 25
DK 1958 Copenhagen, Denmark

ABSTRACT

Recent years have brought a greater awareness of the need for more plentiful as well as more nutritious foods. Discoveries of strains of maize, barley, and other crops having higher levels of essential amino acids have shown the differences in nutritional quality that can occur among strains of crop varieties. Comparisons are made between the total lysine content of common cereals and selected high-lysine mutants. It appears from these comparisons that the total lysine content expressed in percent of protein is very high in some varieties. However, if the digestibility of the individual amino acid components is taken into consideration the picture is somewhat different. Experimental data show that lysine especially has a low availability in several of the cereal grains. It is assumed that this is because lysine is mainly deposited in the protein fractions of lowest digestibility. Based on these observations, the validity of the concept of additivity of gross values can be questioned. It is documented that when barley, rye, wheat, maize, and sorghum are fertilized with increasing amounts of nitrogen more protein will be deposited in the prolamins. As the prolamin fraction is a poor but highly digestible source of lysine, more digestible protein but of lower biological value is obtained. For oats and rice the situation is different as glutelin (relatively rich in lysine) is the main storage protein in these grains. Tannins are present in a number of plant materials. Present work shows that barley also contains significant amounts of tannins. Experiments with rats showed that a highly significant negative correlation exists between the tannin contents of barley and protein digestibility. By adding increasing amounts of tannin to rat diets it was found that tannin has a specific affinity for proline, glycine, and glutamic acid. Protein quality of cereal grains with modified amino acid pattern is discussed and compared with common varieties. The comparison is based mainly on nitrogen-balance experiments with rats. The nutritional superiority of several of these high-lysine varieties is obvious. However, the necessity of taking the availability of the nutrients into consideration in this type of biological study is emphasized. To stress this further, experimental data are given for gross energy and digestible energy in cereal grains. The differences between gross energy and digestible energy vary considerably between different grains. In oats, for instance, only 70% of the energy is digestible, whereas for polished rice almost all the energy is available. It is therefore concluded that in cereal grains neither gross energy values nor crude protein values are additive from a nutritional point of view.

INTRODUCTION

Past research has involved quality evaluations of cereal grains, emphasizing physical properties rather than nutritional quality characteristics. However, recent years have brought a greater awareness of the need for more plentiful, as well as more nutritious, foods. Discoveries of strains of maize, barley, and other crops with higher levels of essential amino acids have shown the differences in nutritional quality that can occur among strains of crop varieties. Discoveries of growth-inhibiting substances in grain and other plant parts have indicated the need to consider both positive and negative factors when working with nutritional quality. Increasing the proportion of essential nutrients is not a sufficient answer; these nutrients must be readily available to the biological system. Therefore, factors affecting the availability of the nutrients must be taken into consideration when judging the nutritional value of a foodstuff.

Considerable attention has been paid to the crude protein and gross energy content in various dietary sources. However, less information is available on the digestibility of the respective protein and energy sources. As there are distinct differences between total and digestible contents from one dietary source to another, the validity of the concept of additivity of gross values can be questioned. Dietary recommendations based on gross values might not have sufficient accuracy. To elucidate the outlined problems the present work is also concerned with the availability of the nutrients to the biological system.

AMINO ACID COMPOSITION AND AMINO ACID DIGESTIBILITY OF CEREAL GRAINS

It is well established that the normal cereal grains are all low in lysine. Therefore, international agencies, plant breeders, biochemists, and so forth, have put much effort into the task of raising the lysine level in cereal protein.

Assuming that the FAO (1973) pattern of 5.2% lysine in the protein is the ideal level of lysine for the infant, we may compare the lysine content of common cereals and selected high-lysine mutants. Such a comparison is made by Mertz (1975) and the data are given in Table I. All these values were obtained in the laboratory at Purdue.

The protein levels of the various cereals are shown in column 1, lysine in % protein in column 2, and % lysine of the ideal FAO level in column 3. Mertz (1975) reports that on the basis of these data, the best of the cereal grains, oats, has about 73% of the ideal level, and the poorest of the grains, sorghum and millet, have 35% and 36%, respectively. The Risö barley mutant contained 5.6% lysine, which is very high. Normal maize contains 52%, whereas Opaque-2 maize, as currently produced in Mexico, contains 87–90% of the ideal level. In contrast, high-lysine sorghum contains nearly twice as much (63%) as normal sorghum. The data also show that wheat contains about 57% and current varieties of rice 71% of the ideal level of lysine.

However, if we take digestibility into consideration, the picture will be somewhat different. Eggum (1975), in an experiment with rats, measured true

Table I. Lysine Content of Cereals and Selected High Mutants

Cereal grain	Protein %	Lysine g/16g N	% of ideal level
Maize 4858[a]	10.5	2.7	52
Maize 4855, high lysine[a]	10.9	4.5	87
Maize 4856, high lysine[a]	10.1	4.7	90
Sorghum, normal[b]	13.1	1.8	35
Sorghum, high lysine[b]	18.5	3.3	63
Barley, normal[c]	19.8	3.3	63
Barley, high lysine[c]	19.4	5.6	108
Rice BB, normal[d]	6.9	3.7	71
Rice BP I 761 high prot.[d]	15.4	3.4	65
Wheat, Genesee, normal[e]	12.1	3.0	58
Wheat, Purdue 4930 high prot.[e]	17.3	2.9	56
Oats, Noble, normal[f]	18.9	3.8	73
Millet[g]	14.5	1.9	36

Source: Mertz (1975).
[a]4858: CIMMYT normal yellow flint synthetic. 4855: CIMMYT yellow hard endosperm Opaque-2 synthetic. 4856: CIMMYT yellow soft endosperm Opaque-2 synthetic. From CIMMYT, Mexico City.
[b]Normal sorghum kernels. High-lysine sorghum: high-lysine (h1 h1 h1) kernels from F_2 segregating heads derived from crosses between "normal" (low-lysine) plants and the high-lysine sorghum line IS 11758.
[c]Normal barley: Bomi barley variety. High-lysine mutant: mutant 1508 from Risö, Denmark.
[d]Normal rice: Blue Bonnet variety. High-protein rice: BPI 761 from IRRI.
[e]Normal wheat: Genesee, variety of New York soft wheat. High-protein wheat: Purdue 4930-A6-28-2-1.
[f]Normal oats: Noble, a Wisconsin variety.
[g]Millet: Finger millet, variety from Uganda supplied by Dr. S. A. Eberhart, Iowa State University, Ames, Ia.

digestibility (TD) of protein in eight different cereal grains and compared these data with the gross values. The results are given in Table II.

It appears from Table II that the differences between total and digestible protein in the cereal grains vary considerably. For rice there is almost no difference between total and digestible protein, whereas in rye this difference is more than 20%. This indicates that crude protein values of rice and rye are not additive from a nutritional point of view irrespective of their amino acid composition. As for the other cereal grains the differences between total and digestible protein are smaller than for rye but nevertheless considerable. For purposes of comparison, the values for soya bean meal are also given. The results show that besides the high-protein content in soya bean meal the protein digestibility is also high. It is a general experience that the digestibility of protein-rich food and foodstuffs is higher than in most cereal grains (Eggum, 1968).

As the protein digestibility in different protein sources varies considerably, it may be assumed that the digestibility of the individual amino acids also will vary in a more or less similar manner.

Table III gives values for lysine in several cereal grains. Digestible amino acids were measured according to the method of Kuiken and Lyman (1948). Although this method is criticized because of microbial activity in the alimentary tract, valuable information can be obtained with this method (Eggum, 1973a).

The differences between values of total and digestible lysine are much more pronounced than for protein. As discussed by Eggum (1973b) this is probably due to the fact that lysine is mainly deposited in the protein fractions of lowest digestibility. In the highly digestible prolamin fraction almost no lysine is found, whereas the glutamic acid content is very high, which explains the high digestibility of glutamic acid, shown in Table IV.

Table II. Total and True Digestible Protein in Eight Cereal Grains

Cereal grain	Total protein in DM[a] (%)	TD protein in DM[a] (%)	Difference (%)
Barley	10.13	8.31	17.96
Oats	10.75	9.04	15.90
Wheat	12.63	11.32	10.37
Rye	9.13	7.03	23.00
Maize	10.06	8.81	12.42
Sorghum	12.54	10.63	15.23
Rice	8.96	8.90	0.66
Triticale	13.07	12.12	7.30
Soya bean meal	53.11	50.35	5.19

[a]DM, Dry matter.

Table III. Total and Digestible Lysine in Cereal Grains

Lysine source	Total lysine in DM (g/16 g N)	Digestible lysine in DM (g/16 g N)	Difference (%)
Barley	3.69	2.80	24.11
Oats	4.03	3.21	20.34
Wheat	2.55	2.02	20.80
Rye	3.67	2.40	26.60
Maize	2.73	2.31	15.38
Sorghum	1.83	1.33	27.30
Rice	3.54	3.51	0.85
Soya bean meal	5.98	5.48	8.30

As expected, the differences between total and digestible glutamic acid are much smaller than for lysine and total protein. These differences are also discussed by Munck (1964), Thomke (1970), Schiller (1971), and Eggum (1973*a*). As for the TD values for the other amino acids, they are all intermediate between lysine and glutamic acid (Eggum, 1973*a*). It should be stressed that aspartic acid, glycine, and alanine have TD values in the lower part of the range, whereas the histidine, arginine, and serine values are in the upper part. This is in agreement with correlation coefficients found by Pomeranz et al. (1973) between lysine and the three amino acids, aspartic acid, glycine, and alanine, whereas the correlation coefficient between lysine and glutamic acid was negative in barley protein.

It is documented that when barley, rye, wheat, maize, and sorghum are fertilized with increasing amounts of nitrogen more protein will be deposited in

Table IV. Total and Digestible Glutamic Acid in Cereal Grains

Glutamic acid	Total glutamic acid in DM (g/16 g N)	Digestible glutamic acid in DM (g/16 g N)	Difference (%)
Barley	25.06	22.90	8.62
Oats	22.10	19.71	10.81
Wheat	35.77	35.41	1.01
Rye	23.62	21.52	8.89
Maize	17.46	16.05	8.08
Sorghum	21.24	19.12	9.98
Rice	17.18	17.18	0.00
Soya bean meal	17.82	17.04	4.38

their prolamin fraction. As this fraction is a poor source of lysine (Pomeranz et al., 1973) but highly digestible (Eggum, 1973*b*), more digestible protein but of lower biological value is obtained (Eggum, 1970*a*; Thomke, 1970; Schiller, 1971; Eppendorfer, 1975). For oats and rice the situation is different as glutelin (relatively rich in lysine) is the main storage protein in these cereal grains (Pomeranz et al., 1973). Juliano et al. (1973) observed a negative correlation between lysine content of protein and protein content of brown and milled rice only in samples with protein below 10%. In further work with rice, Eggum and Juliano (1973) observed that TD and net protein utilization (NPU) were positively correlated with lysine content of rice protein (3.17–4.07 g/16 g N). Utilizable protein ranged from 5.19 to 11.12 and was mainly determined by N content of milled rice (r = 0.988). Digestibility of amino acids of milled rice protein by fecal analysis ranged from 94.1 to 100.0% in samples with 1.38 and 2.74% N, dry basis. According to Eggum and Juliano (1975), an increase in milled rice protein content (N X 6.25) from 9.12 to 11.09 in IR 8 and from 11.09 to 14.56 in IR 480-5-9 owing to N fertilizer application had no significant effect on the lysine content of the protein and had little effect on true digestibility, biological value, and net protein utilization of the protein in growing rats. Maruyama et al. (1975), however, found in rats that increases in protein content were accompanied by an increase in indispensable amino acids.

Mattern et al. (1975) found that the negative correlation between protein and lysine appears to become nonsignificant at higher levels of protein in wheat. However, genetically high-protein wheat has been found to be equal or higher in lysine content as a percentage of protein than are normal wheats grown in the same environment. The amino acid composition of oats is remarkably constant over a wide range of protein content (Bengtsson and Eggum, 1969; Eppendorfer, 1975; Schrickel and Clark, 1975).

The relationship between protein content and protein quality in oats and rye is illustrated by Eppendorfer (1975) (see Fig. 1 and 2).

From Fig. 1 it is evident that the concentrations of lysine in particular, but those of threonine, cystine, and methionine as well, are only slightly decreased with increasing nitrogen content. Consequently, BV almost remains unchanged. TD, however, increases linearly with protein content and consequently NPU.

In Fig. 2 concentrations of lysine, threonine, methionine, and cystine are also shown as a function of N content of grain. This graphic presentation clearly shows that the decrease of the BV is very closely paralleled by decreasing concentrations of those amino acids. Figure 2 is probably representative of similar relationships between protein content and protein quality in barley, wheat, maize, and sorghum.

N applications normally increase yield or protein content, or both, of grain and, therefore, also the production per area of protein and individual amino acids including lysine. A decrease in the nutritional value of protein, whether

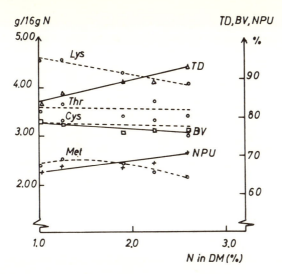

Fig. 1. Relationships between true digestibility (TD), biological value (BV), net protein utilization (NPU), lysine, threonine, methionine, and cystine, and the concentration of nitrogen in grain of oats (var. Selma). (From Eppendorfer, 1975, with permission.)

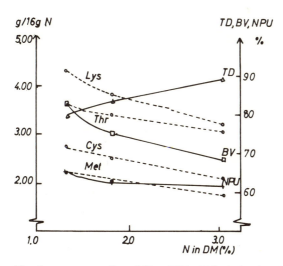

Fig. 2. Relationships between true digestibility (TD), biological value (BV), net protein utilization (NPU), lysine, threonine, methionine, and cystine, and the concentration of nitrogen in grain of spring rye (var. Petkus).

expressed as a reduction in lysine or NPU, will probably always be more than balanced by a larger protein and amino acid production (Eppendorfer, 1975).

THE INFLUENCE OF TANNIN ON PROTEIN UTILIZATION

Tannins are present in a number of plant materials at very high levels, often 10% or more of dry weight (Singleton and Kratzer, 1969). They may be of significance in some common feed- and foodstuffs, such as sorghum grains (Chang and Fuller, 1964) and rape seed meal (Clandinin and Heard, 1968).

Milić et al. (1972) suggest that the tannins affect the rate of methylation and the formation of complexes with the constituents of the feed. Gallic acid and gallotannins possess a distinctive inhibitory effect on the digestive enzymes, forming complexes with the protein part of enzymes or binding the simple constituents of the digested feed into complexes. However, the mode of action of enzyme inhibition by tannin is still uncertain. Furthermore, types of protein and tannin influence the reaction. Axtell et al. (1975) put forward the hypothesis that seed proteins become complexed or bound with tannin compounds of the whole grain, and that the complexed proteins are substantially less available for utilization by monogastric animals.

Experiments with chicks fed tannic acid and other tannins have shown that about 0.5% tannic acid in the diet results in depression of growth and at 5%, high mortality occurs (Vohra et al., 1966). This is in agreement with work of Baelum and Petersen (1964) and Petersen (1969), who found that tannin had a negative effect on feed conversion. Furthermore, chicken fed on diets with added tannin had a significantly lower flavor quality than did those fed diets without tannin.

As mentioned above, tannins are present in a number of plant materials, but at different levels. Barley, the most widespread cereal grain in Denmark, also contains significant amounts of tannins, which might partly explain the relative low digestibility of barley protein (Eggum, 1970b). To evaluate the influence of both protein and tannin content on protein digestibility in barley, 29 samples were tested (Eggum and Christensen, 1975).

As the concentrations of nitrogen and tannin have a detrimental influence on protein digestibility, the relationship between protein digestibility and content of nitrogen and tannin was determined by use of a multiple regression equation, as follows:

$$TD = 82.60 + [3.89 \times N(\%)] - [6.27 \times \text{tannin}(\%)]$$
$$s_{b1} = 0.81; s_{b2} = 2.11; R = 0.72; r_1 = 0.60; r_2 = 0.60; t = 3.0$$

The regression coefficient is significantly different from zero, a t test showing $P < 0.001$. Hence, the nitrogen content has a positive influence on protein digestibility, whereas tannin has a negative influence.

Table V. Influence of Tannin on Protein Utilization in Soya Bean Protein[a]

Tannin supplement (%)	TD (%)	BV (%)	NPU (%)
0	92.9	77.9	72.4
0.5	81.1	77.9	63.2
1.0	78.4	81.3	63.6
1.5	73.2	77.9	57.0

[a]Source: Eggum and Christensen (1975).

To evaluate the effect of tannin on protein utilization, Eggum and Christensen (1975) gave increasing amounts of tannin in diets to rats. Soya bean meal was used as dietary protein. True digestibility (TD), biological value (BV), and net protein utilization (NPU) were employed as biological criteria (see Table V).

It would appear from these results that tannin exerts a severe negative effect on protein digestibility. A supplement of 0.5% resulted in a decrease in TD from 92.9 to 81.1%, whereas 1.5% tannin in the diet reduced TD to 73.2%. The biological value is almost unaffected by tannin. The results do not indicate that methionine is more sensitive to tannin than other amino acids—as has been proposed by other workers (Nelson and Finkel, 1964). If tannin had a specific effect on this particular amino acid, the biological value of soya bean protein would have been reduced by a tannin supplement. This was not the case.

To investigate this aspect of the problem, the availability of the individual amino acids was measured. The group without tannin was compared with the diet supplemented with 1.5% tannin in terms of the TD of the individual amino acids.

Table VI shows that all amino acids in soya bean protein have high availabilities. With tannin in the diet, however, the availability of all amino acids

Table VI. Amino Acid Availability in Soya Bean Protein without and with 1.5% Tannin in the Diet

	0% Tannin TD (%)	1.5% Tannin TD (%)		0% Tannin TD (%)	1.5% Tannin TD (%)
Lys	93.3	81.1	Val	90.0	76.9
Met	91.9	80.6	Iso	90.7	78.1
Cys	94.0	84.7	Leu	90.1	77.6
Asp	93.4	78.7	Tyr	90.6	77.3
Thr	90.4	78.5	Phe	93.3	78.4
Ser	96.6	83.1	His	97.4	75.6
Glu	94.9	68.1	Arg	97.4	75.3
Pro	93.5	0.9	Try	94.2	83.9
Gly	89.3	41.5	NH_3	93.4	64.9
Ala	88.3	75.1			

decreases but to a different degree. As discussed earlier, methionine is not more severely affected than are the other amino acids; in fact, this acid is least affected by the addition of tannins. The availability of some of the other amino acids such as proline, glycine, and glutamic acid is severely reduced. Proline is not absorbed at all, whereas about 60% of the glycine and more than 30% of the glutamic acid are recovered in the feces. As none of these amino acids is essential for rats, this decrease in availability will have no negative influence on BV, in agreement with the results in Table V. The theory of the detoxification effect of methionine—and thereby a higher requirement for this amino acid when tannin is fed—does not apply to the present data. Whether or not proline, glycine, and possibly glutamic acid have a detoxifying effect is unclear. However, these three amino acids in particular are present in very high concentrations in gelatin. As discussed by Van Buren and Robinson (1969), bonding between gelatin and tannin molecules is strong. This could indicate that tannin has a specific affinity for proline, glycine, and glutamic acid.

PROTEIN QUALITY OF CEREAL GRAINS WITH MODIFIED AMINO ACID PATTERN

Maize

In nitrogen balance experiments with samples of Floury-2 and Opaque-2 placed at our disposal by Oliver E. Nelson, TD, BV, NPU, and UP (utilizable protein) were measured in experiments with rats.

Amino acid composition (AAC) together with amino acid availability were also measured. For comparison Table VII also includes values for normal hybrid maize.

The maize varieties Floury-2 and Opaque-2 show considerable possibilities with respect to improved nutritional value and have been the subject of widespread interest. The lysine and tryptophan content of Floury-2 and Opaque-2 are very high compared to the content in hybrid maize. This has resulted in improved BV values—particularly in Opaque-2. As Floury-2 has the highest protein content, UP is highest in this mutant (10.21). It also appears from Table VII that the digestibility is high for all amino acid constituents. The nutritional superiority of Opaque-2-modified maize has been proved by many workers—also by human nutritionists (Pradilla et al., 1975).

Barley

Screening of mutagenically treated materials (Doll et al., 1974) disclosed 14 barley mutants which have from a few to about 40% more lysine in the protein and one mutant with 10% less lysine in the protein than the parent variety.

Table VII. Amino Acid Content: TD, BV, NPU, and UP of Different Maize
Varieties

	Variety					
	Hybrid		Floury-2		Opaque-2	
	g/16 g N	TD (%)	g/16 g N	TD (%)	g/16 g N	TD (%)
Lys	2.74	93.6	3.66	93.0	4.48	92.9
Met	1.88	96.6	2.39	96.4	1.78	94.1
Cys	1.83	97.7	1.84	95.7	2.19	96.1
Thr	3.31	93.7	3.46	92.6	3.46	90.8
Try	0.62	92.3	0.89	93.3	1.07	93.8
Protein in DM	10.19		15.44		12.31	
TD	95.9		95.4		94.1	
BV	59.8		69.3		74.3	
NPU	57.3		66.1		70.0	
UP	5.84		10.21		8.62	

Feeding tests with rats revealed substantial increases in the biological value of
the high-lysine mutant protein. Results from the rat experiments are given in
Table VIII.

The very high lysine content of the mutant 1508 leads to a nearly 20%
increase in the biological value compared with Bomi. However, because of a
reduced true digestibility, the net protein utilization in mutant 1508 is only
improved about 10%. Mutant 29 has about the same improvement in protein
utilization as mutant 1508, but the biological value and digestibility are less
changed in No. 29 than in No. 1508. The lines Hily 71/669 and 82/3 have about
the same increase in protein utilization as the mutants 29 and 1508. It probably
should be stressed here that recent feeding experiments did not disclose any
significant difference between the protein digestibility in the barley mutants and
in the present varieties (Køie et al., 1975). The BV averaged 77 for field-grown
normal lysine barley against 90 for the high-lysine mutant 1508. A marked
negative correlation between BV and percent N in the seed was found for both
Bomi and mutant 1508. This is in agreement with the findings of Rhodes and
Jenkins (1975), but the lysine value, even at the highest protein content, was
still well above the point at which this amino acid would be nutritionally
limiting. These authors, regard Risö 1508 as highly-lysine cultivar which may be
expected to maintain its improved amino acid balance over a wide range of
cultural conditions. Rhodes and Mathers (1974) found that Hiproly deviated
significantly from the negative correlation between essential amino acids and
protein content.

Table VIII. Nutritional Value of High-Lysine
Mutants and Lines, and the Parent Varieties[a]

Variety or line	TD (%)	BV (%)	NPU (%)	Lysine (g/16 g N)
Carlsberg II	78	78	61	(3.90)
Mutant 29	77	87	66	(4.09)
Line 29[x]	75	88	66	(4.19)
Mutant 56	82	79	64	(4.39)
Bomi	83	76	63	(3.73)
Mutant 1508	78	90	70	(5.30)
Hily 71/669	85	83	71	(4.31)
Hily 82/3	84	82	69	(4.32)

[a]Source: Doll et al. (1974).

Rice

Rice protein is among the most nutritious of all cereal proteins. However, the protein content of milled rices is low (7% protein at 14% moisture) (Juliano and Beachell, 1975).

Several semidwarf breeding lines have been developed at the IRRI that appear to have higher protein content than traditionally grown rice. Feeding trials with experimental rats (Bressani et al., 1971) and with human subjects (Clark et al., 1971) confirm the nutritional superiority of higher-protein rice owing to the higher levels of all essential amino acids in the milled rice (Bressani et al., 1971; Clark et al., 1971). Protein digestibility in rats (Eggum, 1969) and humans (Clark et al., 1971) was not affected adversely by the higher protein content of milled rice. This is in agreement with data of Eggum and Juliano (1973). These workers carried out nitrogen-balance studies in rats fed seven milled rice samples with 1.10–2.73% N, dry basis. The results appear in Table IX.

The protein content of milled rice was negatively correlated with the lysine content. The correlation coefficients of protein content with TD, BV, and NPU were negative but not significant. NPU for milled rice samples were positively correlated with TD and BV. The utilizable protein (protein content $\times$ NPU/100) showed a corresponding increase with protein content and the correlation was highly significant. Thus, the protein content of rice is the major influence on the nutritional value of this cereal. In a recent work by Eggum and Juliano (1975) it was found that an increase in milled rice protein (N $\times$ 6.25) from 8.14 to 9.90 (at 12% moisture) in IR 8 and from 9.90 to 13.0% in IR 480-5-9 owing to N fertilizer application had no significant effect on the lysine content of the protein and had little effect on the true digestibility, the biological value, and the net protein utilization of the protein in growing rats.

Table IX. Mean True Digestibility, Biological Value, and Other Properties of
Protein of Rices Differing in Protein Content

Protein source	Protein (DM)	TD (%)	BV (%)	NPU (%)	UP (%)	Lysine (g/16 g N)
Milled rice						
Intan	6.88	100.1	75.2	75.3	5.18	4.07
IR 8	8.50	96.2	73.1	70.3	5.98	3.59
IR 8	11.06	95.4	68.4	65.2	7.21	3.50
IR 22	11.75	98.5	69.7	68.7	8.07	3.87
IR 1103-15-8	13.13	95.9	74.3	71.1	9.34	3.65
IR 480-5-9	13.56	94.5	67.9	64.2	8.71	3.34
BPI 761	17.06	94.4	70.1	66.2	11.29	3.19
Brown rice						
IR 480-5-9	12.38	90.8	70.8	64.2	7.95	3.59

As for the amino acid availability in rice protein, Eggum and Juliano (1973)
found in rats that all amino acids are almost completely available in uncooked
rice. Some Japanese workers (Tanaka et al., 1975), however, did not find that
cooked rice protein was completely available to humans.

Sorghum

Sorghum is similar to the other cereal grains in many of its nutritional
deficiencies, yet it differs in several important characteristics. The protein
quality of sorghum grain is limited by the low lysine content, reflecting the
high-prolamin content of the endosperm and the relatively small embryo size as
a proportion of the mature grain (Axtell et al., 1975).

Singh and Axtell (1973) found in the world sorghum collection two floury
lines of Ethiopian origin, IS 11167 and IS 11758, which were exceptionally high
in lysine at relatively high levels of protein. The average whole-grain lysine
concentration of high lines IS 11167 and IS 11758 was 3.34 and 3.13 (g/100 g
protein) at 15.7 and 17.2% protein, respectively. The major changes were
increased lysine, arginine, aspartic acid, glycine, and tryptophan concentrations
and decreased amounts of glutamic acid, proline, alanine, and leucine in the *hl
hl hl* endosperm.

Based on their improved amino acid composition, the high-lysine sorghum
lines should have higher nutritional value than the average sorghum. Singh and
Axtell (1973) performed nutritional studies of two high-lysine lines, three
normal sorghum lines, and a casein-bearing diet for comparison. All grain rations
were fed as isonitrogenous diets at approximately 10% protein, except for the

casein diet, which was fed at 13.3% protein. Some of the experimental results of Singh and Axtell (1973) are given in Table X.

Data on the chemical composition of whole grain samples, as well as rat weight gain in 28 days and protein efficiency ratio (PER), are given in Table X. Weight gain on the IS 11758 diet was nearly twice that of IS 2319 and three times higher than the average of normal sorghum lines. Weight gain of rats on the IS 11167 ration was 71% of gain on the IS 11758 ration. The PER values for both high-lysine sorghum lines were higher than the average PER for normal sorghum, but were lower than that for casein. Thus, the identification of a high-lysine gene in IS 11167 and IS 11758, represents a significant step toward improvement of the nutritional quality of grain sorghum. It should be added that Eckert and Allee (1974) found in experiments with growing pigs that threonine is the limiting amino acid after lysine.

Wheat

Enhanced value of wheat as a human food encompasses different but related factors, such as grain yield, grain-protein content, and grain-protein quality. Co-operative ARS–University of Nebraska research has demonstrated the feasibility of breeding wheat with 15–25% higher protein content (Johnson et al., 1969). Protein increases are not associated with depressed productiveness or with a less desirable balance of essential amino acids. Analyses of the essential amino acid balance of several high-protein Atlas-66-derived lines indicate that high protein need not be associated with decreased lysine or methionine, two of the three most limiting amino acids found in wheat. This appears from Table XI (Johnson et al., 1969).

As is seen from Table XI some of the high-protein lines possess higher amounts of these amino acids than other varieties. In this study, only threonine among the first three most limiting amino acids failed to have comparable levels in high- and low-protein lines.

In work with the protein-rich Mexican wheat varieties Eggum (1970b) found low lysine and threonine content as a percent of protein. Consequently, the biological values were very low—significantly lower than in a normal Danish variety.

Oats

As mentioned before, the amino acid composition of oats is remarkably constant over a wide range of protein content. Recent analyses on lines from *A. sterilis,* the wild oat from Israel, confirm this point (Table XII).

In addition, Robbins et al. (1971) found only a slight correlation between grain-protein percentage and lysine percentage in the protein. Of the 289 oat

Table X. Nutritional Values of Isonitrogenous
(10% Protein) Diets Prepared with High-Lysine
and Normal Sorghum Lines in a 28-Day
Rat-Feeding Experiment[a]

Source	Protein (%)	Lysine (g/100 g protein)	Weight gain (g)	PER
High-lysine lines				
IS 11167	16.6	3.36	34.5	1.78
IS 11758	18.0	3.38	48.8	2.06
Normal lines				
IS 2319	12.7	2.30	25.3	1.24
IS 2520	13.3	1.85	10.3	0.61
IS 1269	14.8	2.10	14.0	0.74
Mean of normal lines	13.06	2.08	16.5	0.86
Casein	91.0	8.00	85.8	2.20

[a]Source: Singh and Axtell (1973).

samples surveyed the maximum lysine content was 5.2% and the minimum was
3.2%. For threonine the maximum was 3.5% and the minimum 3.0%. Methionine had a maximum of 3.3% and a minimum of 1.0%. The range for threonine
and methionine is apparently limited. Schrickel and Clark (1975) emphasize that
the oat breeder should pay strict attention not only to protein content and the
percentage of lysine, but also to the maintenance of a satisfactory level of the
second and third limiting amino acids, threonine and methionine. Robbins et al.
(1971) found negative correlations for protein with threonine and methionine.

Table XI. Lysine, Methionine, and Threonine Levels in Selected High-Protein
Lines of Atlas-66 × Comanche[a]

Variety	Protein % DWB[b]	Lys % protein	Met % protein	Thr % protein
Comanche	15.0	3.23	1.67	3.54
Atlas	18.0	3.33	1.11	3.35
Atl 66 × cmn 2507	17.7	3.72	1.74	2.62
2509	18.3	3.45	1.83	3.32
2504	17.9	3.38	1.14	3.69
2510	16.5	3.37	1.67	3.22
2499	18.2	3.29	1.68	3.10
2500	18.3	3.20	1.65	3.16

[a]Source: Johnson et al. (1969).
[b]% total dry weight.

Tang et al. (1958) reported that threonine from oat protein was not available to experimental rats. This is not in agreement with work of Eggum (1973a) who measured the availability of threonine in oats to be above 80%.

Triticale

When triticale was fed to rats as the sole source of protein at a 10% protein level, triticale was first-limiting in lysine, second-limiting in threonine, and marginal in sulfur amino acids (Shimada and Cline, 1974). The same order was noted for pigs. Kies and Fox (1970), using the nitrogen-balance method, concluded that lysine was the first limiting amino acid of triticale protein for human adults.

As to the availability of the individual amino acid components, Sauer et al. (1974) found in experiments with pigs (10 kg) that all amino acids in triticale protein were highly available (Table XIII).

In experiments with chicks, rats, and pigs, they further determined metabolizable energy (ME) values of three lines of triticale compared with that of maize. ME values for triticale were lower than those for maize in all species tested despite the fact that the gross energy values of the triticale and maize were almost equal.

GROSS ENERGY CONTRA DIGESTIBLE ENERGY IN CEREAL GRAINS

When discussing whether the cereal plant breeders should put their main efforts into protein or yield improvement it ought to be stressed that more

Table XII. Percentages of Protein and Amino Acids in Grains of *Avena Sterilis* Lines[a]

	Line number (%)		
Component	1	2	3
Protein[b]	17.0	25.1	21.7
Lysine[c]	4.0	3.9	4.1
Threonine	3.3	3.4	3.4
Cystine	1.8	1.7	1.6
Valine	5.7	5.7	5.9
Leucine	7.8	7.8	7.9
Tyrosine	3.3	3.4	3.4
Phenylalanine	5.5	5.5	5.7

[a]Source: Unpublished data, Quaker Oats Company, 1971.
[b]Percentage of dry weight.
[c]Amino acids, percentage of protein.

**Table XIII. Amino Acid Availability of Triticale
Measured in Experiments with Pigs**[a]

	TD(%)		TD (%)
Lysine	86.3	Tyrosine	92.9
Alanine	88.4	Leucine	92.7
Methionine	90.3	Histidine	93.8
Threonine	90.9	Serine	94.2
Aspartic acid	91.0	Arginine	94.5
Isoleucine	91.5	Phenylalanine	94.5
Glycine	92.1	Proline	97.1
Valine	92.4	Glutamic acid	97.6

[a]Source: Sauer et al. (1974).

protein in the grain also means more calories per weight unit. In a series of experiments with barley we found that the relationship between gross energy and nitrogen content in the grain was highly correlated ($r = 0.87$). Twenty samples were evaluated and in Table XIV, data for five of the samples are shown.

It appears clearly from Table XIV that gross energy as well as digestible calories in barley dry matter increase significantly with increasing nitrogen content. The same relationship is also found in experiments with maize. It should be stressed that neither Opaque-2 nor Floury-2 fall outside the regression line for hybrid maize. This indicates that the energy is just as digestible in these mutants as in normal maize. To illustrate the situation for other cereal grains single values are given in Table XV.

As shown in Table XV, the differences between gross energy and digestible energy in the different cereal grains vary considerably. In oats, for instance, only 70% of the energy is digestible, whereas for rice almost all the energy is available. It therefore appears that neither the gross energy values nor crude protein values in cereal grains are additive from a nutritional point of view.

**Table XIV. Nitrogen Content in Barley in
Relationship to Gross Energy and Digestible Energy,
Respectively**

Sample	N in DM (%)	Gross E[a] in DM (gcal/g)	Dig. E (%)	Dig. E in DM (gcal/g)
1	2.51	4501	80.1	3605
5	2.09	4307	79.8	3437
10	1.80	4227	79.3	3352
15	1.68	3903	78.3	3056
20	1.50	3600	80.1	2884

[a]E = energy.

Table XV. Nitrogen and Energy Content in Different Cereal Grains

Sample	N in DM (%)	Gross E. in DM (gcal/g)	Dig. E (%)	Dig. E in DM (gcal/g)	Gross E – Dig. E (gcal)
Barley	1.86	4098	78.9	3233	865
Barley (naked)	2.38	4260	87.1	3710	550
Oats	2.24	4570	70.6	3226	1344
Rye	1.80	4361	85.0	3706	655
Wheat	2.17	4157	86.4	3592	565
Maize	1.60	4382	87.2	3821	561
Rice	1.40	4150	96.3	3996	154

Therefore in dietary recommendations for protein and energy, gross values are not sufficiently accurate. In animal nutrition this has been accepted for years.

CONCLUSION

Comparison of results of chemical assays with assumed human essential amino acid requirements does not take into consideration digestibility of and interactions between amino acids. Furthermore, as indicated by Kies and Fox (1975) amino acid requirements of the human age/sex groups are not well enough established. One must also consider variations due to physiological conditions and genetic background. Until amino acid requirements are better established the plant breeder must continue to base breeding work on improving protein and specific amino acid contents. However, it seems to be generally agreed that cereal grains do not contain enough protein—and that this protein is primarily deficient in lysine and threonine. The tryptophan content in maize is also very low. Furthermore, it appears from this discussion that the availability of the nutrients must be taken into consideration. Observed severe effects of processing on protein quality make it even more urgent to include availability in breeding work. For this purpose, biological experiments with laboratory animals are tremendously useful.

REFERENCES

Axtell, J. D., Oswalt, D. L., Mertz, E. T., Pickett, R. C., Jambunathan, R. and Srinivasan, G. (1975). Components of nutritional quality in grain sorghum. In *High-Quality Protein Maize*, pp. 374–386. Halsted Press, Stroudsburg, Pennsylvania.

Baelum, J. and Petersen, V. E. (1964). II. Forsøg med siagtekyllinger. In *Bilag Landøkonomisk Forsøgslab. efterårsmøde* pp. 311–315. Copenhagen.

Bengtsson, A. and Eggum, B. O. (1969). Virkiningen af stigende N-gødskning på havre og bygproteinets kvalitet. *Tidskr. Plant. 73*:105–114.

Bressani, R. L., Elias, L. G., and Juliano, B. O. (1971). Evaluation of the protein quality of milled rices differing in protein content. *J. Agri. Food Chem. 19*:1028–1034.

Buren, van, J. P., and Robinson, W. B. (1969). Formation of complexes between protein and tannic acid. *J. Agri. Food Chem. 17*:772–777.

Chang, S. I. and Fuller, H. L. (1964). Effect of tannin content of grain sorghums on their feeding value for growing chicks. *Poultry Sci. 43*:30–36.

Clandinin, D. R. and Heard, J. (1968). Tannins in press-solvent and solvent processed rapeseed meal. *Poultry Sci. 47*:688.

Clark, H. E., Howe, J. M., and Lee, C. J. (1971). Nitrogen retention of adult human subjects who consumed a high protein rice. *Amer. J. Clin. Nutrition 24*:324–328.

Doll, H., Køie, B., and Eggum, B. O. (1974). Induced high lysine mutants in barley. *Radiat. Bot. 14*:73–80.

Eckert, E. and Allee, G. L. (1974). Limiting amino acids in milo for the growing pig. *J. Animal Sci. 39*:694–698.

Eggum, B. O. (1968). *Aminosyrekonsentration og Proteinkvalitet.* 99 pp. Stougaards Forlag, Copenhagen.

Eggum, B. O. (1969). Hvedesorter med højt proteinindhold. *Ugeskr. Agronomer 35*: 648–651.

Eggum, B. O. (1970*a*). Über die Abhängigkeit der Proteinqualität von Stickstoffgehalt der Gerste. Ztschr. Tierphysiol. *Tierernährung Futtermittelk, 26*(2):65–71.

Eggum, B. O. (1970*b*). Current methods of nutritional protein evaluation. In *Improving Plant Protein by Nuclear Techniques,* pp. 289–302. International Atomic Energy Agency, Vienna.

Eggum, B. O. (1973*a*). A study of certain factors influencing protein utilization in rats and pigs. thesis. 406. Beretn. Forsøgslab. Copenhagen, 173 pp.

Eggum, B. O. (1973*b*). Biological availability of amino acid constituents in grain protein. pp. 391–408. In *Nuclear Techniques for Seed Protein Improvement,* 422 pp. International Atomic Energy Agency, Vienna.

Eggum, B. O. (1975). The relationship between total and digestible protein (amino acids) and total and digestible energy in cereal grains as determined in experiments with rats. *Xth Int. Congress of Nutrition, Kyoto, Japan, Aug. 3–9, 1975.*

Eggum, B. O. and Christensen, K. D. (1975). Influence of tannin on protein utilization in feedstuffs with special reference to barley. In *Breeding for Seed Protein Improvement using Nuclear Techniques,* pp. 135–143. International Atomic Energy Agency, Vienna.

Eggum, B. O. and Juliano, B. O. (1973). Nitrogen balance in rats fed rices differing in protein content. *J. Sci. Food Agri. 24*:921–927.

Eggum, B. O. and Juliano, B. O. (1975). Higher protein content from nitrogen fertilizer application and nutritive value of milled-rice protein. *J. Sci. Food Agri. 26*:425–427.

Eppendorfer, W. (1975). Effects of fertilizers on quality and nutritional value of grain protein, pp. 213–227. *11th Kolloquium of International Potash Institute, Rønne, Denmark, June 2–5.*

Johnson, V. A., Mattern, P. J., Whited, D. A., and Schmidt, J. W. (1969). Breeding for high protein content and quality in wheat In *New Approaches to Breeding for Improved Plant Protein,* pp. 29–40. International Atomic Energy Agency, Vienna.

Juliano, B. O. and Beachell, H. M. (1975). Status of rice protein improvement. In *High-Quality Protein Maize,* pp. 457–469. Halsted Press, Stroudsburg, Pennsylvania.

Juliano, B. O., Antonio, A. A., and Esmama, B. V. (1973). Effects of protein content on the distribution and properties of rice protein. *J. Sci. Food Agri. 24*:295–306.

Kies, C. and Fox, H. M. (1970). Determination of the first limiting amino acid of wheat and triticale grain for humans. *Cereal Chem. 47*:615–625.

Kies, C. and Fox, H. M. (1975). Techniques in using normal human subjects in the protein bioassay of food products. In *Protein Nutritional Quality of Foods and Feeds,* (Friedman, M. ed.), Part 1, pp. 1–10. Dekker, New York.

Kuiken, K. A. and Lyman, C. M. (1948). Availability of amino acids in some foods. *J. Nutr.* *36*:359–368.

Køie, B., Ingversen, J., Andersen, A. J., Doll, H., and Eggum, B. O. (1975). Composition and nutritional quality of barley protein. *Proceedings IAEA/FAO/GSF Research Co-ordinating Meeting, Hahnenklee, May 5–9.*

Maruyama, K., Shands, H. L., Harper, A. E., and Sunde, M. L. (1975). An evaluation of the nutritive value of new high protein oat varieties (cultivars). *J. Nutr.* *105*:1048–1054.

Mattern, P. J., Johnson, V. A., Stroike, J. E., Schmidt, J. W., Klepper, L., and Ulmer, R. L. (1975). Status of protein quality improvement in wheat. In *High-Quality Protein Maize,* pp. 387–397. Halsted Press, Stroudsburg, Pennsylvania.

Mertz, E. T. (1975). Breeding for improved nutritional value in cereals. In *Protein Nutritional Quality of Foods and Feeds,* (Friedman, Mendel, ed.), Part 2, pp. 1–12. Dekker, New York.

Milić, B. L., Stojanović, S., and Vućrević, N. (1972). Lucerne tannins. II. Isolation of tannins from lucerne, their nature and influence on the digestive enzymes in vitro. *J. Sci. Food Agri.* *23*:1157–1162.

Munck, L. (1964). The variation of nutritional value in barley. I. Variety and nitrogen fertilizer effects on chemical composition and laboratory feeding experiments. *Hereditas* *52*:1–35.

Nelson, R. F. and Finkel, B. J. (1964). Enzyme reactions with phenolic compounds: Effects of O-methyltransferase and high pH on the polyphenol oxidase substrates in apple. *Phytochemistry 3*:321–325.

Petersen, V. E. (1969). A comparison of the feeding value for broilers of corn, grain, sorghum, barley, wheat and oats, and the influence of the various grains on the composition and taste of broiler meat. *Poultry Sci.* *48*:2006–2012.

Pomeranz, Y., Robbins, G. S., Wesenberg, D. M., Hockett, E. A., and Gilbertson, J. T. (1973). Amino acid composition of two-rowed and six-rowed barleys. *J. Agri. Food Chem. 21*:218–221.

Pradilla, A. G., Harpstead, D. D., Sarria, D., Linares, F. A. and Francis, C. A. (1975). Quality protein maize in human nutrition. In *High-Quality Protein Maize,* pp. 27–37. Halsted Press, Stroudsburg, Pennsylvania.

Rhodes, A. P. and Jenkins, G. (1975). The effect of varying nitrogen supply on the protein composition of a high lysine mutant of barley. *J. Sci. Food Agri. 26*:705–709.

Rhodes, A. P. and Mathers, J. C. (1974). Varietal differences in the amino acid composition of barley grain during development and under varying nitrogen supply. *J. Sci. Food Agri. 25*:963–972.

Robbins, G. S., Pomeranz, Y., and Briggle, L. W. (1971). Amino acid composition of oat groats. *J. Agri. Food Chem. 19*:536–539.

Sauer, W. C., Giovannetti, P. M., and Stothers, S. C. (1974). Availability of amino acids from barley, wheat, triticale and soybean meal for growing pigs. *Can. J. Animal Sci. 54*:97–105.

Schiller, K. (1971). Untersuchungen über die Variabilität von Futtergerstenprotein. 2. Mitteilung: Über den Einfluss ökologischer Faktoren auf die Verteilung der Eiweissarten im Protein von Gerstekaryopsen. *Landwirtsch. Forsch. XXIV*(1):15–33.

Schrickel, D. J. and Clark, W. L. (1975). Status of protein quality improvement in oats. In *High-Quality Protein Maize,* pp. 398–411. Halsted Press, Stroudsburg, Pennsylvania.

Shimada, A. and Cline, T. R. (1974). Limiting amino acids of triticale for the growing rat and pig. *J. Animal Sci. 5*:941–946.

Singh, R. and Axtell, J. D. (1973). High lysine mutant gene (hl) that improves protein quality and biological value of grain sorghum. *Crop Sci. 13*:535–539.

Singleton, V. L. and Kratzer, F. H. (1969). Toxicity and related physiological activity of phenolic substances of plant origin. *J. Agri. Food Chem. 17*:497–512.

Tanaka, Y., Hayashida, S., and Hongo, M. (1975). The relationship of the feces protein particles to rice protein bodies. *Agri. Biol. Chem. 39*:515–518.

Tang, J. J., Laudick, L. L., and Benton, D. A. (1958). Studies of amino acid supplementation and amino acid availability with oats. *J. Nutr. 66*:533–543.

Thomke, S. (1970). Über die Veränderung des Aminosäuregehaltes der Gerste mit steigendem Stickstoffgehalt. *Zeit. Tierphysiol. Tierernährung Futtermittelk. 27*(1):23–31.

Vohra, P., Kratzer, F. H., and Joslyn, M. A. (1966). The growth-depressing and toxic effects of tannins to chicks. *Poultry Sci. 45*:135–142.

33

Wheat Protein

V. A. Johnson

USDA Agricultural Research Service
University of Nebraska
Lincoln, Nebraska 68583

ABSTRACT

Results from AID-supported Nebraska research to improve the nutritional quality of wheat indicate that substantial genetic variation for grain protein content exists in wheat. Experimental lines with 5% higher protein in their grain than ordinary varieties have been selected from a high-protein X high-protein cross. Genetic variability for lysine in wheat grain is limited. The genetic component of total lysine variability among 12,600 wheats in the USDA World Collection was only 0.5%. Genetic increases in lysine ranging from 0.4 to 0.7% lysine have been identified in selections from a high-lysine X high-lysine cross. Lysine per unit protein is negatively correlated with protein content. In contrast, lysine per unit weight of grain is positively correlated with protein content suggesting that increasing the protein content of wheat can effectively increase the amount of lysine in the grain. Seed fractionation studies have determined that high protein in whole wheat results mainly from increased protein content of the starchy endosperm. Lysine differences were detected both in the endosperm and non-endosperm fractions. A new productive high-protein hard winter wheat variety derived from Atlas-66, with genetic potential for 2% higher grain protein content was released to growers by the Agricultural Research Service, USDA and the Nebraska Agricultural Experiment Station in 1975.

INTRODUCTION

Cereal grains are the main source of calories and protein for an estimated two-thirds of the world's population. Wheat and rice are the most important food species among the cereals. The average protein content of wheat grain is approximately 12%, higher than the protein contents of rice, maize, or sorghum. The protein content of wheat is strongly influenced by production environment, especially soil fertility, water, and grain yield.

Wheat protein lacks the balance of essential amino acids required for its full utilization when wheat is the sole source of daily nutrition. Lysine is in shortest supply in wheat protein, which is comprised mainly of gliadin and glutenin. These protein fractions, particularly gliadin, are notably poorer in lysine than the albumens and globulins, which constitute only 10–15% of the total protein in wheat grain (Neurath and Bailey, 1954). Differences in the amino acid composition of the cereal grains can be accounted for largely by the proportion of the four solubility fractions that comprise the protein in each.

VARIABILITY

More than 15,000 common wheats (*Triticum aestivum* L.) maintained in the USDA World Wheat Collection were systematically analyzed for protein and lysine contents of their grain at the University of Nebraska. This was done as a part of a research effort to improve the nutritional quality of wheat by breeding. The analyzed seed was produced at Yuma, Arizona, but not all in the same year.

Total protein variation was from 6 to 22% with most of the wheats falling in the 10–16% range (Vogel *et al.*, 1973). Some of the wide variation in protein could be attributed to large differences in seed plumpness among the wheats. More than 600 of the wheats were regrown at Yuma, Arizona in 1972 and 1973. Interyear protein correlations, which ranged from only 0.33 to 0.44 but were highly significant statistically, indicated a substantial portion of the total variation in protein to be nongenetic (Vogel *et al.*, 1975). Our data suggest the genetic component of total protein variability among the World Collection wheats to be no greater than 5%. Protein variability among 3500 durum wheats and 600 spelt wheats in the collection was similar to that of the common wheats.

Lysine values among 15,000 common wheats in the World Collection ranged from 2.2 to 4.2% with a mean of 3.2%. Most of the values were in the 2.8–3.6% range. Correlation of lysine values over years was (0.40) but statistically significant. The genetic component of total lysine variation was approximately 0.5%— far less than the estimated 1.5% increase required to bring lysine into reasonable balance with other essential amino acids in wheat protein.

Failure to detect major genetic variation for lysine among the hexaploid common wheats similar to that found in maize, barley, and sorghum suggested possible genomic masking of genes. However, this was not supported by the results of our analyses of tetraploid *T. durum* wheats and available *T. monoccum* strains in the World Collection. The range of variation for lysine was approximately the same as that demonstrated for the common hexaploid wheats.

RELATIONSHIP OF PROTEIN AND LYSINE

Lysine per unit protein is strongly affected by level of protein (Vogel et al., 1973). The relationship is negative and nonlinear. Increases in grain protein up to approximately 15% are associated with pronounced depression of lysine per unit protein (Fig. 1). Further increases in protein above 15% produce little, if any, further depression of lysine. Fifty-two percent of the variation in lysine per unit protein among 12,600 World Collection common wheats was attributable to variation in protein.

Adjustment of lysine values to a common protein level is necessary to remove the effect of protein content on lysine per unit protein. We use the regression of lysine per unit protein on protein shown in Fig. 1 for the adjustment. Such adjustment permits valid comparisons of lysine values among wheats that differ in protein content. We believe it to be essential in genetic selection for increased lysine. Lysine selection based on unadjusted values would

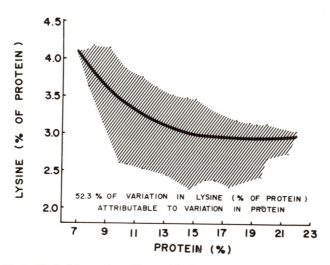

Fig. 1. Marked depression of lysine (% of protein) with increased protein.

likely be ineffective owing to the strong and variable influence of protein content.

Low-protein wheat grain characteristically contains a higher proportion of water- and salt-soluble albumins and globulins in its protein than does high-protein wheat. The albumins and globulins contain significantly more lysine than do glutenin and gliadin. We believe this to largely account for the observed depression of lysine per unit total protein with increased protein content.

The depression of lysine per unit protein with higher protein content in wheat is not proportionate to the increase in protein. This is evident from the relationship of lysine per unit grain weight to protein content shown in Fig. 2. With increased protein content there is significant increase in lysine per weight of grain. Clearly, the amount of lysine in wheat grain can be increased effectively by increasing protein content.

GENETIC SOURCES OF HIGH PROTEIN AND HIGH LYSINE

Genetic potential for elevated grain protein content has been uncovered in numerous wheats. They include

Source		Growth habit
Atlas-50 (CE 12534)		Intermediate
Atlas-66 (CI 12561)		Intermediate
Frondoso (CI 12078)	Probably the	Spring
Frontana (CI 12470)	same genes	Spring
Frontiera (CI 12019)		Spring
Lancota (CI 17389)		Winter
Aniversario (CI 12578)		Spring
Male fertility restorer (Nebr.) NB 542437		Winter
NB/4/Agrus/7*Thatcher/3/2*Hume (So. Dak.)		Winter
Hybrid English (CI 6225)		Winter
Nap Hal (PI 176217)		Spring
Cirpiz (PI 166859)		Winter
Velvet (PI 283864)		Winter

Few wheats with proven potential for elevated lysine have been identified to date. Those most prominently used in the ARS–Nebraska program are

Nap Hal (PI 176217)	Spring
Norin-10/Brevor//50-3 (CI 13449)	Winter
Norin-10/Brevor//25-15//Rex/Rio (CI 13447)	Winter

Nap Hal holds special interest because it combines elevated grain protein and lysine.

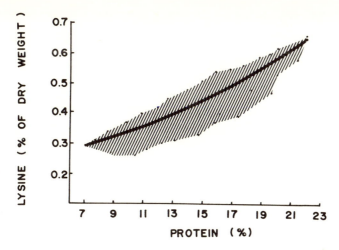

Fig. 2. Relationship of lysine per unit grain weight to protein: increased protein plus increased lysine.

GENETIC MANIPULATION OF PROTEIN AND LYSINE

Protein

Breeding experiments for higher protein content in wheat have involved the use of Atlas-66 most extensively as a genetic source of high grain protein. Atlas-66 is a leaf-rust-resistant soft red winter wheat reported to produce grain with significantly higher protein content than other Eastern soft wheats of the United States (Middleton et al., 1954). Atlas-66 possesses genes for high protein from the Brazilian variety Frondoso. The related Brazilian varieties Frontana and Frontiera are also believed to carry the same genes for high grain protein as Frondoso.

We were able to readily transmit the Atlas-66 protein genes to the progenies of crosses of Atlas-66 with the hard winter varieties Comanche and Wichita (Johnson et al., 1968). Analysis of homozygous leaf-rust-resistant and leaf-rust-susceptible F_6 rows from Atlas-66/Wichita indicated a close genetic linkage between a gene for high protein and the leaf-rust resistance in Atlas-66. We postulated a second major gene for high protein unlinked with leaf-rust resistance in Atlas-66 based on recovery of intermediate protein levels in leaf rust-susceptible and leaf-rust-resistant lines. The ease with which we recovered high-protein lines suggested that the number of major genes for high protein in

Atlas-66 is not large. Through the use of monosomics and whole chromosome substitutions, we have tentatively identified chromosome 5D as carrier of the linked protein gene (Morris et al., 1973). The other group 5 chromosomes may be involved, but their contributions to high protein are unclear as yet.

Analyses of foliage nitrogen content in Atlas-66-derived winter lines throughout the spring growing season at Lincoln, Nebraska demonstrated that high grain protein was not associated with high N content of the plants. This suggested to us that more efficient and complete translocation of nitrogen from the foliage to grain rather than differential N uptake accounts for the high grain protein content of Atlas-66 derivatives. More recently Klepper (1976) of our Nebraska wheat team has demonstrated that Atlas-66 exhibits elevated levels of nitrate reductase activity in its foliage as compared to varieties with ordinary grain protein content. He believes that reduction of NO_3 is a rate-limiting step in plant-nitrogen metabolism and that high-protein varieties must exhibit high capability for NO_3 reduction.

Phenotypic expression of Atlas-66 genes for high protein is not dependent on high soil fertility. We compared the Atlas-66-derived experimental wheat CI 14016 with the Lancer variety (ordinary protein content) at seven different nitrogen fertilizer levels in Nebraska. Yields of the two varieties were similar. With N-fertilizer applications from 0 to 135 kg/ha the grain protein content of CI 14016 increased from 12.5 to 16.3% and Lancer from 10.8 to 14.0% (Johnson et al., 1973a). CI 14016 maintained an approximate 2% protein advantage over Lancer over all fertility treatments (Table I). Performance of Atlas-66 and its derivatives in the International Winter Wheat Performance Nursery supports the Nebraska data (Stroike et al., 1974).

Table I. Mean Yield and Protein Responses of CI 14016 and Lancer Wheats to Nitrogen Fertilizer at Selected Low-Fertility Test Sites in Nebraska in 1969 and 1970

Nitrogen applied (kg/ha)	Grain yield		Protein content	
	Lancer (Q/ha)	CI 14016 (q/ha)	Lancer (%)	CI 14016 (%)
0	25.9	25.8	10.8	12.5
22.5	29.9	27.4	11.2	13.3
45.0	31.4	29.5	11.8	14.0
67.5	31.1	30.6	12.6	14.9
90	31.1	30.3	13.2	15.4
112.5	30.7	30.5	13.6	15.8
135	30.2	31.1	14.0	16.3
$LSD_{0.05}$	1.1	1.1	0.3	0.3

The first high-protein hard red winter wheat, variety Lancota from the ARS-Nebraska wheat nutritional improvement program, was released to producers in four states in 1975. Lancota selected from Atlas-66/Comanche//Lancer has genetic potential for 2% higher protein in its grain than ordinary hard varieties (Table II). It has been equal to or higher in yield than currently grown winter varieties in central United States (Johnson et al., 1976) (Table III). It is field resistant to leaf and stem rust. Its grain has excellent bread-making characteristics. Lancota provides good evidence that genetic increases in grain protein content can be accomplished without sacrifice of productivity and other desirable agronomic and quality traits.

Atlas (high protein) was crossed with Nap Hal (high protein and high lysine). Apparent transgressive segregation for grain protein content was detected among 671 F_2-derived rows grown in the F_3 and F_4 generations at Yuma, Arizona. Lysine content of the F_2 progeny rows was distributed between the lysine means of the parent varieties (Johnson et al., 1973b). We postulated that Atlas-66 and Nap Hal carried different genes for high protein that together produced protein levels in progenies that exceeded either parent. This has been

**Table II. Grain Yield and Protein Content of
Lancota and Centurk in Paired Plot Comparisons,
Lincoln, Nebraska, 1975**

	Lancota		Centurk
Yield q/ha	Protein content (%)	Yield (q/ha)	Protein Content (%)
45.7	16.6	40.7	15.3
40.8	17.6	36.2	15.6
37.7	17.8	37.0	16.1
38.0	17.1	33.8	16.1
33.5	17.9	34.1	16.1
39.2	17.9	36.6	15.3
38.2	17.4	33.2	15.9
35.2	17.1	35.2	15.4
34.9	17.7	35.3	16.0
28.9	17.7	32.4	15.8
43.0	17.7	38.3	15.3
37.3	17.7	35.6	15.6
40.0	17.3	37.9	15.0
36.5	17.6	38.8	15.6
38.7	17.8	37.6	14.9
39.9	17.7	42.9	15.2
37.3	17.6	34.7	16.2
29.9	17.5	25.2	15.6
$\bar{x}$ = 37.5	17.5	35.9	15.6

Table III. Performance of Lancota in Nebraska
Statewide Trials in 1973 and 1974

Variety	CI No.	Grain Yield (q/ha)			Protein content (%)[a]		
		1973	1974	2-yr x̄	1973	1974	2-yr x̄
Lancota	17389	28.6	32.6	30.6	15.5	15.0	15.3
Centurk	15075	29.3	32.6	31.0	13.9	13.7	13.8
Scout-66	13996	29.3	31.3	30.3	13.9	13.8	13.9

[a]Dry-weight basis.

substantiated in selections grown in the F_5-F_6 generations in Arizona in 1973 and 1974 (Tables IV and V).

Protein and lysine values for the parents and selected F_6 progeny rows of Nap Hal/Atlas-66 are plotted against the World Collection regression of lysine on protein to show the magnitude of protein advances achieved from this cross (Fig. 3). It is readily apparent that Nap Hal and Atlas-66 possess different genes for high protein that function additively when combined. Furthermore, the protein advances appear to be possible without sacrificing the lysine advantage of Nap Hal.

Grain yield and protein content of some of the Nap Hal/Atlas-66 selections grown at Yuma, Arizona in 1975 in a replicated yield trial are shown in Table VI. A few of the selections with exceptionally high grain protein approached the Atlas-66 parent variety in yield, and all were more productive than Nap Hal.

We have been able to combine protein genes from different sources to achieve exceptionally high levels of grain protein in productive winter-hardy experimental winter wheats. A particularly promising group of selections from

Table IV. F_5 Selections from the Cross Nap Hal/Atlas-66 Grown
at Yuma, Arizona in 1973 That Exhibit Promising Levels of Grain Protein

Variety	Row No.	Protein[a] (%)	Lysine/protein (%)	Adjusted lysine/protein (%)
Nap Hal	x̄ of 9 rows	20.0	3.1	3.3
Atlas-66	x̄ of 9 rows	19.9	2.8	3.0
Nap Hal/Atlas-66 (F_5)	15,138	24.2	2.8	3.0
	14,169	23.7	2.9	3.1
	15,164	23.7	2.9	3.0
	11,602	23.4	3.1	3.2
	11,444	23.2	3.1	3.3
	12,926	22.5	3.0	3.2

[a]Dry-weight basis.

Table V. F_6 Rows from Nap Hal/Atlas-66 Grown at Yuma, Arizona
in 1974 That Exhibit Very High Protein Combined with the Nap Hal
Level of Lysine

Name or pedigree	1974 Row No.	Protein (% dwb)	Lysine per unit protein	
			Unadj.	Adjusted[a]
Nap Hal (parent)	$\bar{x}$ of 17 rows	14.1	3.3	3.4
Atlas-66 (parent)	$\bar{x}$ of 17 rows	14.6	3.0	3.1
Centurk (check)	$\bar{x}$ of 17 rows	12.3	3.1	3.1
Nap Hal/Atlas-66 (F_6)	7,453	19.8	3.2	3.4
	6,349	19.1	3.2	3.4
	7,227	18.7	3.1	3.3
	6,645	18.5	3.0	3.3
	7,107	18.4	3.2	3.4
	7,128	17.8	3.2	3.4
	10,234	17.0	3.2	3.4

[a]Adjusted to 13% protein.

the complex cross Favorit/5/Cirpiz/Jang Kwang//Atlas-66Cmn/3/Velvet grown
in 1975 at Lincoln, Nebraska is characterized in Table VII.

LYSINE

CI 13449 produced the highest lysine value among 12,600 common wheats
from the World Collection. On an adjusted basis, its lysine value was 0.5% above

Table VI. Performance of Nap Hal/Atlas-66
Lines in the 1975 Yuma High-Protein–
High-Lysine Wheat Nursery

Entry	Protein (%)	Adjusted lysine per unit protein (%)	Yield (q/ha)
Nap Hal	14.7	3.3	27.4
Atlas-66	14.9	3.1	44.5
Centurk	11.7	3.1	55.0
Nap Hal/At-66 292	19.0	3.1	35.7
297	17.8	3.2	32.9
232	17.8	2.9	43.1
296	17.6	3.2	34.9
285	17.0	3.2	33.2
185	16.1	3.2	35.7
$LSD_{0.05}$	1.3	0.1	15.3

Table VII. Promising High-Protein Experimental Winter Wheats Grown in Unreplicated Plots at Lincoln, Nebraska in 1975

Pedigree or name	Plot No.	Plant height (in.)	Seed rating[a]	Grain yield (q/ha)	Grain protein content (%)
Centurk (check)	x̄ of 18 plots	40	G	35.9	15.6
Lancota (check)	x̄ of 18 plots	38	VG	37.5	17.5
Favorit/5/Cirpiz//Jang Kwang/4/					
Atl 66/Cmn/3/Velvet	11,345	34	VG	39.6	19.1
	12,288	33	VG	41.4	18.9
	12,291	32	G–VG	41.0	19.8
	12,293	33	VG	41.1	19.3
	12,297	32	VG	42.0	19.1
	12,312	32	VG	39.0	19.1
	12,327	34	VG	41.0	18.7
	12,332	33	VG	41.6	18.9
	12,335	34	Exc.	41.9	18.5

[a]G, VG, and Exc. = good, very good, and excellent, respectively.

expectation according to the regression of lysine on protein (Vogel et al., 1975). CI 13449 is an experimental winter variety that has below-normal grain protein content.

F_2 progeny rows from the cross Nap Hal/CI 13449 grown in Arizona in the F_3 generation had an adjusted lysine frequency distribution that exceeded the parent varieties (Johnson et al., 1973b). Lysine analyses of F_4 and F_5 selections further substantiated F_3 evidence of transgressive segregation for high lysine in the cross (Tables VIII and IX). In several lines, very high lysine was combined with the Nap Hal level of grain protein.

Table VIII. F_4 Selections from the Cross Nap Hal/CI 13449 Grown at Yuma, Arizona That Exhibit Promising Combined High Levels of Protein and Lysine in Their Grain

Variety	Row No.	Protein[a] (%)	Lysine/protein (%)	Adjusted lysine/protein (%)
Nap Hal	x̄ of 26 rows	17.5	3.2	3.4
CI13449	x̄ of 2 rows	15.5	3.1	3.3
Nap Hal/CI13449 (F_4)	16,900	19.4	3.4	3.6
	16,927	17.8	3.4	3.6
	16,921	17.7	3.4	3.6
	18,640	16.8	3.4	3.6
	17,330	16.2	3.6	3.8
	16,442	15.3	3.5	3.7

[a] Dry-weight basis.

Table IX. F_5 Rows from Nap Hal/CI 13449 Grown at Yuma, Arizona in 1974 That Exhibit Promising Combined High Levels of Protein and Lysine

| | | | Lysine per unit protein (%) | |
Variety	Row No.	Protein (%)	Unadj.	Adjusted[a]
Nap Hal (parent)	x̄ of 39 rows	14.4	3.3	3.4
CI 13449 (parent)	x̄ of 8 rows	11.2	3.5	3.3
Centurk (check)	x̄ of 38 rows	12.5	3.1	3.1
Nap Hal/CI 13449 (F_5)	11,635	15.8	3.4	3.6
	10,866	15.0	3.4	3.6
	12,582	14.9	3.5	3.7
	13,140	14.6	3.5	3.6
	14,177	14.1	3.6	3.7
	10,841	13.6	3.5	3.6
	11,668	13.6	3.5	3.6

[a]Adjusted to 13% protein.

CI 13449 is a productive semidwarf winter wheat. The productiveness of CI 13449 together with high protein from Nap Hal and exceptionally high lysine were transmitted to F_6 lines from Nap Hal/CI 13449 evaluated in a replicated nursery at Yuma, Arizona in 1975 (Table X). Lysine and protein values for parents and the best of the Nap Hal/CI 13449 F_5 lines grown in 1974 are plotted against the World Collection regression of lysine per unit protein on protein in Fig 4. The protein level of Nap Hal was generally maintained or exceeded in lines higher in lysine than either Nap Hal or CI 13449.

Table X. Performance of Nap Hal/CI 13449 Lines in the 1975 Yuma High-Protein–High-Lysine Wheat Nursery

Entry	Protein (%)	Adjusted lysine per unit protein (%)	Yield (q/ha)
Nap Hal	14.7	3.3	27.4
CI 13449	10.9	3.3	67.8
Centurk	11.7	3.1	55.0
Nap Hal/CI 13449 248	13.3	3.3	63.6
245	12.9	3.6	70.4
305	12.7	3.5	57.2
253	12.5	3.4	87.5
247	12.2	3.5	71.0
205	12.2	3.5	65.5
$LSD_{0.05}$	1.3	0.1	15.3

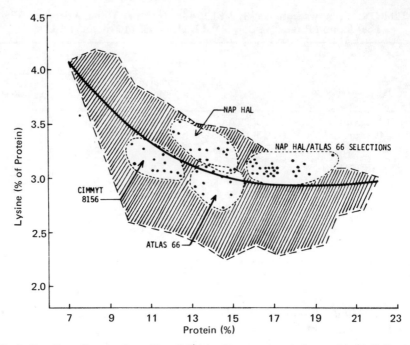

Fig. 3. Breeding advances from Nap Hal/Atlas-66 cross in relation to World Collection lysine–protein regression.

SEED-FRACTIONATION STUDIES

In many countries wheat is milled into white flour comprised entirely of starchy endosperm. Protein and lysine analyses of whole-ground grain provide no information on the site of the high-protein and high-lysine effects in the wheat kernel. These effects would be of most value if they resided in the starchy endosperm. If in the bran fraction (this includes the aleurone layer and embryo in our analyses), they would be useful only if the whole grain is consumed.

The varieties Atlas-66, CI 13449, Nap Hal, and Centurk were cleanly separated into starchy endosperm and bran fractions. Whole ground grain and the two fractions of each variety were separately analyzed for protein and lysine. The data are summarized in Table XI. In Atlas-66, the high-protein trait appears to reside entirely in the starchy endosperm. In contrast, the high protein of Nap Hal results from elevated protein both in the starchy endosperm and bran fractions. The high lysine content of CI 13449 was detectable mainly in the starchy endosperm fraction, whereas in Nap Hal it was confined to the bran fraction. Our data further indicate that the high protein content of the Nap Hal bran results from the very high protein content of the aleurone layer. As aleurone protein is rich in lysine, this could largely explain the elevated whole-grain lysine content of Nap Hal.

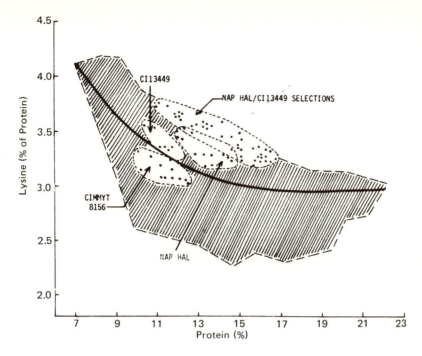

Fig. 4. Breeding advances from Nap Hal/CI 13449 cross in relation to World Collection lysine–protein regression.

Table XI. Protein and Lysine Contents of Whole Grain, Endosperm,
and Nonendosperm Fractions of Four Wheat Varieties Grown at Yuma,
Arizona in 1973

Variety	Protein content[a] (%)			Lysine content (% protein)		
	Whole grain	Endosperm fraction	Nonendosperm fraction	Whole grain	Endosperm fraction	Nonendosperm fraction
Nap Hal	19.6	18.9	24.5	3.1	2.5	4.6
Atlas-66	19.4	19.3	19.8	2.8	2.5	4.4
CI 13449	15.5	14.5	19.6	3.1	2.8	4.4
Centurk	15.4	15.0	19.6	3.0	2.5	4.5
$LSD_{0.05}$	1.0	0.9	1.0	ns	ns	ns

[a]Dry-weight basis.

We have determined that whole-grain analyses of protein reliably reflect protein differences in the starchy endosperm and can be utilized for selection purposes (Vogel et al., 1976). This is because the starchy endosperm comprises as much as 85% of whole seed weight. Large differences in whole-seed protein content not involving the starchy endosperm are unlikely. In contrast, wheats with elevated whole-seed lysine content do not always have high-endosperm lysine; hence, whole-grain analyses would not reliably identify endosperm lysine differences.

OUTLOOK

Much genetic variability for grain-protein content is present in wheat. Our data indicate that grain-protein potential can be increased by 5%. High-yield potential and high-protein potential are compatible in the common wheats. The frequently encountered suggestion that high grain yield results in depressed protein content of the grain in some production situations is true. However, the more relevant question is whether high-yielding varieties can be developed that, in a given production situation, are capable of producing grain with substantially higher protein content than other equally productive varieties. Our data clearly indicate that they can.

Genetic variability for lysine identified to date is limited. We believe it to be of sufficient magnitude to be useful for breeding. Our data suggest that lysine potential can be increased from 0.5 to 0.7%. This increase would more than overcome the depression of lysine per unit protein encountered as protein is increased. Productive varieties with 15%-or-more protein in their grain and with actual lysine per unit protein fully comparable to the level of lysine in low-protein wheats are possible.

ACKNOWLEDGMENT

This research was funded in part since 1966 by the Agency for International Development, U.S. Department of State under Contract Numbers AID/csd-1208 and AID/ta-c-1093.

REFERENCES

Johnson, V. A., Schmidt, J. W. and Mattern, P. J. (1968). Cereal breeding for better protein impact. *Econ. Bot. 22*:16–25.
Johnson, V. A., Dreier, A. F. and Grabouski, P. H. (1973*a*). Yield and protein responses to nitrogen fertilizer of two winter wheat varieties differing in inherent protein content of their grain. *Agron. J. 65*:259–263.

Johnson, V. A., Mattern, P. J. Schmidt, J. W. and Stroike, J. E. (1973*b*). Genetic advances in wheat protein quantity and composition. *Proc. 4th Int. Wheat Genet. Symp., Missouri Agr. Exp. Sta., Columbia, Mo.*

Johnson, V. A., Mattern, P. J. Stroike, J. E. and Wilhelmi, K. D. (1976). Breeding for improved nutritional quality in wheat. *Proc. 2nd Int. Winter Wheat Conf., Zagreb, Yugoslavia.*

Klepper, L. A. (1976). Nitrate assimilation enzymes and seed protein in wheat. *Proc. 2nd Int. Winter Wheat Conf., Zagreb, Yugoslavia.*

Middleton, G. K., Bode, C. E., and Bales, B. B. (1954). A comparison of the quantity and quality of protein in certain varieties of soft wheat. *Agron. J. 46*:500–502.

Morris, R., Schmidt, J. W., Mattern, P. J., and Johnson, V. A. (1973). Chromosomal locations of genes for high protein in the wheat cultivar Atlas 66. *Proc. 4th Int. Wheat Genet. Sympos., Missouri Agr. Exp. Sta., Columbia, Mo.*

Neurath, H. and Bailey, K. (1954). *The Proteins—Chemistry, Biological Activity and Methods* (Neurath, H. and Bailey, K., eds.), Vol. 2, Part A, p. 493. Academic Press, New York.

Stroike, J. E., Johnson, V. A., Schmidt, J. W., Mattern, P. J., and Wilhelmi, K. D. (1974). Results of the fourth international winter wheat performance nursery. *Nebraska Res. Bull. 265,* 159 pp.

Vogel, K. P., Johnson, V. A., and Mattern, P. J. (1973). Results of systematic analyses for protein and lysine composition of common wheats (*Triticum aestivum* L.) in the USDA World Collection. *Nebraska Res. Bull. 258,* 27 pp.

Vogel, K. P., Johnson, V. A., and Mattern, P. J. (1975). Re-evaluation of common wheats from the USDA World Wheat Collection for protein and lysine content. *Nebraska Res. Bull. 272,* 36 pp.

Vogel, K. P., Johnson, V. A., and Mattern, P. J. (1976). Wheats from the USDA World Wheat Collection. *Crop Sci. 16*:655–660.

34

Improving Protein Content and Quality in Legumes

D. Boulter

Department of Botany
University of Durham
Durham, England DH1 3LE

ABSTRACT

Methods suitable for screening protein content in legumes are identified, including dye-binding, infrared (IR) reflectance, air-gap electrode, and micro-Kjeldahl with automatic nitrogen determination. Consideration is given to protein quality, because a smaller content of high-quality protein may be a more desirable breeding objective than a larger amount of less nutritious protein. Chemical assay and rat-feeding trials of seed meals of *Vigna unguiculata* and *Phaseolus vulgaris* lead to the conclusion that it is necessary to monitor both the sulfo-amino acids, cysteine and methionine. Total sulfur is suggested as a suitable measure of these after prior removal of sulfur-containing soluble components, such as *S*-methyl-L-cysteine. The importance of considering legume protein modification in relationship to diet and not in isolation is emphasized. Legume seeds contain many different proteins which for present purposes may be classified into (1) those which are of interest insofar as they can be manipulated to increase protein content or quality in seed meals; (2) those which are antimetabolites; and (3) those which may afford protection against pests or diseases. This classification is discussed subsequently. The special position of storage protein in relationship to nutritional improvement is stressed in terms of the process of protein biosynthesis in seeds.

SCREENING METHODS

Yield, stability of yield, and pest and disease resistance are the primary objectives of most breeding programs for improved grain legumes. However, protein content and quality should also be monitored in elite materials derived from such breeding programs, as these may be of considerable importance in some diets, as discussed later.

About 20 species of legumes are commonly used as human food; Roberts (1970) lists six of these as being of particular importance. As is well known, grain legumes are high-protein crops; different species and varieties usually have between 20 and 50% protein in their seeds. Because it is necessary in breeding programs to screen large numbers of samples (of the order of tens to one-hundred thousands according to the purpose), satisfactory screening methods are those which require small amounts of material, are simple and fast, and do not use expensive equipment. Such methods already exist for protein content, e.g., dye-binding (Mossberg, 1968; Evans and Boulter, 1974), IR reflectance (Rosenthal, 1971), the air-gap electrode (Ruzicka and Hansen, 1974), and micro-Kjeldahl with automatic nitrogen determination (Evans and Boulter, 1974). The first two methods are the fastest, as they do not involve a digestion step. Of the two, dye-binding requires the less sophisticated apparatus, but because it records the basic amino acid content as a measure of protein content (and this may change in different samples), a secondary screen using micro-Kjeldahl is required once the large numbers of samples have been reduced to a reasonable number. These methods work satisfactorily with several legumes and are probably of general application, but they may need some modification for use with a particular legume.

Consideration should be given not only to protein content, but also to its quality, because for certain diets and usage, lines with a smaller content of high-quality protein may be more suitable than ones with a larger amount of less nutritious form of protein. Generally, the first-limiting amino acids of legumes are the sulfo-amino acids (FAO, 1970). Tables I and II give the amino acid composition of, and the results of rat-feeding trials on, representative seed meal samples of *Vigna unguiculata* (cowpea) and *Phaseolus vulgaris* (dry bean). The major conclusion from the cowpea experiment is that cysteine rather than methionine is first-limiting in these experiments, and that it is necessary, therefore, to consider both sulfo-amino acids, cysteine and methionine, when attempting to establish the nutritional status of the protein of a legume meal (Boulter et al., 1973).

Total sulfur has been suggested as a possible measure of the sulfo-amino acids as a primary screen for the coarse-ranking of breeding materials (Boulter et al., 1973; Porter et al., 1974). For many legumes it is necessary to remove S-methyl-L-cysteine before analysis, although this may not be necessary for some legumes where relatively little of this compound occurs, e.g., peas, pigeon

Table I. Amino Acid Compositions of Seed Meals of
Vigna unguiculata and *Phaseolus vulgaris*[a]

Amino acid	g/16 g N	
	Vigna unguiculata[b]	*Phaseolus vulgaris*[c]
Asp	10.91	11.97
Thr	3.81	3.98
Ser	4.77	5.55
Glu	16.54	14.78
Pro	5.83	3.57
Gly	3.60	3.79
Ala	4.03	4.19
Val	4.24	4.59
Met	1.48	1.06
Ile	3.81	4.19
Leu	7.10	7.62
Tyr	2.97	2.53
Phe	5.62	5.22
His	3.18	2.83
Lys	6.99	7.20
Arg	6.36	5.68
Cys H	1.20	0.85
Total	92.44	89.60
Total nitrogen (g/100 g meal)	3.54	3.54

[a] Tryptophan and ammonia were not determined, cyst(e)ine as cysteic acid after performic acid oxidation.
[b] Average or extrapolated values for 22-, 48-, and 72-h hydrolysis.
[c] Mean values for duplicate 22-h hydrolysis.

pea, field bean, broad bean, soya bean, lupin, and yam beans (Evans and Boulter, 1975). In these latter cases, however, other soluble non-amino acid sulfur compounds may interfere; before this strategy can be accepted as firmly established, further work needs to be done with other legumes, particularly on lines that show a greater range of sulfo-amino acid content than those tested so far.

TYPES OF SEED PROTEIN AND THE IMPORTANCE OF STORAGE PROTEINS

Legume seeds contain several thousand different proteins (see, for example, Thurman, 1971; Boulter and Derbyshire, 1971). Of direct interest for the present purposes are (1) those which may be altered to increase protein content

Table II. Digestibility, Biological Value, and Net Protein Utilization
of Seed Meals of *Vigna unguiculata* and *Phaseolus vulgaris*[a,b]

	True digestibility (% ± SE)[c]	Biological value (% ± SE)	Net protein utilization (% ± SE)
8% Albumin	99.14 ± 0.33	97.08 ± 1.11	96.24 ± 0.91
Cowpea meal	85.44 ± 0.45	57.88 ± 1.19	49.42 ± 1.17
Cowpea + cystine (0.2305%)	85.53 ± 1.33	95.73 ± 1.46	81.89 ± 1.49
Cowpea + cystine (0.2305%) + methionine (0.0825%)	86.21 ± 0.90	96.01 ± 1.97	82.76 ± 1.16
8% Albumin	99.42 ± 0.21	100.30 ± 0.59	99.71 ± 0.17
Phaseolus meal	80.28 ± 1.78	48.90 ± 6.77	38.97 ± 5.06
Phaseolus + methionine to level of both sulfo-amino acids in albumen	82.16 ± 0.60	83.78 ± 2.75	68.75 ± 1.91

[a]Both *Vigna* and *Phaseolus* seeds were cooked prior to rat-feeding trials.
[b]Data from Boulter et al. (1973) and A. Thompson and D. Boulter (unpub.).
[c]SE = standard error.

or quality in seed meals; (2) those which have antimetabolic activity; and (3) those which may afford protection against pests or diseases. With regard to the first group of proteins, the question may be asked, How are improved lines most likely to be constituted, by a change in the proportion of some proteins, or by a change in the amino acid composition of particular proteins? Apparently, in cereals the former possibility is the more likely (Nelson and Burr, 1973). In considering which proteins are of potential interest, we can eliminate most of the enzymes of the central metabolic pathways on an individual basis, because these occur in small amounts that will not vary greatly in different lines, as they are normally constitutive and not under synthetic regulatory control; their activities, but not their synthesis, are controlled by inhibitory/activating mechanisms. Therefore, any increase in the sulfo-amino acid content of one of these enzymes would have a negligible effect on the seed meal composition overall, apart from the fact that such changes in amino acid composition are likely to be rare (Nelson and Burr, 1973). However, whereas enzyme proteins of the central metabolic pathways are unlikely to be of significance individually, as a class the enzymes (albumins), are higher in essential amino acids than are the legume storage proteins (globulins) (Boulter and Derbyshire, 1971). They also occur in greater amounts in the embryo axis than in the cotyledons, and screening lines for those with a higher proportion of embryo axis to cotyledons might be feasible.

Generally speaking, it is the storage proteins of legumes, of which there are several, on which most effort should be concentrated. These are synthesized on polysomes of rough endoplasmic reticulum, which is assembled at the appropriate time in large amounts during seed development (Millerd, 1975; Boulter,

1976). They are deposited in membrane-bound vesicles for storage until required during germination; these particular proteins are synthesized, or have the potential to be, in large amounts. As can be seen from representative examples given in Table III, the amino acid composition of different storage proteins differs significantly nutritionally; results using a variety of different legumes have indicated that the different storage proteins are under separate genetic control (Wright and Boulter, 1972; Millerd, 1975). That a change in the proportions of the storage proteins is still compatible with seed viability can be inferred from the fact that different species of legumes contain very different proportions of equivalent storage proteins (Derbyshire et al., 1976). These facts suggest that lines with changed proportions of storage proteins probably can be generated by breeding programs and that some of these lines may have improved protein content and quality.

A negative correlation has been found between protein sulfo-amino acid content and percentage protein content in legume seeds (Evans and Boulter, 1974); this finding has important implications for screening strategy (Evans and Boulter, 1974). The negative correlation is probably explained by the fact that

Table III. Amino Acid Compositions (g/100 g) of Some Proteins and Protein Fractions of *Phaseolus vulgaris* and *Vicia faba*

	Phaseolus vulgaris			*Vicia faba*	
	Glycoprotein II[a]	Legumin[b]	Trypsin inhibitor[c]	Vicilin[d]	Legumin[e]
Asp	12.4	8.6	16.7	12.3	10.6
Thr	3.4	3.9	7.1	2.62	3.40
Ser	6.7	5.0	12.9	4.77	4.24
Glu	15.1	12.8	9.4	17.1	15.7
Pro	2.9	3.8	6.6	6.25	6.38
Gly	2.7	3.6	1.8	2.98	3.43
Ala	3.0	3.8	3.3	2.65	3.23
Val	5.2	5.5	1.8	5.35	4.38
Met	0.7	1.4	1.5	0.20	0.38
Ile	5.6	4.5	4.8	5.73	4.27
Leu	9.1	7.7	3.4	9.71	7.27
Tyr	3.5	3.7	2.3	4.10	4.90
Phe	6.6	5.2	2.0	6.83	4.55
His	2.6	3.2	5.1	2.72	2.87
Lys	5.6	7.9	5.8	8.25	4.73
Arg	5.0	5.9	5.4	9.21	9.64
Trp	0.8	1.0	1.6	0.0	1.13
Cy H	0.3	0.5	14.5	0.13	1.26

[a] Pusztai and Watt (1970).
[b] Derbyshire and Boulter (1976).
[c] Pusztai (1966).
[d] Bailey and Boulter (1972).
[e] Bailey and Boulter (1970).

storage proteins, which are relatively low in sulfo-amino acids, are laid down later in development; high-protein-containing seeds will have higher proportions of these nutritionally inferior storage proteins. However, this negative correlation would not hold in lines in which higher sulfo-amino-acid-containing storage proteins predominate.

Exactly how many storage proteins there are, whether counterparts of each are present in all crop legumes, and their exact nutritional status, are questions for which there are only partial answers. However, suitable methods designed to answer these questions are now available (see, for example, Derbyshire et al., 1976), and a considerable effort should now be expended on extending our basic knowledge of these important proteins.

Information on proteins belonging to groups 2 and 3 are also very limited and again more information is sorely needed (see, for example, Bressani et al., 1973). One interpretation of the difference between the results obtained in Table II in rat-feeding trials with *Vigna* and *Phaseolus* for example, may be a reflection of the fact that there appear to be no heat-labile antimetabolites in cowpeas, whereas there may be in *Phaseolus*. The possible protective role of some proteins (group 3) against pests and diseases is discussed by Ryan (1973).

It would also appear possible, on a limited scale, to screen lines from breeding programs for particular proteins, either by using one of the gel electro- phoretic methods, e.g., sodium dodecyl sulfate—acrylamide gel electrophoresis, or serologically, and in this way to identify lines with higher concentrations of nutritionally or otherwise desirable proteins or those with lower levels of anti- metabolic proteins.

DIETARY CONSIDERATIONS

If improved lines with changed proportions of major seed proteins are forthcoming from breeding programs, it may be possible to predict the diets in which particular lines should be most usefully employed, because in the final analysis it is diet deficiencies that have to be corrected. For example, Table III gives the amino acid composition of two of the storage proteins, legumin and glycoprotein II, of *Phaseolus vulgaris,* the latter being the major storage protein (Barker et al., 1976). It can be seen that legumin contains about twice as much sulfo-amino acids as does glycoprotein II and also more lysine. *Phaseolus* is often used in diets in which maize is the main staple, and diets with some proportion of maize to beans are lysine- rather than methionine-deficient (Bressani et al., 1973). Changing the overall amino acid composition of the diet by using *Phaseolus* lines with a higher proportion of legumin/glycoprotein II (vicilin) would be satisfactory in these diets whether the proportions of maize were such as to make them limiting in lysine or in sulfo-amino acids. This situation can be contrasted with the use of *Vicia faba* in otherwise similar diets in which legumin, although it contains much more sulfo-amino acids than does vicilin, has a lower lysine content.

It is also interesting to note the very high levels of sulfo-amino acids, especially cysteine in trypsin inhibitor (Table III). Because trypsin inhibitors are usually inactivated by normal cooking procedures, the question is raised as to whether it is advantageous or disadvantageous to have high contents of trypsin inhibitor in seeds (Jaffe, 1950; Kakade et al., 1969; Seidl et al., 1969), especially if they are eventually shown to have a protective role (see Ryan, 1973).

It was recently pointed out that protein and calorie deficiency usually go together (Waterlow and Payne, 1975), and that it is normally more food that is needed rather than more protein per se. However, there are many diverse diets in the world, and the exact dietary situations is usually not known, so that generalizations should be treated cautiously. Diets in which legumes may be of particular importance as high-protein crops are those in which the main staples are root crops, such as cassava. As the world population increases, the dietary pattern of a root crop combined with a legume may become of increasing importance, since root crops are a more efficient source of calories per hectare than cereals. In some cases, agronomic considerations may favor this combination; in such diets sulfo-amino acids will be first-limiting.

PLANT ARCHITECTURE AND PROTEIN YIELD

Jain (1971) has pointed out that the relatively low yields of legumes (see FAO, 1972) can be partly explained by the fact that normally they are given less management and are grown on less fertile land than are cereals. Furthermore, relatively little breeding improvement has been carried out to transform them from their wild state with relatively low harvest index, which offers no particular advantage when the plant grows in nature.

Several authors (e.g., Adams, 1973; Evans, 1973; Wallace, 1973) have described bean plant ideotypes that should be selected in breeding for higher yield, although it would be fair to say that there is not a firm consensus of opinion on all the characteristics such an ideotype should possess, or whether it is possible to consider one ideotype satisfactory for a wide range of different agroecological situations (Evans, 1973). As pointed out by Wallace (1973), efficient breeding of higher-yielding varieties requires an understanding of the processes leading to the phenotypic expression of yield. When considering protein as a measure of economic yield, major components of importance are pathways of nitrogen uptake, transport and protein synthesis, repartitioning of photosynthate into storage protein, as well as photosynthate accumulation and photosynthate partitioning.

Sinclair and de Wit (1975) have carried out an interesting analysis of the photosynthate and nitrogen requirements for seed production by various crops.

Their calculations indicate that nitrogen requirements of legumes are so great, that in order to sustain seed growth, continued nitrogen translocation from vegetative tissues is necessary. This process may eventually induce senescence in these tissues and this would further restrict nitrogen uptake because nitrogen fixation is dependent on a supply of photosynthate from the leaves. The net result is a serious limitation in seed yield.

From this point of view, breeding for protein lines with a lower level of nitrogen-rich amino acids, i.e., amides and basic amino acids, which occur in large amounts in some legume-storage proteins (Boulter and Derbyshire, 1971), would appear a desirable strategy. However, the extent to which it is possible to change the amino acid composition of storage proteins and still retain seed viability is determined by various possible constraints (see Derbyshire et al., 1976).

ENERGY CONSIDERATIONS

Protein synthesis is a relatively energy-demanding process (Sinclair and De Wit, 1975), but the energy required is approximately the same for proteins with good and bad amino acid profiles. From this consideration, breeding for protein quality is an important objective.

Because one unit of glucose can give rise to 0.83 units of carbohydrate but only 0.4 units of protein, under some circumstances there is a trade-off between seed protein content and yield. This is clearly seen in the cereals where the harvest index is high and where an increased protein content is likely to depress yield, unless high-protein lines also generate an increased partitioning of photosynthate into their seeds. In legumes, with the possible exception of soya bean, the harvest index is such as to suggest that we have not reached the point where increasing protein content necessarily decreases yield, although initially high-protein lines are likely to be of lower yield.

In conclusion then, there is every reason to be optimistic that it will be possible, with better management and with breeding programs, to increase yield, protein yield, and protein content of legumes. It should also be possible to improve protein quality, but the extent of improvement is difficult to forecast in the absence of reliable data on the variation found in this character in the world germ plasm collections of legumes.

ACKNOWLEDGMENTS

Financial assistance of the Ministry of Overseas Development is gratefully acknowledged, and thanks are also due to E. Derbyshire for suggestions on the manuscript.

REFERENCES

Adams, M. W. (1973). Plant architecture and physiological efficiency in the field bean. In *Potentials of Field Beans and Other Food Legumes in Latin America,* pp. 266–278. Series Seminars No. 2E, Centro Internacional de Agricultura Tropical, Cali, Colombia.

Bailey, C. J. and Boulter, D. (1970). The structure of legumin, a storage protein of broad bean (*Vicia faba*) seed. *Eur. J. Biochem. 17*:460–466.

Bailey, C. J. and Boulter, D. (1972). The structure of vicilin of *Vicia faba. Phytochemistry 11*:59–64.

Barker, R. D. J., Derbyshire, E. Yarwood, A., and Boulter, D. (1976). Purification and characterisation of the major storage proteins of *Phaseolus vulgaris* L. seeds, and their intracellular and cotyledonary distribution. *Phytochemistry 15*:751–757.

Boulter, D. (1976). Protein synthesis in the cytoplasm. In *Cellular and Molecular Plant Physiology* (Smith, H., ed.). Blackwell Scientific Publications Ltd., Oxford.

Boulter, D. and Derbyshire, E. (1971). Taxonomic aspects of the structure of legume proteins. In *Chemotaxonomy of the Leguminosae* (Harborne, J. B., Boulter, D., and Turner, B. L., eds.), pp. 285–308. Academic Press, London and New York.

Boulter, D., Evans, I. M., and Thompson, A. (1973). Protein quality. *Proc. 1st Int. Inst. Tropical Agri. Grain Legume Improvement Workshop, Ibadan, Nigeria, 29th Oct.-2nd Nov., 1973,* pp. 239–248.

Bressani, R., Flores, M. and Elias, L. G. (1973). Acceptability and value of food legumes in the human diet. In *Potentials of Field Beans and Other Food Legumes in Latin America.* pp. 17–48. Series Seminars No. 2E, Centro Internacional de Agricultura Tropical, Cali, Colombia.

Derbyshire, E., and Boulter, D. (1976). Isolation of legumin-like protein from *Phaseolus aureus* and *Phaseolus vulgaris. Phytochemistry 15*:411–414.

Derbyshire, E., Wright, D. J., and Boulter, D. (1976). Legumin and vicilin, storage proteins of legume seeds. *Phytochemistry 15*:3–24.

Evans, A. M. (1973). 1. Commentary upon: Plant architecture and physiological efficiency in the field bean. In *Potentials of Field Beans and Other Food Legumes in Latin America,* pp. 279–286. Series Seminars No. 2E, Centro Internacional de Agricultura Tropical, Cali, Colombia.

Evans, I. M. and Boulter, D. (1974). Chemical methods suitable for screening for protein content and quality of cowpea (*Vigna uniguiculata*) meals. *J. Sci. Food Agri. 25*: 311–322.

Evans, I. M. and Boulter, D. (1975). S-methyl-L-cysteine content of various legume meals. *Qual. Plant.–Plant Foods Hum. Nutr. XXIV,* 257–261.

Food and Agriculture Organization of the United Nations. (1970). *Amino-Acid Content of Foods and Biological Data on Proteins.* Nutritional Studies No. 24, Rome.

Food and Agriculture Organization of the United Nations. (1972). *Production Yearbook,* Vol. 26. FAO, Rome.

Jaffe, W. G. (1950). Protein digestibility and trypsin inhibitor activity of legume seeds. *Proc. Exp. Biol. Med. 75*:219.

Jain, H. K. (1971). New types in pulses. *Indian Farming,* November 1971.

Kakade, M. L., Arnald, R. L., Liener, I. E., and Warbel, P. E. (1969). Unavailability of cystine from trypsin inhibitors as a factor contributing to the poor nutritive value of navy beans. *J. Nutr. 99*:34.

Millerd, A. (1975). Biochemistry of legume seed proteins. *Annu. Rev. Plant Physiol. 26*:53–72.

Mossberg, R. (1969). Evaluation of protein quality and quantity by dye-binding capacity: A tool in plant breeding. In *New Approaches to Breeding for Improved Plant Protein,* pp. 151–160. International Atomic Energy Agency, Vienna.

Nelson, O. E., Jr. and Burr, B. (1973). Biochemical genetics of higher plants. *Annu. Rev. Plant Physiol. 24*:493–518.

Porter, W. M., Maner, J. H., Axtell, J. D. and Keim, W. F. (1974). Evaluation of the nutritional quality of grain legumes by analysis for total sulfur. *Crop Sci. 14*:652–654.

Pusztai, A. (1966). The isolation of two proteins, Glycoprotein I and a trypsin inhibitor, from the seeds of kidney bean (*Phaseolus vulgaris*). *Biochem. J. 101*:379–384.

Pusztai, A. and Watt, W. B. (1970). Glycoprotein II. The isolation and characterization of a major antigenic and nonhaemagglutinating glycoprotein from *Phaseolus vulgaris*. *Biochim. Biophys. Acta 207*:413–431.

Roberts, L. M. (1970). The food legumes: Recommendations for expansion and acceleration of research. Rockefeller Foundation, New York. (*Mimeogr. report.*)

Rosenthal, R. D. (1971). Introducing: The Grain Quality Analyzer. A rapid and accurate means of determining the percent moisture, oil and protein in grain and grain products. *Ann. Meeting Kansas Assoc. of Wheat Growers and the Kansas Wheat Commission, Dec. 10, 11, 1971, Neotec Instruments, Md. 20852.*

Ruzicka, J. and Hansen, E. H. (1974). A new potentiometric gas-sensor—the air-gap electrode. *Anal. Chim. Acta 69*:129–141.

Ryan, C. A. (1973). Proteolytic enzymes and their inhibitors in plants. *Annu. Rev. Plant Physiol. 24*:173–196.

Seidl, D., Jaffe, M., and Jaffe, W. G. (1969). Digestibility and proteinase inhibitory action of a kidney bean globulin. *J. Agri. Food Chem. 17*:1318.

Sinclair, T. R., and de Wit, C. T. (1975). Photosynthate and nitrogen requirements for seed production of various crops. *Science 189*:565–567.

Thurman, D. A. (1971). Comparative studies of legume enzymes. In: Chemotaxonomy of the *Leguminosae* (Harborne, J. B., Boulter, D., and Turner, B. L., eds.), pp. 463–483. Academic Press, London and New York.

Wallace, D. H. (1973). II. Commentary upon: Plant Architecture and physiological efficiency in the field bean. In *Potentials of Field Beans and Other Food Legumes in Latin America,* pp. 287–295. Series Seminars No. 2E.

Waterlow, J. C. and Payne, P. R. (1975). The protein gap. *Nature. (London) 258*:113–117.

Wright, D. J. and Boulter, D. (1972). The characterisation of vicilin during seed development in *Vicia faba* (L.). *Planta (Berlin) 105*:60–65.

35

The Variability of Free Amino Acids and Related Compounds in Legume Seeds

E. A. Bell, M. Y. Qureshi, B. V. Charlwood,
D. J. Pilbeam, and C. S. Evans

Department of Plant Sciences
King's College
London, England SE24 9JF

ABSTRACT

Legume seeds are an important source of protein for humans and domestic animals. The Leguminosae contain more than 700 genera and 25,000 species, yet fewer than 20 of these are grown as major world crops. The nutritional value of legume seeds is frequently less than ideal, however, because their proteins contain lower concentrations of certain "essential" amino acids than do animal proteins. The fact that "free" amino acids frequently constitute more than 10% of the weight of legume seeds is often overlooked when considering their nutritional value, as free amino acids tend to be lost in traditional methods of cooking. Toxins, such as the alkaloids, cyanogenic glycosides, and certain of the "nonprotein" amino acids are also found in the seeds of numerous legumes. An understanding of their nature, concentration, and distribution is necessary if we are to exploit the great potential food reserve represented by the thousands of legume species that have never been brought into cultivation or used for the improvement of established crop species. During the past few years we have studied the free amino acids in the seeds of more than 1500 legume species representing 300 of the 700 known genera, and in time propose to make a complete survey of the family. For ease of retrieval, we are assembling analytical data on magnetic tape in a computer bank. Complementary information on the presence of alkaloids, cyanogenic glycosides, toxic amino acids, and physiologically active amines in these seeds is also being accumulated, and we are presently seeking funds to extend this work and determine the protein content and composition of the seeds of this unique collection.

INTRODUCTION

Seeds of the Leguminosae are a major source of food for man and his domestic animals in many parts of the world. The family contains more than seven hundred genera and well over 25,000 species. Of these species, the seeds of fewer than 20 are cultivated as major world crops, though many others are used locally, either as a normal part of the diet or as "famine foods."

Frequently, the nutritional value of legume seeds is less than ideal, however, because their proteins contain lower concentrations of certain "essential" amino acids (those amino acids which must be provided in the human or animal diet) than do animal proteins. The sulfur-containing amino acids methionine and cysteine are usually the limiting amino acids in legume proteins, although the level of other "essential" amino acids, such as lysine and tryptophan, may be important if the other constituents of a mixed diet are deficient.

That free amino acids often constitute more than 10% of the weight of legume seeds frequently has been overlooked when considering their nutrient value. These free amino acids, nevertheless, represent an enormous potential store of nourishment for man and animals, particularly if the free amino acid pool is rich in one or more essential amino acids or contains a precursor that will give rise to an essential amino acid after being ingested.

Free amino acids, it may be argued, are of little value in human nutrition as they are likely to be leached out and lost in the course of cooking. If, however, we are aware of the presence of high concentrations of a free essential amino acid in a particular species, appropriate precautions can be taken to minimize cooking losses, or in the case of large-scale processing to recover the amino acid from the water used in their preparation. These difficulties do not arise in the same way with animal feeds, as the whole uncooked seed meal usually is supplied to the animals.

Among the wild legumes there may be many species with favorable characteristics (in terms of free or protein-bound amino acids, or both) which could contribute directly or indirectly (as a source of genes for plant breeding programs) to the world's food supply. A search for such legumes among those species that grow naturally in regions of the world that are suffering from chronic food shortages, or which are unsuitable for raising soya beans or other cultivated legumes, would seem a matter of urgency.

The qualitative and quantitative determination of free essential amino acids in the seeds of species and varieties of legumes already used as human and animal foods may also indicate ways in which the processing of seed crops can be modified to provide a greater yield of essential nutrients. A good legume source of methionine, for example (free or bound), which could be used to supplement a lysine-rich cereal diet, would be very welcome in many areas.

In addition to the common amino acids—those 25 to 30 found universally as protein constituents (e.g., alanine and lysine) or as metabolic intermediates (e.g., ornithine and homoserine)—legume seeds frequently contain high concentrations of uncommon amino acids (e.g., canavanine, I, and homoarginine, II). The presence of these "uncommon" amino acids (and of other secondary compounds

$$H_2NC(:NH)NHOCH_2CH_2CH(NH_2)COOH$$

[I]

$$H_2NC(:NH)NHCH_2CH_2CH_2CH_2CH(NH_2)COOH$$

[II]

such as alkaloids and cyanogenic glycosides) has a direct bearing on the possible use of the seeds for human and animal food, and on the resistance of the seeds to destruction by insects and other organisms (animals, molds, etc.). It is clear, then, that a knowledge of the distribution, concentration, physiological activity, and variability of uncommon amino acids and other secondary compounds, no less than a knowledge of the distribution, concentration, and variability of essential amino acids, is of vital importance when the development of new legume crops or the improvement of old ones is being considered.

In addition to our studies of the free amino acids and related compounds in the seeds of genera which are already of economic importance, our laboratory is making a major collection of legume seeds from all over the world (to date we have analyzed 1500 species, representing 270 of the 700 known genera), and are using this collection to determine the distribution and concentration of free amino acids ("common" and "uncommon") in species throughout the family. We are now extending this survey to the protein content and composition of the seeds as well. The data on essential, nonessential, protein, and nonprotein amino acids in the free amino acid pool of the seeds will, we believe, provide a guide for the better use of species already under cultivation, as well as for the selection of species and genera which may be developed as new food crops, or used as a source of genes for the improvement of existing cultivated species by appropriate interbreeding. To facilitate the acquisition, storage, and retrieval of data, the output of our automatic amino acid analyzer is being fed directly onto magnetic computer tape. The computer provides calculating and storage capacity. From the completed bank of information it will be possible, for example, to retrieve information immediately as to which species or genera are rich in a specific essential amino acid, or are rich in physiologically active or toxic amino acids such as L-dopa, III, or mimosine, IV. It will also be possible to compare with equal facility the amino acid profile of a newly analyzed seed with the profiles

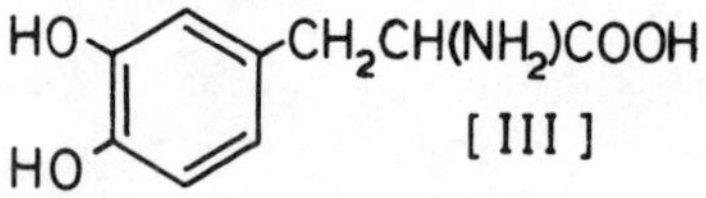

HO—⟨ ⟩—CH$_2$CH(NH$_2$)COOH

[III]

HO

O=⟨ ⟩NCH$_2$CH(NH$_2$)COOH

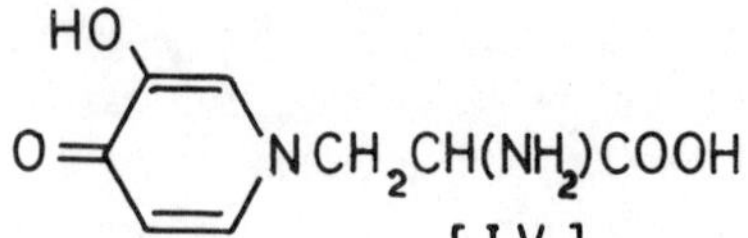

[IV]

of all species of seed previously analyzed. In this way, we shall be able to place the newly analyzed species with other species sharing a common amino acid pattern (free and protein bound). Information on the nutritional value of any one species of such a related group clearly will be of significance when considering the potential of the others.

As little is known of the nutritive value to humans and higher animals of most of the uncommon amino acids, these are being isolated (when sufficient seed is available) in quantities which will permit appropriate evaluations to be made. L-Homoarginine, which occurs in some legumes, is capable of replacing lysine in the mammalian diet (Stevens and Bush, 1950); it is possible that other nonprotein acids may be of similar potential importance.

In addition to free amino acids, many legume seeds accumulate free amines which are detected during the preliminary screening of extracts by high-voltage electrophoresis on paper. The distribution of these amines, including vaso- and psychoactive ones, such as tyramine, V, 5-hydroxytryptamine (5-HT), VI (serotonin) and *N*-dimethyl-5-hydroxytryptamine (bufotenin, VII) are being deter-

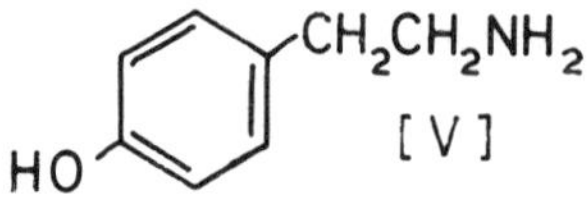

CH$_2$CH$_2$NH$_2$

[V]

HO

HO

CH$_2$CH$_2$NR$_2$

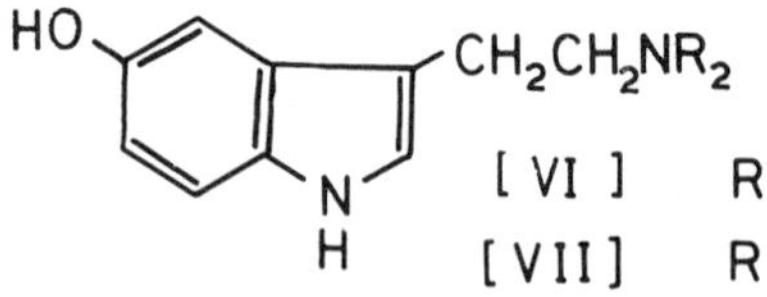

[VI]   R = H

[VII]   R = Me

mined. Each species of seed is being routinely tested for the presence of alkaloids and cyanogenic glycosides.

It is our ultimate intention to provide comprehensive data on the content and composition of the free amino acid pool, the content and composition of the protein reserves, and the presence or absence of potential toxins for seeds of species from virtually all genera of the Leguminosae. These data, stored in our computer bank, will allow the rapid identification of species with the characteristics required to meet specific nutritional needs in particular parts of the world for the human population and its domesticated animals. The information also will be of value in identifying those seed constituents which deter potential predators—animals, insects, or microorganisms.

ESTABLISHMENT OF PRIORITIES

The program outlined in the Introduction is a long-term project which will take some years to complete; clearly some parts of it will have more immediate relevance to developing world food resources than will others.

In selecting genera for detailed study in the past, we chose those which are important as sources of food to man and his domestic animals or have been implicated as causes of disease in man or animals. Such considerations led to our work on distribution of toxic amino acids in the seeds of *Lathyrus*; subsequent studies of *Vicia, Phaseolus,* and *Vigna* (Bell, 1964, 1971, 1973), and *Crotalaria* and *Acacia* are among those being studied at present.

In choosing these genera we benefited from the advice of workers interested in the implications of our work to their own fields for whose help we are grateful; we would welcome further collaboration, particularly with scientists in the developing countries where basic knowledge of legume chemistry may be of importance in selecting wild species for cultivation or in improving established crops.

QUALITATIVE VARIATION IN AMINO ACID COMPOSITION

Between Genera

Some legume genera apparently are unique in their capacity to synthesize and store a particular amino acid. All species of *Mucuna,* but of no other genera examined (see Table I), accumulate high concentrations of L-3,4-dihydroxy-phenylalanine (III) in their seeds (Bell and Janzen, 1971). Similarly, the seeds of *Griffonia* species are exceptional in containing high concentrations (7–14%) of 5-hydroxy-L-tryptophan, VIII (Bell et al., 1976). Canavanine, on the other hand, is found as the principal seed amino acid in species of many different genera. All

$$HO-\text{(indole ring)}-CH_2CH(NH_2)COOH \qquad [VIII]$$

these genera are members of the Papilionoideae, however, which suggests that the biosynthetic pathway to canavanine arose since this subfamily became separated from the Minosoideae and Caesalpinoideae.

Table I. Variation in Concentration of
L-Dopa in Individual Seeds of *Mucuna* Species

Species	% L-Dopa in seed (excluding seed coat)
M. andreana	8.9
	6.8
	6.3
M. deeringiana	6.0
	5.7
	4.7
M. gigantea	10.5
	5.9
	5.4
M. glabriata	7.6
M. holtoni	7.3
	6.8
	6.2
	10.9
M. mutisiana	7.4
	7.3
M. poggei	5.5
M. pruriens	7.9
	6.4
	5.9
	4.4
M. sloanei	9.0
	8.7
M. urens	7.4
	6.4
M. utilis	9.7
	7.3
	7.2
	6.5
	5.1

The seeds of some genera can be identified, not by the presence of a single major free amino acid, but by associations of free amino acids which occur in relatively high concentration and appear as a characteristic pattern of ninhydrin-reacting spots after paper chromatography or electrophoresis. Pipecolic acid, IX, and γ-glutamyl-*S*-methylcysteine, X, for example, form such an association in the *Phaseolus* seeds which we have analyzed (unlike *Vigna* seeds, some of which accumulate γ-glutamyl-*S*-methylcysteine but not pipecolic acid). This difference is shown in Table II (see also Casimir and LeMarchand, 1966).

[IX]

$$\text{HOOCCH(NH}_2\text{)CH}_2\text{CH}_2\text{CONHCHCOOH}$$
with side chain $\overset{\text{CH}_2\text{SCH}_3}{|}$ on the CH

[X]

Table II. Differences in Principal Free Amino Acids of *Phaseolus* and *Vigna* Seeds[a]

Species	Arginine	Glutamic acid	Aspartic acid	γ-Glutamyl-S-methylcysteine	Pipecolic acid
Phaseolus gonospermus	++	+	+	++	++
P. acutifolius	+	+	+	++	++
P. caffer	T	+	+	++	++
P. multiflorus	T	+	+	++	++
P. tuberosus	+	+	+	++	++
P. vulgaris	+	+	+	++	++
P. cerasifolius	+	+	+	++	++
P. ricciardianus	+	+	+	++	++
P. semierectus	T	+	+	++	++
P. coccineus	+	+	+	++	++
P. calcaratus	+	+	+	++	++
P. hysterinus	T	+	+	++	++
P. lunatus	+	+	+	+	++
Vigna machrorhyncha	+	+			
V. kirkii	+	+	+		
V. luteola	T	T	T		
V. pilosa	+	T	T		
V. vexillata[b]	+	+	+	T	
V. schimperi	+	T	+	+	
V. oblongifolia	+	T	T	+	
V. parviflora	++	+	+	+	
V. heterophylla	+	+	T	+	
V. membranacea	+	++	++	++	
V. gracilis	+	++	+	+	
Vigna (Phaseolus) aurea[c]	+	+	+	+	
V. (Phaseolus) mungo[c]	T	+	+	+	
V. (Phaseolus) grandis[c]	+	+	+	T	
V. (Phaseolus) aconitifolia[c]	+	T	T		
V. (Phaseolus) tenuifloria[c]	+	+	T	T	

[a](++) Strong, (+) medium, (T) trace.
[b]Also contains *paraaminophenylalanine* (Dardenne et al., 1972).
[c]Species once considered to be *Phaseolus* but now included in *Vigna*.

Within Genera

In some genera all species accumulate the same amino acids in their seeds; in others there is much more variability. In *Lathyrus* not all species accumulate α-amino-β-oxalylaminopropionic acid, XI (the toxin responsible for neuro-lathyrism in humans), nor do all species of *Vicia* accumulate the cystathionase inhibitor β-cyanoalanine, XII (Bell, 1971). Variation within *Lathyrus* is illustrated in Table III.

$$HOOCCONHCH_2CH(NH_2)COOH$$
$$[XI]$$

$$NCCH_2CH(NH_2)COOH$$
$$[XII]$$

Within Species

The existence of distinct "chemical races" of particular plant species is well known, and it is possible that some legume species may show more variability in their amino acid biochemistry than they do in their morphology. In our experience, however, the seeds of a single wild species collected from different areas show the same amino acid patterns, even though the relative concentrations of the accumulated amino acids may vary with the environment. Preliminary results suggest that greater variation (even qualitative) may occur between varieties of a cultivated species.

QUANTITATIVE VARIATION IN SEED AMINO ACIDS

In the foregoing discussion of qualitative differences in amino acid accumulation, no mention has been made of the common amino acids. The reason for this is that virtually all the common amino acids can be detected in any seed extract, provided it is concentrated enough. In extracts of legume seeds, however, certain common amino acids—aspartic acid, glutamic acid, asparagine, glutamine, and arginine—are almost always found in readily detectable concentrations. Proline, alanine, and others occur more occasionally as principal constituents of the amino acid pool. When dealing with a common amino acid, it is not always easy to decide whether a high concentration in a seed is a genetically controlled characteristic of the species or whether it is attributable to environmental factors which have favored its synthesis and accumulation in a particular plant. When seeds of a species collected at different times and from different environments all show such an accumulation then we can be more certain of genetic control.

Table III. Amino Acids and Related Compounds in Seeds of *Lathyrus* Species

Group	Species[a]	Compound present[b]											
		B_1	B_2	B_3	B_4	N_1	N_2	A_1	A_2	A_3	A_4	Lat.	Arg.
1	*aurantius*		++										T
	luteus		++										T
	laevigatus sp. *aureus*		++										T
	sylvestris		++				T	+	+	T			+++
	latifolius		++					+	+	T			++
	heterophyllus		++					+	+	T			++
	gorgoni		++					+	+	T			T
	grandiflorus		++					+	+	T			T
	cirrhosus		++					+	+	T			+
	rotundifolius		++				T	+	+	T			+
	tuberosus		++					T	+	T			+
	multiflora		++				T	T	+	T			+
	undulatus		++				+	T	++	T			+
2	*alatus*	++						++					
	articulatus	++						++					
	arvense	++					T	++					
	setifolius	++						+++					
	pannonicus	++						++					
	ochrus	++						++					
	clymenum	++						++					
	sativus	++						T					
	megallanicus	++						T					
	quadrimarginatus	++						T					
	cicera	++						T					

(contd.)

Table III. (*contd.*)

Group	Species[a]	Compound present[b]											
		B_1	B_2	B_3	B_4	N_1	N_2	A_1	A_2	A_3	A_4	Lat.	Arg.
3	*pratensis*	++										T	
	laevigatus sp. *occidentalis*	T										T	
	varius	+										+	T
	niger	+										+	T
	machrostachys	+										+	T
	maritimus	+									+	++	T
	aphaca	+		+							+	+	T
	sphaerious	+		+								++	T
	tingitanus	+		+++								+++	T
	cyanus	+		++								++	T
	alpestris	+			+		++				T	++	
	variegatus	+			+		++				T	+++	
	venetus	+			+		++				T	++	
	inconspicuous	+									++	T	
	incurvus	++									++	T	
4	*vernus*	+++					+++				T	+	
	montanus	+++					++						
	palustris	++					+						+
	aureus	+++					++						T
	neurobolus	++					+						T
	nissolia	++					+						T

5	roseus			T
	hirsutus		+	T
	odoratus	+	+	T
	pisiformis²	T		T
	annuus²	T		T
	angulatus²	T	+	T
	laetiflorus	T	+++	
	venosus	+		T

^{a}These three species contained low concentrations of amino acids and were not assigned to the previous groups; *L. laetiflorus* contained a neutral compound and *L. venosus* a basic compound not seen in other species. All species contained traces of glutamic acid and aspartic acid. ^{b}T = trace; B_1 = homoarginine (II); B_2 = α, γ-diaminobutyric acid (XIII); B_3 = γ-hydroxyhomoarginine (XVII); B_4 = unidentified; N_1 = β(γ-glutamylamino)propionitrile (XIV); N_2 = γ-hydroxynorvaline (tentative identification); A_1 = α-amino-β-oxalylaminopropionic acid (XI); A_2 = α-amino-γ-oxalylaminobutyric acid (XVIII); A_3 = α-amino-γ-oxalylamino-γ-aminobutyric acid (XIX); A_4 = γ-methylglutamic acid (XX); Lat. = lathyrine (XXI); Arg. = arginine.

H$_2$NCH$_2$CH$_2$CH(NH$_2$)COOH

[XIII]

NCCH$_2$CH$_2$NHOCCH$_2$CH$_2$CH(NH$_2$)COOH

[XIV]

H$_2$NC(:NH)CH$_2$CH$_2$CH$_2$CH$_2$CH(NH$_2$)COOH

[XV]

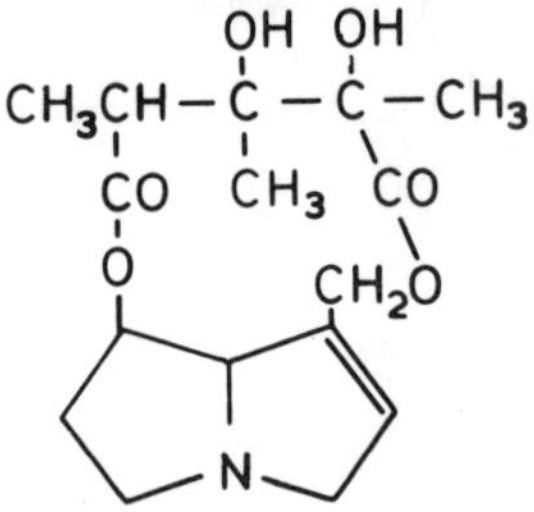

[XVI]

H$_2$NC(:NH)NHCH$_2$CH$_2$CH(OH)CH$_2$CH(NH$_2$)COOH

[XVII]

HOOCCONHCH$_2$CH$_2$CH(NH$_2$)COOH

[XVIII]

H$_2$NCH$_2$CH$_2$CH(NHOCCOOH)COOH

[XIX]

HOOCCH(CH$_3$)CH$_2$CH(NH$_2$)COOH

[XX]

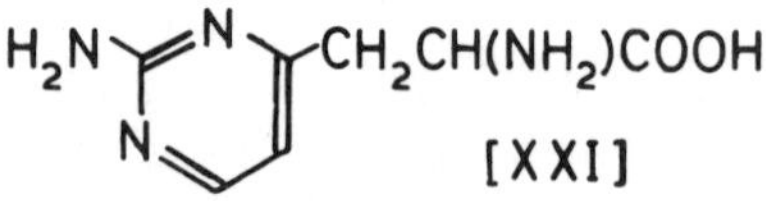

[XXI]

An example of this is seen in the genus *Erythrina* in which high concentrations of histidine clearly characterize the seeds of some species (Romeo and Bell, 1974).

No general rules can be made concerning the quantitative variability of the uncommon amino acids. Canavanine is found as the principal free amino acid in the seeds of some species, but only in trace amounts in others; this is true of very many such compounds.

As would be expected, much more uniformity is found in the concentrations of a single amino acid determined in individual seeds of a single species. Nevertheless, variation does occur, even when the plants have been grown under the same conditions, and it is clear that natural or artificial selection could lead to varieties containing greater or lesser amounts of these compounds.

QUALITATIVE VARIATION AND TOXICITY

The toxicity of certain amino acids to humans and higher animals is well known. α-Amino-β-oxalylaminopropionic acid in *Lathyrus* has been referred to. Various species of the same genus also contain α,γ-diaminobutyric acid, XIII, which inhibits ornithine transcarbamylase of mammalian liver, and γ-glutamyl-β-aminopropionitrile, XIV, which causes skeletal deformation and aortic aneurisms in experimental animals. The selenoamino acids of some *Astragalus* species (the "locoweeds" of the American West) are extremely toxic to horses (Shrift, 1972), whereas mimosine of *Leucaena leucocephala* causes the loss of wool in sheep (Hegarty et al., 1964), and indospicine, XV, of *Indigofera spicata* is both hepatotoxic and teratogenic if ingested by grazing animals (Hegarty and Pound, 1970). These and other toxic amino acids present in legumes have been discussed more fully elsewhere (Bell, 1972), but the examples given here emphasize the need to understand and appreciate the practical consequences of the chemical variability which exists between and sometimes within the genera of this family.

QUANTITATIVE VARIATION AND TOXICITY

It is obviously preferable to cultivate species that do not contain uncommon amino acids or other secondary compounds toxic to humans or domesticated animals, or both. If, however, a species is very suitable in other respects and is widely cultivated already it may be easier to select and propagate strains with successively decreasing toxin content than to replace the species with another which may not be so easy to grow or which is not acceptable to the local population. Our observations on variability within species suggest that this approach might be used to reduce the toxin concentration to insignificant amounts even if it failed to produce a toxin-free variety.

VARIATION AND NUTRITIVE VALUE

Reference has already been made to the ability of L-homoarginine to replace lysine in the mammalian diet; clearly, the selection of species synthesizing this uncommon amino acid would be equivalent to breeding lysine-rich varieties. The nutrient value (and indeed the toxicity) of most of the uncommon amino acids has yet to be determined, but it is possible that others of these may also prove to be precursors of the essential amino acids. One of the objectives of our present survey of free amino acids in the family is to ascertain which, if any, genera or species are particularly rich in one or more essential amino acids. The uncommon amino acids have taken most of our efforts so far, however, and distribution patterns for the essential amino acids are not yet available.

VARIATION AND RESISTANCE TO PREDATORS

A species that diverts 10% of its resources, biosynthetic capacity, and storage space to the accumulation of a compound that is not required for its primary metabolic processes is not going to survive in competition with seemingly less prodigal species in the same environment unless the uncommon amino acid or other secondary compound confers some selective advantage on the plant which contains it.

Preliminary experiments have shown (Rehr et al., 1973*a,b*) that some of the uncommon amino acids in legume seeds are toxic to the larvae of seed beetles and other insects. This raises the possibility that it is insect predation that has in some instances exercised the environmental pressure which has led to the natural selection of species with seeds containing high concentrations of these compounds. In other instances, selection may have resulted from pressures exerted by animals or microorganisms to which certain of these compounds are also toxic. If these hypotheses are correct, and if the predator or predators which exercised the pressures are still part of the ecosystem, then an artificial selection of toxin-low varieties might prove self-defeating. That is to say, the nonpoisonous crop might be destroyed by caterpillars or other predators before it could be harvested. If, however, the toxin is still a deterrent to insects (or microorganisms or rodents) at concentrations that no longer affect humans, or if the toxin is toxic to the predators and not to humans, then either the development of toxin-low varieties or the cultivation of new species containing selective toxins could provide more food for man without necessarily providing more for the insects or molds.

VARIATION AND HYBRIDIZATION

It has been noted (Bell and Fowden, 1964) that *Lathyrus* species showing dissimilar amino acid patterns do not produce viable hybrids. It has also been shown that some uncommon amino acids of the Leguminosae can promote the growth of pollen tubes in species which synthesize them while inhibiting the growth of pollen tubes in species that do not (Simola, 1967). This finding, which indicates that uncommon amino acids can act as chemical barriers to hybridization, suggests that more information on the distribution and physiological activity of these compounds might be helpful to those selecting species for breeding programs.

OTHER SECONDARY COMPOUNDS

Many of the considerations concerning uncommon amino acids also apply to alkaloids, cyanogenic glycosides, and other secondary compounds. It is interesting, moreover, that alkaloids and cyanogenic glycosides appear to replace physiologically active uncommon amino acids in some genera or subgenera. In *Crotalaria*, for example, some species accumulate alkaloids, such as monocrotaline, whereas others accumulate the neurotoxin α-amino-β-oxalylaminopropionic acid.

CONCLUSION

If the full food potential of the Leguminosae is to be realized, phytochemists must coordinate their efforts to provide to geneticists and plant breeders an overall picture of the nutrients and toxins synthesized and accumulated by different genera and species of the family. At the same time, geneticists and plant breeders must realize that phytochemists are frequently unfamiliar with the problems of raising and developing new crops or improving old ones. It is therefore very necessary that phytochemists and plant biochemists be told where their help is likely to be most useful.

ACKNOWLEDGMENTS

We thank the Science Research Council for financial support, and Dr. B. A. Krukoff for invaluable help in obtaining seeds.

REFERENCES

Bell, E. A. (1964). Relevance of biochemical taxonomy to the problem of Lathyrism. *Nature, (London) 203*:378–380.
Bell, E. A. (1971). Comparative biochemistry of "non-protein amino acids". In *Chemotaxonomy of the Leguminosae* (Harborne, J. B., Boulter, D., and Turner, B. L., eds.), pp. 179–206. Academic Press, London and New York.

Bell, E. A. (1972). Toxic amino acids in the Leguminosae. In *Phytochemical Ecology* (Harborne, J. B., ed.), pp. 163–177. Academic Press, London and New York.

Bell, E. A. (1973). Non-protein amino acids and nitriles. In *Toxicants Occurring Naturally in Foods,* pp. 153–169. National Academy of Sciences, National Research Council, Washington, D.C.

Bell, E. A. and Fowden, L. (1964). Studies on amino acid distribution and their possible value in plant classification. In *Taxonomic Biochemistry and Serology.* (Leone, C. A., ed.), pp. 203–223. Ronald Press, New York.

Bell, E. A. and Janzen, D. H. (1971). Medical and ecological considerations of L-dopa and 5-HTP in seeds. *Nature (London) 229*:136–137.

Bell, E. A., Fellows, L. E., and Qureshi, M. Y. (1976). 5-Hydroxy-L-tryptophan; taxonomic character and chemical defense in *Griffonia* Baill. *Phytochemistry 15*:823.

Casimir, J. and Le Marchand, G. (1966). Répartition et importance systématique des acides amines et des peptides libres des Phaseolinae. *Bull. Jard. Bot. Brux. 36*:53–56.

Dardenne, G. A., Marlier, M., and Casimir, J. (1972). Un nouvel acid amine dans les graines de *Vigna vexillata. Phytochemistry 11*:2567–2570.

Hegarty, M. P. and Pound, A. W. (1970). Indospicine, a hepatotoxic amino acid from *Indigofera spicata:* Isolation, structure and biological studies. *Aust. J. Agri. Res. 23*: 831–842.

Hegarty, M. P., Schinkel, P. G., and Court, R. D. (1964). Reaction of sheep to the consumption of *Laucaena glauca* Benth. and its toxic principle mimosine. *Aust. J. Agri. Res. 15*: 153–167.

Rehr, S. S., Bell, E. A., Janzen, D. H., and Feeny, P. P. (1973a). Insecticidal amino acids in legume seeds. *Biochem. Syst. 1*:63–67.

Rehr, S. S., Janzen, D. H., and Feeny, P. P. (1973b). L-dopa in legume seeds: a chemical barrier to insect attack. *Science 181*:81–82.

Romeo, J. T. and Bell, E. A. (1974). Distribution of amino acids and certain alkaloids in *Erythrina* species. *Lloydia 37*:543–568.

Shrift, A. (1972). Selenium toxicity. In *Phytochemical Ecology* (Harborne, J. B., ed.), pp. 145–161. Academic Press, London and New York.

Simola, L. K. (1967). The effect of some non-protein amino acids on pollen germination and pollen-tube growth in five species of the Vicieae. *Planta 77*:287–297.

Stevens, C. M. and Bush, J. A. (1950). New synthesis of α-amino-ε-guanidino-*n*-caproic acid (homoarginine) and its possible conversion *in vivo* into lysine. *J. Biol. Chem. 183*: 139–147.

36

A Genetic Approach to the Increase of Methionine Content in Legume Seeds

Donald E. Foard

Biology Division
Oak Ridge National Laboratory
Oak Ridge, Tennessee

In many developing counties legumes contribute a significant part of dietary protein. Total protein consumed is small in instances of low food intake (e.g., in children), and any nutritional deficiency of that protein prevents its complete utilization. As recently reemphasized by Boulter (1975) and others, an improvement of protein quality is essential in such a situation, whether the diet be cereal- or legume-based.

In the seed proteins of legumes generally, methionine occurs in small amounts, and is usually considered to occur in limiting amounts for the nutrition of monogastric animals. Research aimed at the question of whether it might be possible to alter this condition, principally by genetic means, is in progress in several laboratories worldwide, e.g., at the John Innes Institute by Davies and colleagues on garden peas and at the Division of Protein Chemistry, CSIRO, in Australia by Blagrove and Gillespie (1975) on lupins. In order to determine whether a genetic program to increase the methionine content of the soybean (*Glycine max* L.) is feasible, we have begun to investigate the occurrence of methionine in mature seeds. The variety chosen is Tracy, bred by Hartwig and co-workers to produce a high percentage of protein under the agricultural and climatic conditions of the southern United States.

First, we have confirmed earlier work by Kasai et al. (1970) on a different variety, that methionine does not occur as a free amino acid in mature seeds. Second, we have found, as determined previously (Wolf, 1972), that the globular proteins of the 7 S and of the 11 S fractions, which together constitute approximately 68% of the total in the seed, contain only about 0.4% and 1% (w/w) methionine, respectively, compared with about 1.5% methionine in total seed protein. Presumably, therefore, a high-methionine protein does exist, most likely among proteins of the 2 S fraction. After confirmation that such a protein (or proteins) exists, the question would arise as to whether it occurs in a quantity sufficient to have an enhancing effect on methionine content of seed proteins, were it to be increased relative to other proteins. Finally, we would need to devise an appropriate quantitative assay for the high-methionine protein in the large numbers of plants necessary in such an investigation.

Up to this point in our studies we have found that fractionation of soybean extracts on Sephadex G-100 and G-75, followed by DEAE cellulose chromatography, yields fractions with high contents of methionine and half-cystine (Hwang and Foard, 1976). Currently we are purifying these fractions to characterize them further and to develop, if possible, a quantitative immunological assay to detect elevated levels of these proteins having a high amount of sulfur-containing amino acids in seeds of genetically diverse or segregating populations. The high content of half-cystine suggests that these fractions may contain trypsin-inhibitor activities, a possibility we are currently investigating.

ACKNOWLEDGMENT

This work was supported by Union Carbide for the U.S. Energy Research and Development Administration.

REFERENCES

Blagrove, R. J. and Gillespie, J. M. (1975). Isolation, purification and characterization of the seed globulins of *Lupinus angustifolius. Aust. J. Plant Physiol.* 2:13–27.
Boulter, D. (1975). Breeding for protein yield and quantity. *Nature (London) 256*: 168–169.
Hwang, D. L.-R. and Foard, D. E. (1976). Protein fractions with high content of sulfur-containing amino acids in soybean seeds. *Plant Physiol. 57*:36.
Kasai, T., Sakamura, S., Ohashi, S., and Kumagai, H. (1970). Amino acid composition of soybean V. Changes in free amino acids, ethanolamine, and two γ-glutamyl peptides content during the ripening period of soybean. *Agri. Biol. Chem. 34*:1848–1850.
Wolf, W. J. (1972). What is soy protein? *Food Technol. 26*:44–54.

VII

Genetic Manipulation in Cell Cultures

37

Prospects for Crop Improvement through Plant Tissue Culture

W. R. Scowcroft

Division of Plant Industry, CSIRO
Canberra, Australia

ABSTRACT

The threat of severe malnutrition for much of the world's population can only be mitigated if food production can be increased and sustained at an annual rate of 3.5%. Upgrading the efficiency of plant improvement will be of utmost importance in this quest. More efficient genetic manipulation in plants could result from the development and applicaton of new techniques of plant cell and tissue culture.

Cells of many plant species can be cultured under defined conditions, and for some species whole plants can be differentiated from cultured cells. Moreover, techniques exist for the production of haploid plants and cell lines. These features provide several potential advantages for plant improvement. First, large numbers of cells can be screened in culture for gene functions which can be defined biochemically. Second, the production of haploid plants by pollen culture greatly facilitates the selection of favorable gene combinations. Third, plant cell protoplasts can be isolated and cultured, and will undergo fusion. Plant cell hybridization could lead to a means of transferring valuable genetic information across species barriers. Plant cell culture studies have already provided information which might lead to the development of nonlegume crops which are less dependent on nitrogen fertilizers. Strategies whereby this might be achieved involve interactive research between plant cell culture and biological nitrogen-fixing microorganisms.

INTRODUCTION

The interim report of the World Food and Nutrition Study (1975) pointed out that the effective demand for food in the developing countries during the 1960s increased at an average annual rate of about 3.5%. This was partly satisfied within the developing countries by increased acreages (accounting for approx. 0.9%) and an average annual yield increase per hectare of 1.9%. This yield increase, which was an all-time high for any decade, was partly the result of the high-yielding wheat and rice varieties produced by the International Research Institutes. The shortfall of about 0.7%/year was met by food imports. To maintain food parity with the current population growth, yield increases in developing countries must be sustained at a demanding 2.5%/year during the coming decades. This does not allow for developing countries to achieve self-sufficiency or for increased per capita consumption. Moreover, world food reserves (measured as days of world grain consumption) have been decreasing at an average rate of 5 days/year for the period 1961–1975 (Brown, 1975). To offset these features an impossible 3–4% annual increase in food production is required in the developing countries.

Yield increases can only occur through substantial capital investment in land development, machinery, irrigation, fertilizer plants, etc., or through skillful plant improvement. Developing countries cannot meet the current and future costs of capital investment and so must rely on plant improvement.

The skill of the plant breeder depends first on his ability to define and assemble the requisite genetic variability necessary to achieve his objective. Having done so, his second task is then to recombine this genetic material and extract from the gene pool those gene combinations which yield superior genotypes. There are two major constraints which limit the progress in plant improvement. First, the recurrent cycle of hybridization and selection under field conditions is time- and resource-consuming. Second, the range of genetic variability is restricted usually to that of the species of interest.

Recent developments in plant tissue culture have attracted considerable attention because they offer a supplemental technology which may mitigate these constraints. Of particular importance is the development of somatic cell genetics of plants. This is seen as providing a vehicle for translating the conceptual and, in some cases, experinental methodology of molecular biology to plant genetic systems and ultimately to plant improvement. This expectation is founded on the basis that plant cells can be cultured under defined conditions; biochemical mutants can be isolated; plant cells (as protoplasts) can be fused with the consequent potential for somatic hybridization; haploid cell lines or plants, or both, can be obtained; and cell cultures can be induced to regenerate fertile plants. This last feature allows genetic modifications at the cellular level to be evaluated in mature plants. Herein lies the possible value of cell culture to plant improvement.

PLANT CULTURE AND CELLULAR CLONING

To varying degrees of efficiency, cells of numerous species of higher plants can be cultured on defined media consisting of inorganic salts, trace elements, some organic constituents, a carbon source for energy and plant growth regulators. The methodology of plant cell culture has been adequately covered by Kruse and Patterson (1973), Street (1973), and Gamborg and Wetter (1974). Many plant species can be cultured in liquid suspensions as well as on agar-based media, thereby providing large populations of physiologically homogeneous cells derived from a given genotype.

The advantage of plant cell cultures for genetic studies with eukaryotes is the ability to regenerate mature plants. The number and diversity of plant species in which this can be achieved has increased substantially in recent years (Murashige, 1974). From a relatively few species, such as tobacco, carrot, orchids, and sugar cane, from which entire plants could be successfully and efficiently regenerated, the list has now expanded to include *Brassica* species (Baroncelli et al., 1973), major cereal species, such as rice (Nishi et al., 1973), maize (Green and Phillips, 1975), and barley (Cheng and Smith, 1975), and a tropical legume *Stylosanthes hamata* (Scowcroft and Adamson, 1976). It is less than satisfactory that successful regeneration can be achieved only by empirical methods, i.e., the modification of culture conditions. Light- and electron-microscopy as well as cytological analysis (Street and Withers, 1974) have failed to provide any predictive insight with regard to the triggering of the differentiation process. Regeneration studies which have employed different genotypes of maize (Green and Phillips, 1975), *Brassica oleracea* (Baroncelli et al., 1973) and in our own laboratory, barley and attempts with *Vigna unguiculata* (J. D. Pagan, personal communication), indicate that there are genetic differences in the capacity of cell cultures to undergo differentiation. Since there is as yet no defined control over the process of differentiation, nor an adequate means for monitoring induction, success in achieving regeneration may be enhanced by using material with a wide genetic base.

The ability to clone plant species through tissue culture is currently utilized in the genetic improvement of sugar cane (Nickell and Heinz, 1974), the production of virus-free plants of vegetatively propagated species, and the cloning of sterile hybrids (Murashige, 1974).

HAPLOID CELL CULTURE

Plant cell culture is not restricted to the somatic cells of plants but can include the male gametophyte. The technique of anther culture which gives rise to haploid plants either directly, or through the formation of haploid callus, was pioneered by Guha and Maheshwari (1964) in Datura, and extensively developed by Nitsch (1972) in tobacco. Haploid plants can be produced from anther culture of many species (McComb, 1974; Kasha, 1974; Smith, 1974) including several important crop species such as wheat (Ouyang et al., 1973), rice (Niizeki and Oono, 1968), and barley (Clapham, 1973). Extensive studies (Sunderland and Dunwell, 1974) have shown that under appropriate culture conditions pollen maturation is arrested just after the mitosis that gave rise to the vegetative and generative cells. The normally quiescent vegetative cell (and in some cases the generative cell) divides to form an embryoid, or callus, with the gametic number of chromosomes. In species where anther culture gives rise to callus rather than embryoids, difficulty has been encountered in maintaining the gametic number of chromosomes. A way of favoring the growth of haploid callus is required. The initial indication that p-fluorophenylalanine would inhibit the growth of diploid, but not haploid, callus (Gupta and Carlson, 1972) cannot be sustained (Dix and Street, 1974) or at best is not very reproducible (Chaleff and Carlson, 1974).

The potential value of haploid plants to plant improvement was recognized following the first reports on the spontaneous occurrence of haploid plants (see Kimber and Riley, 1963). The development of an *in vitro* extraction procedure to produce numerous haploids has reemphasized their value. In a breeding program designed to produce pure-line varieties in a self-fertilized crop, or in the production of inbreds for hybrid production, the advantage of haploids is obvious. Homozygous diploids can be produced by doubling the chromosome constitution of the haploids with colchicine. In a conventional breeding program 5–6 generations of selfing are required to produce a homozygous line from a genetically heterogeneous population. Inbreeding depression, which leads to inviability or sterility in many of the lines, is a cost that may not appear until the third or fourth generation of selfing. The use of the doubled haploid technique automatically selects against any inviable gene combinations and immediately exposes mutations causing sterility.

The use of haploids can also lead to greater efficiency in recurrent selection programs. Where recessive genes are involved, the expected proportion of the homozygous recessive genotype in F_2 is 1 in 4^n, where n is the number of heterozygous loci. In contrast, the proportion of gametes which carry all the recessive alleles at these n loci is 1 in 2^n. Therefore, the production of haploids from these gametes improves the efficiency of producing homozygous recessive genotypes by a factor of 2^n. This approach is already being used in tobacco breeding programs for the isolation of disease (blue mold, black shank) resistant segregants (Nakamura et al., 1974; Wark, 1975, and personal communication). Similarly, haploids have also been used for the genetic analysis of flower color (Melchers, 1972) and alkaloid content (Collins et al., 1974) in tobacco.

The doubled haploid technique also has considerable advantage in recurrent selection programs where inheritance is not particulate. Griffing (1975) compared the efficiency of the standard recurrent method with one which included the use of doubled haploids for several models with varying levels of heritability.

Where plant numbers are restricted, which is true for all breeding programs, the efficiency of selection, measured as genetic gain per cycle of selection is enhanced by the inclusion of the haploid technique. Clearly, the development of rapid haploid extraction procedures can improve the rate of genetic gain per year.

MUTANT ISOLATION AND SELECTION

A cornerstone of genetic manipulation is the ability to recognize and select rare genotypes which occur naturally in the gene pool or which result from genetic modification or mutagenesis. The recovery of rare genetic variants in whole plants usually requires expensive resources. In cell cultures it is relatively easy to screen very large numbers of cells, and therefore theoretically possible to isolate biochemical mutants. Mutant selection techniques, developed for microbial genetic systems, have been applied to plant cell cultures with varying degrees of success.

Plant cell clones have been recovered which are resistant to such drugs as streptomycin (Maliga et al., 1973a), 5-bromodeoxyuridine (Maliga et al., 1973b), 8-azaguanine (Lescure, 1973; Bright and Northcote, 1975), and to various amino acid analogs (Widholm, 1974; Chaleff and Carlson, 1975). We have recently isolated tobacco resistant to the arginine analog, canavanine, which occurs naturally in many legumes and in high concentrations in *Canavalia ensiformis.* Among the most thoroughly studied analog-resistant mutants are those isolated by Widholm (see Widholm, 1974) which were resistant to the tryptophan analog, 5-methyltryptophan (5-MT). Some of these mutants have an altered enzyme, anthranilate synthetase, in the tryptophan biosynthetic pathway which was no longer sensitive to analog or tryptophan inhibition. Such mutants may have up to 14 times as much tryptophan in the free amino acid pool as normal cell lines. Similar mutants in carrot cell lines have been selected that are resistant to the phenylalanine analog, p-fluorophenylalanine (Palmer and Widholm, 1975). An alternative form, resistant to p-fluorophenylalanine, as found in tobacco, involves mutations which restrict the uptake of the analog.

The isolation of mutants which have increased levels of cellular amino acids may be valuable for upgrading the nutritional status of important crops. Brock and Langridge, 1973 (see Chapter 12, this volume) have discussed this particular emphasis on using the lysine analog, S-(β-aminoethyl)-cysteine, to recover barley mutants that overproduce lysine. Of possible relevance to this is the recovery of rice cell clones resistant to this analog (Chaleff and Carlson, 1975). Although few experimental details were given it appeared that these resistant mutants had increased levels of several other amino acids in addition to lysine. Plants have not yet been regenerated from these clones; it is not known what effect such mutations have on the grain-storage proteins.

The use of cell cultures as a means of isolating mutants which are of direct value to plant improvement is a desideratum. Already evidence is accumulating that this is possible. Carlson (1973*a*) was able to isolate mutants in tobacco cultures which were resistant to methionine sulfoximine, a presumed analog of the toxin produced by wildfire disease (*Pseudomonas tabaci*). Plants regenerated from methionine sulfoximine-resistant clones were less susceptible to the wildfire pathogen. Interestingly, these mutant cells also had elevated levels of free methionine.

Helgeson et al. (1976) have also found that cell cultures can be used to screen for resistance to the causal agent of black shank in tobacco (*Phytophthora parasitica* var. *nicotianae*). They showed that callus derived from resistant plants inhibited growth in culture of the causal fungus. A mechanism has not been ascribed to this resistance.

Apart from disease resistance, other traits relevant to plant improvement are amenable to genetic studies in tissue culture. Yield potential of many agricultural lands, particularly irrigated areas, is restricted because of salinity. This is particularly true of some agricultural land in Pakistan. It was recently shown that salt-tolerant lines of tobacco can be recovered that are resistant to four times the salt concentration that normally inhibits growth (Nabors et al., 1975). The success of this approach depends on the as yet unknown tolerance of plants regenerated from resistant cell clones.

The yield potential of plants depends in large measure on their net photosynthetic capacity. Net photosynthesis is likely to increase if the rate of photorespiration (oxidation of photosynthate) can be reduced. Zelitch (1975) and Carlson and Polacco (1975) argue that tissue culture may provide a means of altering the genetic regulation of photorespiration and thus increase the rate of net photosynthesis. Generally, plant cells require a carbon source for sustained growth, although some reports (see Zelitch, 1975) suggest that this requirement may not be absolute. Recently, Berlyn and Zelitch (1975) described sustained photoautotrophic growth of tobacco callus. The growth rate under these conditions was only 12–20% of callus grown with sucrose. However, as predicted by Carlson and Polacco (1975), the opportunity is now available to attempt the recovery of genetic variants in which the regulation of photorespiration is altered.

SOMATIC HYBRIDIZATION

Species preserve their genetic integrity because of reproductive mechanisms which prevent interspecific hybridization. The usual mode for preventing interspecific hybridization in plants is to preclude fertilization and zygote formation, although postzygotic mechanisms may operate to reinforce sexual isolation. If an alternative to sexual hybridization can be developed, valuable genetic information may be transferred from one species to another beyond the range of sexual hybridization. This would be of significance for the introduction of disease resistant genes to susceptible crop species and may even allow the transfer of special characteristics, such as the ability to fix atmospheric nitrogen or improved photosynthetic capacity. Apart from interspecific hybridization, somatic hybridization may prove a valuable means of introducing more genetic variability into asexually reproducing economic species, such as bananas, sugar cane, and fruit trees.

The opportunity for somatic hybridization came with the development of techniques for the large scale isolation of protoplasts by the enzymatic digestion of cell walls (Cocking, 1972). Protoplasts can be isolated from a wide range of species (Nickell and Heinz, 1974), and whereas it is possible to produce cell colonies from protoplasts of a number of species, regeneration of entire plants has only been accomplished for a few species. The technology of protoplast production has grown apace (for example, see Eriksson et al., 1974; Shephard and Toten, 1975; Watts and King, 1973), yet the overriding problem is the undefined difficulties associated with culture and regeneration of protoplasts. There are, for example, no reported cases of plant regeneration of protoplasts from cereal or legume species.

Protoplast fusion can occur spontaneously, but the frequency can be increased by several methods including the use of $NaNO_3$ (Power et al., 1970), Ca^{2+} at high pH (Keller and Melchers, 1973) or polyethyleneglycol (Kao and Michayluk, 1974). A comparative evaluation of these methods (Burgess and Fleming, 1974) indicated that the polyethyleneglycol treatment was preferable.

Protoplast fusion has been induced fairly extensively and in some cases repeated division of fused heterokaryocytes to form small calli have been observed (Kao et al., 1974). Some of the difficulties of identifying hybrid calli with inadequate genetic tools have been demonstrated (Power et al., 1975). That protoplast fusion can be employed to produce hybrids has been reasonably well established both at the interspecific (Carlson et al., 1972) and intraspecific levels (Melchers and Labib, 1974). Both cases depended on the use of a selection system which favored the growth of the hybrid clones over either of the parental cells.

The technology of protoplast production and fusion has to some extent lost sight of the objectives of somatic hybridization, namely as an alternative where sexual hybridization cannot be used to exchange genetic information. The frequency of protoplast fusion that has occupied most of the research effort to date, appears somewhat irrelevant to the author. The critical feature is the frequency of genetic exchange resulting from such fusions. I am using genetic exchange in its broadest sense to include chromosome addition(s), chromosome substitution(s), somatic recombination (either spontaneous or induced), and meiotic recombination. For genetic exchange to occur nuclear fusion must take place. The only sufficient test for a true genetic hybrid is segregation of parental characteristics. The only case where this has been satisfied is that of Melchers and Labib (1974) involving intraspecific hybridization with two tobacco mutants.

In the first instance, the identification of a presumptive hybrid depends on the joint expression in the somatic hybrid of specific gene differences of both parental species, i.e., genetic complementation. This of course can be used, and for the sake of efficiency is a prerequisite, to provide a basis for selecting and maintaining the hybrid cells. The limitation of genetic complementation to identify and select somatic hybrids is that their origin may have a trivial explanation, e.g., chimerical association, cross feeding, and so forth. Genetic complementation was used in the isolation of hybrid calli resulting from fusion between two closely related species of tobacco (Carlson et al., 1972). The basis for identifying and selecting the hybrid calli in this case depended on a knowledge of the culture conditions which favored growth of callus from the extant sexual hybrid. This was an ingenious approach, but as Carlson himself has pointed out, somatic hybridization is of potential value only when the sexual hybrid cannot be produced.

Therefore, interspecific somatic hybridization has not yet been evaluated as a means of transferring genetic information between sexually isolated species. This awaits the development of adequate genetic markers for the recognition and selection of presumptive hybrid cells. Beyond this is the problem associated with the regeneration of plants from hybrid clones to test for genetic segregation. The solution of this problem will depend on the success of straightforward regeneration studies with plant cell cultures. Only when these requirements have been met can we judge whether somatic hybridization will be of value in extending the range of germ plasm for plant improvement.

HETEROSPECIFIC TRANSFORMATION

In bacterial systems, DNA from one species (usually in the form of a plasmid) can be employed to genetically modify another species. For example, *Escherichia coli,* which cannot fix atmospheric nitrogen, will accept and integrate into its own chromosome the nitrogen-fixing genes of *Klebsiella pneumoniae* and this confers on *E. coli* the ability to fix atmospheric nitrogen (Cannon et al., 1974). In plants it has been shown that radioactively labeled bacterial DNA is probably incorporated into the DNA of germinating seedlings and it is claimed that these bacterial nucleotide sequences are replicated and transmitted to the next generation (Ledoux, 1971). More recently, Ledoux and Huart (1974) claimed that a thiamine deficiency in *Arabidopsis* can be corrected with DNA isolated from bacteria prototrophic for thiamine. Additional genetic evidence is presented by Ledoux (Chapter 38 in this volume.) However, recent studies with several plant species (Kleinhoffs et al., 1975; Lurquin and Hotta, 1975) have been unable to confirm Ledoux's high levels of covalent binding of foreign bacterial DNA to the DNA of the treated recipient plants.

Studies with plant cell cultures suggest that viral (Carlson, 1973*b*) and bacterial genes (Doy et al., 1973) can be expressed in plant cells. Johnson et al.

(1973) were initially able to confirm the result of Doy et al. (1973) that plant cells, normally unable to utilize lactose as a carbon source, apparently grew following treatment with a bacteriophage carrying the gene for lactose utilization. However, subsequent experiments in Smith's laboratory (Grierson et al., 1975) have been unable to demonstrate any bacterial β-galactosidase activity in their treated sycamore cells. The question of whether plant cells can take up and express bacterial genes is unresolved.

In cooperation with J. B. Langridge, the author is attempting to transform tobacco cells with bacterial DNA. We are using as a model system R plasmid DNA isolated from *E. coli* and which has, as a part of its genetic complement, a gene for resistance to the antibiotic kanamycin. We have established that tobacco cells are sensitive to concentrations of kanamycin as low as 25 μg/ mliter. In several experiments with untreated tobacco cells we have seen no evidence of phenotypic adaptation or of genetic resistance to kanamycin (100 μg/mliter). In *E. coli* this plasmid confers resistance to concentrations of 1.2 mg/liter. Therefore, in our transformation experiments we are seeking an efficiency of transcription and translation of approximately 8–10% to confer resistance on the tobacco cells. Our initial experiments on treating plant cells with this plasmid have been conducted under conditions that minimize the degradation of the plasmid by plant nucleases, conditions which fortunately do not impair the growth of tobacco cells on normal media. At this stage we are unable to report any successful transformation.

It is not known whether bacterial RNA sequences can use plant DNA polymerase for replication, or plant RNA polymerase for transcription. There is some evidence however that the RNA translating mechanism of plant organelles is not unlike that of the bacterial system. Dr. Brock (Chapter 12, this volume) has mentioned parallel work with the double-stranded DNA virus, cauliflower mosaic virus. Current and future experiments are using enzymatic techniques (Chang and Cohen, 1974; Kedes et al., 1975) to construct hybrid DNA molecules between CMV and specific bacterial DNA sequences. In this way we hope to endow the specific bacterial gene with a replicative, and possibly RNA polymerase, function that will allow this gene to be expressed in a plant cell.

PLANT CELL-CULTURE–NITROGEN-FIXATION INTERFACE

Biological nitrogen fixation exists only in prokaryotes. Fortunately, some plant species, the legumes, have evolved a symbiotic association with one prokaryote species *Rhizobium.* The advantage that this confers on the legumes is also highly desirable for the cereal crops. Increasing the extent of biological nitrogen fixation is one of the keys to solving the world food problem (Hardy and Havelka, 1975).

A number of recent scientific discoveries increase the optimism that biological nitrogen fixation can be developed in nonlegume crops. The genetic regulation of the primary enzyme in nitrogen fixation, nitrogenase, is now well understood, at least in *Klebsiella* (Shanmugam and Valentine, 1975). The genes for nitrogen fixation can be mobilized and transferred between bacterial species (Cannon et al., 1974; Dunican and Tierney, 1974). With respect to plants utilizing the products of microbial nitrogen fixation, functional associations between plants and bacteria are not restricted to the legume/rhizobia symbiosis. A naturally occurring association exists between the nitrogen-fixing *Spirillum* and the roots of forage grasses and maize (Bülow and Döbereiner, 1975; Döbereiner, Chapter 30, this volume). Also, an experimentally contrived association has been developed between the nitrogen fixing *Azotobacter* and carrot cells (Carlson and Chaleff, 1974).

We have been directly involved in experiments which have shown the legume/rhizobia association to be less rigid than previously assumed. Rhizobia can fix nitrogen when cultured in association with nonlegume plant cells (Child, 1975; Scowcroft and Gibson, 1975). We then demonstrated that the induction of nitrogen fixation was the result of an undefined diffusate from the plant cells. From this point, it was a short step to develop the cultural conditions which would allow rhizobia to fix nitrogen independently of the host plant (Pagan et al., 1975), a result which was simultaneously confirmed by others (see Scowcroft, 1975). These results prove, in contrast to previous beliefs, that at least some strains of rhizobia have all the genetic information necessary for the biosynthesis of nitrogenase and, moreover, that a nonlegume plant cell environment is compatible with nitrogen fixation. More recently Drs. Pagan, Gibson, and the author have gained some insight into the genetic and physiological regulation of nitrogenase synthesis and activity. The regulation appears to be quite different to that which applies to *Klebsiella* nitrogenase since we have been unable to demonstrate any correlation between altered rates of nitrogenase activity and presumed functioning of the enzymes involved in ammonia assimilation.

While the technology that would be necessary to develop nitrogen fixation in nonlegumes is little short of formidable, research in the immediate past has removed the conceptual constraints on achieving this end. Plant cell culture has figured prominently in this phase and will undoubtedly contribute to future exciting developments.

CONCLUSION

The theme of this volume is to probe and discuss the latest developments in the field of crop improvement. The pragmatic consequences of these developments will have a bearing on the capacity to feed an already undernourished world population. Novel and alternative technologies will be necessary, and amongst these plant cell culture is perhaps one of the more promising.

Somatic cell genetics should not be envisaged as a panacea for plant breeding, but rather as part of an interdisciplinary effort involving cellular and whole plant biology. The gain to plant improvement will depend on the ease with which economic species can be established in culture, and plants regenerated from such cell lines. Relevant genetic modification at the cellular level will depend on the degree to which physiological and agronomic parameters may be defined in cellular or biochemical terms, or both.

The successes of plant breeding have depended on the use of novel genes and gene combinations. Developments in somatic cell genetics should be geared to increase the efficiency with which valuable genetic information can be identified, isolated and recombined into relevant crop species. These developments are still in their infancy and therefore increases in plant productivity will depend for some time on conventional plant breeding. It is to be hoped that plant cell culture will become increasingly relevant to the task of expanding the world's food-producing capacity.

REFERENCES

Baroncelli, S., Buiatti, M., and Bennici, A. (1973). Genetics of growth and differentiation "*in vitro*" of *Brassica oleracea* var. *botytis*. I. Difference between six inbred lines. *J. Plant Breed. 70*:99–107.

Berlyn, M. B. and Zelitch, I. (1975). Photoautotrophic growth and photosynthesis in tobacco callus cells. *Plant Physiol. 56*:752–756.

Bright, S. W. J. and Northcote, D. H. (1975). A deficiency of hypoxanthine phosphoribosyltransferase in sycamore callus resistant to azaguanine. *Planta 123*:79–89.

Brock, R. D. and Langridge, J. (1973). Prospects for genetic improvement of seed proteins in plants. In *Breeding for Seed Protein Improvement Using Nuclear Techniques*, pp. 3–13. Int. Atomic Energy Agency, Vienna.

Brown, L. R. (1975). The world food prospect. *Science 190*:1053–1059.

von Bülow, J. F. W. and Döbereiner, J. (1975). Potential for nitrogen fixation in maize genotypes in Brazil. *Proc. Natl. Acad. Sci. USA 72*:2389–2393.

Burgess, J. and Fleming, E. N. (1974). Ultrastructural studies of the aggregation and fusion of plant protoplasts. *Planta 118*:183–193.

Cannon, F. C., Dixon, R. A., Postgate, J. R., and Primrose, S. B. (1974). Chromosomal integration of Klebsiella nitrogen fixation genes in *Escherichia coli. J. Gen. Microbiol. 80*:227–239.

Carlson, P. S. (1973*a*). Methionine sulfoximine resistant mutants of tobacco. *Science 180*:1366–1368.

Carlson, P. S. (1973*b*). The use of protoplasts for genetic research. *Proc. Natl. Acad. Sci. USA 70*:598–602.

Carlson, P. S. and Chaleff, R. S. (1974). Forced association between higher plant and bacterial cells *in vitro. Nature (London) 252*:393–394.

Carlson, P. S., and Polacco, J. C. (1975). Plant cell cultures: Genetic aspects of crop improvement. *Science 188*:622–625.

Carlson, P. S., Smith, H. H., and Dearing, R. D. (1972). Parasexual interspecific plant hybridization. *Proc. Natl. Acad. Sci. USA 69*:2292–2294.

Chaleff, R. S., and Carlson, P. S. (1974). Somatic cell genetics of higher plants. *Annu. Rev. Genet. 8*:267–278.

Chaleff, R. S., and Carlson, P. S. (1975). Higher plants as experimental organisms. In *Modification of the Information Content of Plant Cells* (Markham, R., Davies, D. R., Hopwood, D. A., and Horne, R. W., eds.),pp. 197–214. North-Holland, Amsterdam.

Chang, A. C. Y., and Cohen, S. N. (1974). Genome construction between bacterial species *in vitro:* Replication and expression of *Staphylococcus* plasmid genes in *Escherichia coli. Proc. Natl. Acad. Sci. USA 71*:1030–1034.

Cheng, T-Y., and Smith, H. H. (1975). Organogenesis from callus culture of *Hordeum vulgare. Planta 123*:307–310.

Child, J. J. (1975). Nitrogen fixation by *Rhizobium* sp. in association with non-leguminous plant cell cultures. *Nature (London) 253*:350–351.

Clapham, D. (1973). Haploid hordeum plants from anthers *in vitro. Z. Pflanz. 69*:142–155.

Cocking, E. C. (1972). Plant cell protoplasts—isolation and development. *Annu. Rev. Plant Physiol. 23*:29–50.

Collins, G. B., Legg, P. D., and Kasperbauer, M. J. (1974). Use of anther-derived haploids in Nicotiana. I. Isolation of breeding lines differing in total alkaloid content. *Crop. Sci. 14*:77–80.

Dix, P. J., and Street, H. E. (1974). Effects of *p*-fluorophenylalanine (PFP) on the growth of cell lines differing in ploidy and derived from *Nicotiana sylvestris. Plant. Sci. Lett. 3*:283–288.

Doy, C. H., Gresshoff, P. M., and Rolfe, B. H. (1973). Biological and molecular evidence for the transgenosis of genes from bacteria to plant cells. *Proc. Natl. Acad. Sci. USA 20*:723–726.

Dunican, L. K. and Tierney, A. B. (1974). Genetic transfer of nitrogen fixation from *Rhizobium trifolii* to *Klebsiella aerogenes. Biochem. Biophys. Res. Commun. 57*:62–72.

Eriksson, T., Bonnett, H., Glimelius, K., and Wallin, A. (1974). Technical advances in protoplast isolation, culture and fusion. In *Tissue Culture and Plant Science* (H. E. Street, ed.), pp. 213–232. Academic Press, London.

Gamborg, O. L. and Wetter, L. R., eds. (1974). *Plant Tissue Culture Methods.* National Research Council of Canada, Ottawa.

Green, C. E. and Phillips, R. L. (1975). Plant regeneration from tissue cultures in maize. *Crop Sci. 15*:417–421.

Grierson, D., McKee, R. A., Attridge, T. H., and Smith, H. (1975). Studies on the uptake and expression of foreign genetic material by higher plant cells. In *Modification of Information Content of Plant Cells* (Markham, R., Davies, D. R., Hopwood, D. A., and Horne, R. W., eds.) pp. 91–99. North-Holland, Amsterdam.

Griffing, B. (1975). Efficiency changes due to use of doubled-haploids in recurrent selection methods. *Theoret. Appl. Genet. 46*:367–386.

Guha, S. and Maheshwari, S. C. (1964). *In vitro* production of embryos from anthers of Datura. *Nature (London) 204*:497.

Gupta, N. and Carlson, P. S. (1972). Preferential growth of haploid plant cells *in vitro. Nature (London) 239*:86.

Hardy, R. W. F. and Havelka, U. D. (1975). Nitrogen fixation research: A key to world food. *Science 188*:633–643.

Helgeson, J. P., Haberlach, G. T., and Upper, C. D. (1976). A dominant gene conferring disease resistance to tobacco plants is expressed in tissue cultures. *Phytopathology 66*: 91–96.

Johnson, C. B., Grierson, D., and Smith, H. (1973). Expression of λplac5 DNA in cultured cells of a higher plant. *Nature New Biol. 244*:105–107.

Kao, K. N. and Michayluk, M. R. (1974). A method for high-frequency intergeneric fusion of plant protoplasts. *Planta 115*:355–367.

Kao, K. N., Constabel, F., Michayluk, M. R., and Gamborg, O. L. (1974). Plant protoplast fusion and growth of intergeneric hybrid cells. *Planta 120*:215–227.

Kasha, K. J., ed. (1974). *Haploids in Higher Plants–Advances and Potential.* Univ. of Guelph, Ontario.

Kedes, L. H., Chang, A. C. Y., Houseman, D., and Cohen, S. N. (1975). Isolation of histone genes from unfractionated sea urchin DNA by subculture cloning in *E. coli. Nature (London) 255*:533–538.

Keller, W. A. and Melchers, G. (1973). The effect of high pH and calcium on tobacco leaf protoplast fusion. *Z. Naturforsch. 28*:737–741.

Kimber, G. and Riley, R. (1963). Haploid angiosperms. *Bot. Rev. 29*:490–531.

Kleinhoffs, A., Eden, F. C., Chilton, M. -D., and Bendich, A. J. (1975). On the question of integration of exogenous bacterial DNA. *Proc. Natl. Acad. Sci. USA 72*:2748–2752.

Kruse, P. F. and Patterson, M. K., eds. (1973). *Tissue Culture: Methods and Applications.* Academic Press, New York.

Ledoux, L. ed. (1971). *Informative Molecules in Biological Systems.* North-Holland, Amsterdam.

Ledoux, L. and Huart, R. (1974). DNA-mediated genetic correction of thiamineless *Arabidopsis thaliana. Nature (London) 249*:17–21.

Lescure, A. M. (1973). Selection of markers for resistance to base-analogues in somatic cell cultures of *Nicotiana tabacum. Plant. Sci. Lett. 1*:375–383.

Lurquin, P. F. and Hotta, Y. (1975). Reutilization of bacterial DNA by *Arabidopsis thaliana* cells in tissue culture. *Plant Sci. Lett. 5*:103–112.

Maliga, P., Sz-Breznovits, A., and Marton, L. (1973a). Streptomycin-resistant plants from callus culture of haploid tobacco. *Nature New Biol. 244*:29–30.

Maliga, P., Marton, L., and Sz-Breznovits, A. (1973b). 5-Bromodeoxyuridine-resistant cell lines from haploid tobacco. *Plant Sci. Lett. 1*:119–121.

McComb, J. A. (1974). New techniques for plant breeding. *J. Aust. Inst. Agri. Sci. 40*:3–10.

Melchers, G. (1972). Haploid higher plants for plant breeding. *Z. Pflanz. 67*:19–32.

Melchers, G. and Labib, G. (1974). Somatic hybridization of plants by fusion of protoplasts. I. Selection of light resistant hybrids of "Haploid" light sensitive varieties of tobacco. *Mol. Gen. Genet. 135*:277–194.

Murashige, T. (1974). Plant propagation through tissue cultures. *Annu. Rev. Plant Physiol. 25*: 135–166.

Nabors, M. W., Daniels, A., Nadolny, L., and Brown, C. (1975). Sodium chloride tolerant lines of tobacco cells. *Plant Sci. Lett. 4*:155–159.

Nakamura, A., Yamada, T., Kadotani, N., Itagaki, R., and Oka, M. (1974). Studies on the haploid method of breeding in tobacco. *SABRAO J. 6*:107–131.

Nickell, L. G., and Heinz, D. J. (1974). Potential of cell and tissue culture techniques as aids in economic plant improvement. In *Genes, Enzymes and Populations.* (Srb, A. M., ed.), pp. 109–128. Plenum Press, New York.

Niizeki, H. and Oono, K. (1968). Induction of haploid rice plant from anther culture. *Proc. Jap. Acad. 44*:554–556.

Nishi, T., Yamada, Y., and Takahashi, E. (1973). The role of auxins in differentiation of rice tissue cultures *in vitro. Bot. Mag. Tokyo 86*:183–188.

Nitsch, J. P. (1972). Haploid plants from pollen. *Z. Pflanz. 67*:3–18.

Ouyang, T., Hu, H., Chuang, C., and Tseng, C. (1973). Induction of pollen plants from anthers of *Triticum aestiuum* L. cultures *in vitro. Sci. Sin. 16*:79–95.

Pagan, J. D., Child, J. J., Scowcroft, W. R., and Gibson, A. H. (1975). Nitrogen fixation by *Rhizobium* cultured on a defined medium. *Nature (London) 256*:406–407.

Palmer, J. E. and Widholm, J. (1975). Characterization of carrot and tobacco cell cultures resistant to *p*-fluorophenylalanine. *Plant Physiol. 56*:233–238.

Power, J. B., Cummings, S. E., and Cocking, E. C. (1970). Fusion of isolated plant protoplasts. *Nature (London)* 225:1016–1018.

Power, J. B., Frearson, E. M., Hayward, C., and Cocking, E. C. (1975). Some consequences of the fusion and selective culture of petunia and parthenocissus protoplasts. *Plant Sci. Lett.* 5:197–207.

Scowcroft, W. R. (1975). The potential use of somatic cell genetics in plant improvement. *SABRAO J.* 7:147–158.

Scowcroft, W. R. and Adamson, J. A. (1976). Organogenesis from callus cultures of the legume, *Stylosanthes hamata. Plant Sci. Lett.* 7:39–42.

Scowcroft, W. R. and Gibson, A. H. (1975). Nitrogen fixation by *Rhizobium* associated with tobacco and cowpea cell cultures. *Nature (London)* 253:351–352.

Shanmugam, K. T. and Valentine, R. C. (1975). Molecular biology of nitrogen fixation. *Science 187*:919–924.

Shephard, J. F. and Totten, R. E. (1975). Isolation and regeneration of tobacco mesophyll cell protoplasts under low osmotic conditions. *Plant Physiol.* 55:689–694.

Smith, H. H. (1974). Model systems for somatic cell plant genetics. *Bioscience 24*:269–276.

Street, H. E., ed. (1973). *Plant Tissue and Cell Culture.* Blackwell Scientific Publications, Oxford.

Street, H. E. and Withers, L. A. (1974). The anatomy of embryogenesis in culture. In *Tissue Culture and Plant Science 1974* (Street, H. E., ed.), pp. 71–100. Academic Press, London.

Sunderland, N. and Dunwell, J. M. (1974). Pathways in pollen embryogenesis. In *Tissue Culture and Plant Science 1974* (Street, H. E., ed.), pp. 141–168. Academic Press, London.

Wark, D. C. (1975). Tobacco breeding and genetics. In *Genetics Report 1975,* pp. 43–46. Division of Plant Industry, CSIRO, Canberra.

Watts, J. W. and King, J. M. (1973). The use of antibiotics in the culture of non-sterile plant protoplasts. *Planta 113*:271–277.

Widholm, J. M. (1974). Selection and characteristics of biochemical mutants of cultured plant cells. In *Tissue Culture and Plant Science* (Street, H. E., ed.), pp. 287–300. Academic Press, London.

World Food and Nutrition Study: Interim Report. (1975). *NRC Study on World Food and Nutrition.* National Academy of Sciences, Washington, D.C.

Zelitch, I. (1975). Improving the efficiency of photosynthesis. *Science 188*:626–633.

38

Biophysical and Genetic Evidence for Transformation in Plants

L. Ledoux

Centre d'Etudes de l'Energie Nucléaire, Mol
and
Université de Liège
Liège, Belgium

ABSTRACT

In thiamine mutants of Arabidopsis, genetic corrections have been obtained by treatment with DNA bearing a thiamine information. When correction is attempted under selective conditions, about 0.7% of the treated plants grow and set fruit. Their progeny and the following ones, obtained by selfing, behave as homozygotes. Segregation of characters is found only when correction is attempted under nonselective conditions or when the correcting genes were of plasmidian origin. The correction is hereditary; results of backcrosses and test crosses indicate that it is dominant, nuclear, and strongly bound to the genome. The corrective factor appears to be added to the mutated genome and not substituted for the mutation, as it can be suppressed by outcrossing with the wild type or with a plant corrected by another DNA.

INTRODUCTION

A complete survey of the fate of foreign DNA in a living organism should include an analysis of (1) the DNA uptake process, (2) the possible survival of fragments either in a free form or bound to the genome, (3) the possible replication of the foreign structures, (4) biological parameters concerned with its expression in the host cell (transcription, traduction), and (5) the inheritance and transmission of the foreign information to the progeny.

Each of these steps can, of course, correspond to a dead end for the foreign molecule in the material used. For instance, several systems such as tobacco cells in tissue culture (Bendich and Filner, 1971), callus from tobacco (Lurquin and Kado, 1976), Arabidopsis (Lurquin and Hotta, 1975), or soya (Luyindula et al., unpublished results) degrade a DNA present in the incubation medium. Other systems take up the DNA but later destroy it and reuse its components for *de novo* synthesis—barley coleoptile (Ledoux and Huart, 1969) and Chlamydomonas (Lurquin and Behki, 1975). In other systems, reasonably sized pieces of foreign DNA appear to survive as such for several hours, days, or even weeks: barley seedlings (Ledoux and Huart, 1969, 1968), Arabidopsis (Ledoux et al., 1971), Sinapis (Coumanne et al., 1971; Ledoux, 1975), Matthiola (Hemleben et al., 1975), tomato shoot (Stroun et al., 1967), cell protoplasts (Ohyama et al., 1972; Hoffman and Hess, 1973) and pollen grains (Hess, 1975).

In a few cases, indications have been obtained of a binding of the foreign DNA to the recipient DNA. These came from experiments from labeled exogenous DNA with a density differing from that of the recipient, in which an analysis of CsCl density gradients showed the appearance of molecules that were denser than the recipient DNA, and behaved as "hybrid" macromolecules. They indeed had the unique property to be split by sonication into two components, the densities of which were close to that of the recipient and the donor DNA, respectively (Ledoux and Huart, 1968, 1969; Ledoux et al., 1971; Hemleben et al., 1975; Stroun et al., 1967). Centrifugation in an alkaline CsCl gradient did not produce heterogeneity in the population and the observed increment of density suggested that the two populations freed by sonication were actually covalently jointed (Ledoux and Huart, 1969; Stroun et al., 1967; Fox and Ayad, 1972; Ledoux et al., 1971; Hemleben et al., 1975).

Hybrid macromolecules were obtained in different plant materials: barley roots (Ledoux and Huart, 1968, 1969; Hotta and Stern, 1971), tomato shoots (Stroun et al., 1967), Arabidopsis tissues (Ledoux et al., 1971), and Matthiola seedlings (Hemleben et al., 1975) using labeled bacterial or plant isologous DNA. Indications of a replication of such hybrid molecules were obtained only in barley (Ledoux and Huart, 1968, 1969), in tomato shoots (Stroun et al., 1967), and in the offspring of treated Arabidopsis (but not in the treated plants themselves; Brown et al., 1971; Ledoux et al., 1972). In contrast, Kleinhoffs et al. (1975) brought along very contradictory results: the authors claimed that no replicating hybrid band was to be found in different DNA-treated systems (including tomato) except those caused by contamination or artifacts generated by the technique used to prepare the plant DNA. Shortly after this work was reported, Hanson and Chilton (1975) reconsidered the problem and showed that peculiar "hybrid" satellites, splitting on sonication, could indeed be found in axenic conditions and in plant DNA prepared by various techniques, in addition to the one condemned by Kleinhoffs et al. (1975). Hanson and Chilton were unable to reassociate the hybrid material with DNA of the donor type, but were able to do so with the recipient DNA.

This reassociation of the hybrid with the recipient DNA only is a significant point, suggesting that such hybrid band material might be a plant satellite, the production of which is initiated by the donor DNA. It is unfortunate, in this view, that Hanson and Chilton did not use alkaline CsCl gradients, nor did they verify that, as shown by Stroun et al. (1967), such a hybrid was specific for the DNA species used and did not appear at the same density when tomato shoots were treated with other DNAs. An endogenous satellite specifically initiated by a given foreign DNA species would indeed constitute an interesting material for further investigation.

Another possibility, however, is that the lack of reassociation between the "hybrid" material and the donor DNA is caused by artifacts of the reassociation technique. This could, for instance, be the result of modification of the intruding foreign DNA by a host restriction–modification system leading to decreased T_m and/or to poor hybrid formation.

We are presently exploring this possibility while analyzing further, by reassociation kinetics, the nature of hybrid molecules obtained in barley treated with *M. lysodeikticus* or by other bacterial DNA. Indeed, in barley, where no natural heavy satellite DNA has yet been observed, hybrid DNA can be obtained in axenic conditions, and in well-defined physiological conditions. The actual density appears to depend on the nature of the DNA used. In contrast, as previously shown (Ledoux, 1975; Hess, 1969), an analysis of hybridization products in CsCl gradients indicated that they could reassociate with the donor DNA. The method used was supposedly less specific than the reassociation kinetics indicated and a definite conclusion has to be postponed. Whatever the size of the exogenous molecule and the difficulty of pinpointing it in the recipient cells, the expression of foreign information in the receptor could be, in itself, a sufficient criterion for transfer of genetic information from a donor to a recipient plant.

DNA-mediated transformation in higher organisms has been reported in animal cells in tissue culture (Merril et al., 1971), in insects (Fox et al., 1971), and in plants (Ledoux et al., 1972, 1974, 1975; Hess, 1969, 1973; Ledoux and Jacobs, 1969; Turbin et al., 1975; Doy et al., 1973a,b; Smith et al., 1975; Rédei, 1970, 1975). Phage-mediated transformations have also been reported (Merril et al., 1971; Doy et al., 1973a,b; Smith et al., 1975). With Dr. M. Jacobs (Vrije Universiteit, Brussels) we used Arabidopsis mutants characterized by a deficiency of thiamine metabolism. In such plants we could follow the fate of labeled bacterial DNA and recover molecules with a hybrid behavior (Ledoux et al., 1971). However, it was impossible to find evidence for the replication of this population. Only in the progeny of DNA-treated plants was it possible to observe a heterogeneity of the plant DNA (Brown et al., 1971;

Ledoux et al., 1972. These Arabidopsis mutants are strict conditional lethal mutants (Rédei, 1970, 1975). One locus (*py*) controls the synthesis of the pyrimidine moiety of thiamine, locus *tz* controls the synthesis of the thiazole half of the vitamin, and two genes are concerned with intermediate steps between these two precursors and thiamine. The frequency of spontaneous reversion at the *py* locus has been estimated to be lower than 5×10^{-5} (Rédei, 1975). Low concentrations of thiamine ($10^{-5} - 10^{-6}M$) allow a normal growth of all mutants.

The DNA treatment has been described elsewhere (Ledoux et al., 1974, 1975). Treated plants were grown on perlite moistened with a mineral solution (in Brussels) or in test tubes containing agar dissolved in a mineral nutrient (in Mol). Plants were kept under continuous illumination at $24°C$. All mutant seedlings grown on mineral medium died within 15–20 days. A few plants among the DNA-treated mutants grew at a slow rate with a more-or-less normal green color, and eventually set flowers. About one third of them produced fertile siliques. Only these were considered as "corrected."

A series of DNAs were used. They were freshly prepared, cleaned in CsCl gradients, had a molecular weight $> 10^7$ and did not contain appreciable amounts of single strand breaks. All DNA batches (1 mg/ml, 0.01 M NaCl) were independently used in Brussels and in Mol, Belgium. Results were pooled. Corrections could be obtained with a relatively high frequency (0.1–0.7%). Controls were obtained by treating mutant seeds with 0.01 M NaCl, with DNA from thiamine-deficient bacteria or phages containing normal or abnormal bases, and with DNase-treated DNA. A total of 34 corrected plants were obtained and their lines were propagated by selfing. All plants corrected in selective conditions produced progenies with a constant "corrected" phenotype; no segregation could be found in their offspring, although they frequently showed a variegated pattern of chlorophyll pigmentation with light discoloration at the base of the limb. In practically all cases, the average fresh and dry weight of the corrected types grown on mineral medium could be enhanced by the addition of $10^{-4} M$ thiamine. In that way also, corrected pyrimidine or thiazole mutants specifically responded to the addition of pyrimidine or thiazole and showed improved growth. Therefore, the correction did not always restore 100% of the wild-type properties. That the progenies of corrected plants behave as true-breeding homozygotes was verified by crossing them with the mutant parent. The F_1 progeny was normal and segregation obtained in F_2 showed that the correction was dominant.

When performed in nonselective conditions (in the presence of thiamine) the DNA treatment leads to plants which either produce a mutant progeny or show drastic segregation in their offspring (Ledoux et al., 1975; Ledoux et al., in preparation). This suggests that the occurrence of corrected homozygotes under selective conditions could be due to selective advantages conferred on the gametes by the information encoding the foreign thiamine.

Table I. Summary of Results Obtained[a]

Treatment

m $\xrightarrow{\text{DNA}}$ chimera F₁ mC (34 established lines)

m $\xrightarrow{\text{DNA + thiamine}}$ F₁ mC + m

Selfing

mC × mC $\xrightarrow{}$ F₁, F₂, F₃, . . . N

Example.[b]

                 76 : 6 : 17 (116)

tzBS   25 : 65 : 10 (202)

                 76 : 24(131)

Outcrosses

I

  a mC × m $\xrightarrow{}$ F₁ N $\xrightarrow{}$ F₂ N : Lk : m $\xrightarrow{\text{F}_3}$ N : Lk : m ; N : m

                         90 : 9 : 1 (163)

                         22 : 70 : 8 (198)

                         96 : 2 : 2 (198)

  b m × mC $\xrightarrow{}$ F₁ N

II

  mC × wt $\xrightarrow{}$ F₁ N $\xrightarrow{}$ F₂ N : Lk : m $\xrightarrow{\text{F}_3}$ N : Lk : m ; N : Lk : m

Cross between two corrected parents

tzEC × tz′EC $\xrightarrow{}$ F₁ N $\xrightarrow{}$ F₂ N   100 :(73)

tzBS × tzEC $\xrightarrow{}$ F₁ N $\xrightarrow{}$ F₂ N : m   97 : 0 : 3 (144)

[a]In all outcrosses, the addition of thiamine F₂ F₃ N. m = mutant genotype; mC = corrected mutant genotype; wt = wild-type genotype; N = normal phenotype; Lk = Leaky phenotype (limited growth; white patches on leaves, white stems); tzBS = tz mutant corrected by B. subtilis DNA; EC = E. coli DNA.
[b]Numbers refer to the last row of the schema presented: 76 : 6 : 17 (116) corresponds to percentage of classified types N : Lk : m. Between brackets, the number of plants used.

In another series of experiments, the DNA used was prepared from *E. coli thiA* bacteria (requiring thiazole for growth), harboring an F' thi^+ plasmid. The strain used was *recA−* to prevent recombination of the plasmid with the bacterial genome. This DNA contained about 5% of plasmid DNA. It proved very efficient in correcting different mutants (Ledoux et al., 1975). (However, when these corrected plants were selfed and the progenies grown on mineral medium, only about 50% of them appeared to be of the mutant type, as compared with the 100% mutant progeny we found with plants corrected with "plain" bacterial DNA). Reciprocal crosses between the corrected mutants and the lethal ones indicate that the correction can be transmitted through the male as well as through the female gamete, and therefore does not appear to be due to a cytoplasmic factor (Ledoux et al., 1975).

When crossing corrected plants with the wild type, a segregation was observed in the F_2 or F_3 progeny. It appears, therefore, that recombination is implicated in these crosses, so that the genome site or sites occupied by the donor-plant DNA do not correspond, homologously, with the locus containing the mutant defect. (Correction being dominant, the recessive mutation is not expressed unless the correction is masked or lost as, probably, in crossing with a wild-type plant not provided with the correcting fragment).

Recent results show that crosses between two corrected plants can lead also to segregation in the F_2 progeny, especially when the plants were corrected by DNA of different origins (Ledoux et al., in preparation). All these genetical results are summed up in Table I, where numerical examples are also given.

ACKNOWLEDGMENTS

Thanks are due to the Fonds de la Recherche Fondamentale Collective, to the Ministère de l'Education Nationale, and to the Institut pour l'Encouragement de la Recherche Scientifique dans l'Industrie et l'Agriculture for financial support.

REFERENCES

Bendich, A. J. and Filner, P. 1971. Uptake of exogenous DNA by pea seedlings and tobacco cells. *Mutat. Res. 13*:199–214.

Brown, J., Huart, R., Ledoux, L., and Swinnen, J. (1971). High specific radioactivity of a heavy DNA fraction in progeny of Arabidopsis treated by *M. lysodeikticus* DNA. *Arch. Int. Physiol. Biochim. 79*:820–821.

Coumanne, C., Jacqmard, A., Kinet, J. M., Bodson, M., Ledoux, L. and Huart, R. (1971). Translocation and distribution of bacterial DNA in Sinapis alba. *Arch. Int. Physiol. 79*:823–824.

Doy, C., Gresshoff, P. M., and Rolfe, B. (1973a). Transgenous of bacterial genes from *E. coli* to culture of lycopersiconese and haploid Arabidopsis thaliana. In *Plant Cells in*

Biochemistry of Gene Expression in Higher Organisms, (Pollack, R., and Lee, L., eds.) pp. 21–37. New Zealand Book Co., Sydney.

Doy, C. M., Gresshoff, P. M., and Rolfe, B. (1973*b*). Biological and molecular evidence for the transgenosis of genes from bacteria to plants. *Proc. Natl. Acad. Sci. USA 70:* 723–726.

Fox, A. S., Yoon, S. B., Duggleby, W. F., and Gelbart, W. M. (1971). Genetic transformation in Drosophila. In *Informative Molecules in Biological Systems* (Ledoux, L., ed.), pp. 313–333. North-Holland, Amsterdam.

Fox, M. and Ayad, S. R. (1972). Uptake and integration of exogenous DNA by lymphoma cells. In *Uptake of Informative Molecules by Living Cells* (Ledoux, L., ed.), pp. 295–326. North-Holland, Amsterdam.

Hanson, R. S. and Chilton, M. D. (1975). On the question of integration of *A. tumefaciens* DNA by tomato plants. *J. Bacteriol. 124*:1220–1224.

Hemleben, V., Ermisch, N., Kimmich, D., Leber, B., and Peter, G. (1975). Studies on the fate of homologous DNA applied to seedlings of *Matthiola incana. Eur. J. Biochem. 56*:403–410.

Hess, D. (1969). Versuche zur Transformation an höheren Pflanzen: Induktion und konstante Weitergabe der Anthocyansynthese bei Petunia hybrida. *A. Pflanz. 60*:348–358.

Hess, D. (1973). Transformationsversuche an höheren Pflanzen: Untersuchungen zur Realization des Exosomen-Modells der Transformation bei Petunia hybrida. *Z. Pflanz. 68*:432–440.

Hess, D. (1975). Uptake of DNA and bacteriophage into pollen and genetic manipulation. In *Genetic Manipulations with Plant Material* (Ledoux, L., ed.), pp. 519–538. Plenum Press, New York.

Hoffman, F. and Hess, D. (1973). Die Aufnahme radioaktiv markierter DNS in isolierte Protoplasten von Petunia hybrida. *Z. Pflanz. 69*:81–83.

Hotta, Y. and Stern, H. (1971). Uptake and distribution of heterologous DNA in living cells. In *Informative Molecules in Biological Systems* (Ledoux, L., ed.), pp. 176–186. North-Holland, Amsterdam.

Kleinhoffs, A., Eden, F., Chilton, M. D., and Bendich, A. (1975). On the question of integration of exogenous bacterial DNA into plant DNA. *Proc. Natl. Acad. Sci. USA 72*:2748–2751.

Ledoux. L. (1975). Fate of exogenous DNA in plants. In *Genetic Manipulations with Plant Materials* (Ledoux, L., ed.), pp. 479–498. Plenum Press, New York.

Ledoux, L. and Huart, R. (1968). Integration and replication of DNA of *M. lysodeikticus* in DNA of germinating barley. *Nature (London) 218*:1256–1259.

Ledoux, L. and Huart, R. (1969). Fate of exogenous bacterial DNA in barley seedlings. *J. Mol. Biol. 43*:243–262.

Ledoux, L. and Huart, R. (1975*a*). Importance of DNA size for integration in plant materials. *Arch. Int. Physiol. Biochim. 83*:194–195.

Ledoux, L. and Huart, R. (1975*b*). Integration and replication of DNA in barley root cells. *Arch. Int. Physiol. Biochim. 83*:196–197.

Ledoux. L. and Jacobs, M. (1969). Rédistribution, lors de la floraison, des DNA exogènes absorbés par des graines d'Arabidopsis thaliana. *Arch. Int. Physiol. Biochim. 77*: 568–569.

Ledoux. L., Huart, R. and Jacobs, P. (1971). Fate of exogenous DNA in Arabidopsis thaliana. *Eur. J. Biochem. 23*:96–108.

Ledoux, L., Brown, J., Charles, P., Huart, R., Jacobs, M., Remy, J., and Watters, C. (1972). Fate of exogenous DNA in mammals and plants. *Adv. Biosci. 8*:347–367.

Ledoux. L., Huart, R., and Jacobs, M. (1974). DNA-mediated genetic correction of thiamineless Arabidopsis thaliana. *Nature (London) 249*:17–21.

Ledoux. L., Huart, R., Mergeay, M., Charles, P., and Jacobs, M. (1975). DNA-mediated genetic correction of thiamineless Arabidopsis thaliana. In *Genetic Manipulations with Plant Material* (Ledoux, L., ed.), pp. 499–517. Plenum Press, New York.

Ledoux, L., Huart, R., and Jacobs, M. *In preparation.*

Lurquin, P. and Behki, R. M. (1975). Use of molecular sieving on agarose gels to study DNA uptake by *Chlamydomonas reinhardi. Mutat. Res. 29*:35–38.

Lurquin, P. and Hotta, Y. (1975). Reutilization of bacterial DNA by Arabidopsis cells in tissue culture. *Plant Sci. Lett. 5*:103–112.

Lurquin, P. and Kado, C. (1976). Studies on *A. tumefaciens:* Fate of exogenously added bacterial DNA in *Nicotiana tabacum. Physiol. Plant. Pathol. 8*:73–82.

Luyindula, N., Lurquin, P., and Ledoux, L. (unpublished results).

Merril, C., Geier, M., and Petricciani, J. (1971). Bacterial virus gene expression in human cells. *Nature (London) 233*:398–400.

Ohyama, K., Gamborg, O. L., and Miller, R. A. (1972). Uptake of exogenous DNA by plant protoplasts. *Can. J. Bot. 50*:2077–2080.

Rédei, G. (1970). Arabidopsis thaliana. A review of the genetics and biology. *Biblio. Genet. 20*:20 pp.

Rédei, G. (1975). Induction of auxotrophic mutations in plants. In *Genetic Manipulations with Plant Material* (Ledoux, L., ed.), pp. 329–350. Plenum Press, New York.

Smith, H., McKee, R. A., Attridge, T. H., and Grierson, D. (1975). Studies on the use of transducing bacteriophages as vectors for the transfer of foreign genes to higher plants. In *Genetic Manipulations with Plant Material* (Ledoux, L., ed.), pp. 551–564. Plenum Press, New York.

Stroun, M., Anker, P., and Ledoux, L. (1967). DNA replication in *Solanum lycopersicum* after absorption of bacterial DNA. *Curr. Mod. Biol. 1*:231–234.

Turbin, N. V., Soyfer, V. N., Kartel, N. A., Chekalin, N. M., Dorokov, Y. L., Titov, Y. B., and Cieminis, K. K. (1975). Genetic modification of the waxy character in barley under the action of exogenous DNA of the wild variety. *Mutat. Res. 27*:59–68.

39

Tissue Culture Studies on *Amaranthus viridis*

M. Zain-ul-Abedin, Amtul Nafees, and A. Mahmood

Biological Research Center
Tissue Culture Laboratory, University of Karachi
Karachi, Pakistan

ABSTRACT

Amaranthus viridis is a plant that is very widely distributed in our country, grows easily, and is eaten by low-income groups. It has been found that the proteins of this plant, like most other plants, are deficient in some essential amino acids. We were able to develop cultures from the cut-end parts of this plant tissue. The commonly used media were modified to achieve good and fast growth. Results have been obtained on the techniques, histology, chromosomal, and biochemical studies which indicate that the plant could be useful as a research tool to study problems in crop improvement at the cellular level.

INTRODUCTION

One of the alarming situations created by the increase in growth rate of the world population is the problem of food shortage. In addition to carbohydrate deficiency, there is also a great insufficiency of dietary protein which is very essential for normal growth and development. This problem is compounded by the fact that the staple cereal crops are generally low in protein content and are also deficient in certain essential amino acids. This problem is more prevalent in developing countries where average protein intake is very low (Scrimshaw, 1963a,b). Nutritional surveys have indicated that protein malnutrition is also widespread in Pakistan (National Survey of Pakistan, U.S. Department of Health,

Education, and Welfare, Washington, D.C., March, 1962, and Jan., 1964). Arable land is limited and attempts are being made to increase crop productivity through plant breeding and genetics, pest control, and agronomy.

In recent years the techniques of cell and tissue culture have been explored as a potential tool for crop improvement. Significant developments include:

1. The regeneration of plants from callus and cell cultures. This has been accomplished with enough species to consider it theoretically possible to culture almost any tissue from any plant (Murashige, 1974).
2. The production of haploids by anther culture. This can improve the efficiency of genetic analysis and speed up the approach to homozygosity.
3. Meristem culture which allows rapid clonal multiplication.
4. Cell hybridization by protoplast fusion. This may provide a means for gene transfer between species which cannot hybridize sexually.

This chapter reports the successful culture stem callus of a local edible plant *Amaranthus viridis* (commonly called cholai). All the parts of the plant including the leaves, the tender shoots, and immature spikes are edible. The biochemical and nutritional studies on this plant (Kidwai et al., 1969) indicate a high protein content (N $\times$ 6.25 = 38%) with reasonably good biological value, N balance, and digestibility when fed to rats at a 10% level. However, with a biological value of 76, compared to 90 for egg albumen, this protein like many other plant proteins is deficient in some essential amino acids. These factors encouraged us to initiate tissue culture studies on this plant with the intention of improving its productivity and protein quality and quantity.

EXPERIMENTAL

Plant Material

Amaranthus viridis is an herbaceous annual and grows up to 120 cm in height. It takes 1–2 months to attain maturity from the time of sowing. It is widely distributed and can be grown without much effort.

Tissue Culture

Explants were initially obtained from stems and roots, and in some cases anthers were also used. The tissue was washed, the surface sterilized with 0.1 N sodium hypochlorite for 1 min and rinsed thoroughly two or three times with sterile distilled water. The exposed cut end was discarded and the remainder cut into 1.5- to 2.0-cm pieces. The upper part of each piece was cut vertically and one to three explants transferred to a 100-ml Erlenmeyer flask containing the growth medium. The cultures were incubated in the dark at 25°C and subcultured to fresh medium when necessary. Samples were taken weekly for histology. Two- to 3-week-old samples were used for chromosome studies and 4- to 5-week-old samples were used for biochemical studies.

Development of a Medium

The inorganic salts, vitamins, and growth regulators (giberellic acid, indoleacetic acid, 2,4-dichlorophenoxyacetic acid, naphthalene acetic acid, benzyladenine, kinetin) of several media (Gamborg et al., 1968; Nitsch and Nitsch, 1969; Welander, 1974) were modified. This provided two combinations of nutrients which gave 100% callus formation.

Histological Studies

Small pieces of tissue were fixed in Formalin, 70% ethanol, and acetic acid (90 : 5 : 5), dehydrated in a butanol series, and embedded in paraffin wax (56–58) for section cutting. The sections were dewaxed and stained in safranin and fast green for microscopic examination.

Chromosomal Studies

Two- to 3-week-old callus tissue was treated with $0.002 M$ 8-hydroxyquinoline to contract the chromosomes. The tissue was fixed (Stringam, 1970), hydrolyzed in $1 N$ HCl at 60°C for 20 min, washed thoroughly with water, and transferred to Feulgen stain for 4 h. The tissues were later kept overnight in acetoorcein. Immediately before making the squash preparation, the tissue was dipped for 1 min in 1% picric acid in ethanol to remove the stain from organelles other than the nuclei and chromosomes.

Biochemical Studies

Carbohydrates were determined by the anthrone method (Fales, 1951) and protein by determination of nitrogen by direct nesslerization (Hawk et al., 1954) after digestion. This value was multiplied by 6.25 for protein content. Lipids were extracted by chloroform : methanol (2 : 1) and triglycerides determined by the method of Stern and Shapiro (1953). Lipid components and phospholipids were separated by micro-TLC (Neuhoff, 1973); RNA and DNA were estimated by orcinol and diphenylamine (DPA) reactions, respectively (Dische, 1955). The biologically active carotenes were separated by the solvent partition method (*Methods of Vitamin Assay*, 1951) and read against standard β-carotene at 450 nm. Iron was estimated on the ashed sample by the dipyridyl method (Ramsay, as cited in Bothwell and Finch, 1962). Moisture content was computed by difference between the wet and dry weights.

RESULTS AND DISCUSSION

Amaranthus viridis has not so far been cultured in any laboratory. Our initial attempts have been to develop a growth medium so that the explants of this plant could successfully be cultured in the laboratory. For our initial studies we selected several well-defined media developed for other plant tissues. In two of these media (Murashige and Skoog, 1962; Gamborg et al., 1968) the frequency of callus formation was low from stem or root explants and anthers (23–29%), and subsequent callus growth rate was exceedingly slow. However, in medium H for tobacco (Nitsch and Nitsch, 1969) and that for *Beta vulgaris* (Welander, 1974), the frequency of callus formation improved considerably, but the growth was still meager. The addition of NH_4NO_3 (10 nmoles) in place of urea, sucrose to 2.5%, benzyladenine (BA), and 2,4-dichlorophenoxyacetic acid (2-4-D), each at 1 mg/liter, or indoleacetic acid (IAA) and kinetin (K), each at 5 mg/liter, gave improved callus initiation and growth rate. Among the vitamin mixtures the combinations of Gamborg et al. (1968) and Nitsch and Nitsch (1969) were tested and the latter was preferred (Table I). Callus grew within 1 or 2 weeks and roots emerged soon after.

The growth rate of *Amaranthus* callus in comparison to similar studies on other plant calli is shown in Fig. 1. Although the callus of this plant grew fairly well, there is a higher percentage of aneuploids (Table II) and it is therefore necessary to improve the medium particularly to bring down this abnormal condition.

The callus was formed on the cut surface mostly in the region of the pith in the first week. However, after 3–4 weeks callus formation was noticed also in the cambial region. The newly formed callus cells were very small in size and increased in size gradually from 14 to 38 μm by the 5th week, whereas the original size of the pith cells was about 54 μm, but in the presence of IAA and K or 2-4-D and BA they enlarged to 80 μm within 5 weeks.

The squash preparation of the callus indicated that 53% of the cells counted in a new callus were aneuploid. Among the 47 euploid cells 39 were diploid, five were tetraploid, two hexaploid, and one octaploid. Among the aneuploids the number of chromosomes varied from 28 to 163; most (84%) fell within the range $2n–7n$. Such variability in the chromosome number is not unusual among plant tissue culture studies. Shimada and Tabata (1967) attributed this to the artificial growth media. However, the precise mechanism and the component(s) in the medium responsible for this is not known.

Table I. Growth Medium Developed for
Amaranthus viridis Explants

	Minerals	
NH_4NO_3	800[a]	
KNO_3	900	
$MgSO_4 7H_2O$	100	
Na–Fe–EDTA	40	Sucrose 2.5% (w/v)
$MnSO_4$	15	Agar 2%
$ZnSO_4 \cdot 7H_2O$	10	
H_3BO_3	10	pH adjusted to 5.6
KH_2PO_4	50	$25° \pm 2°C$
$Na_2MoO_4 2H_2O$	0.25	
KI	0.5	
$CaSO_4 2H_2O$	0.02	
$Ca(NO_3)_2 \cdot 4H_2O$	30	
$Mg(NO_3)_2 6H_2O$	10	
$Na_2H PO_4 2H_2O$	15	
$CoCl_2$	150	
$CuSO_4 5H_2O$	0.025	
Growth substances		
Kinetin	5	
IAA	5	
or		
BA	1	
2,4-D	1	
Vitamins		
Same as described for medium H[b]		

[a]mg/liter.
[b]Nitsch and Nitsch (1969).

Biochemical studies were carried out on the explants as well as callus to follow the changes during growth, and to identify some possible biochemical markers. The moisture content of the newly formed tissue was higher (86%) than that of the explant (75%). Apparently the fresh tissue contains more water than the older tissues. Moreover, the newly formed callus cells are rather small and loosely packed and hence may contain some intercellular fluid. This is also indicated by a slight fall in the DNA content in the callus tissue. Despite the increase in the water content of callus, the concentration of soluble proteins, soluble carbohydrates, triglycerides, and RNA were increased considerably, which indicates that the newly formed tissue is metabolically more active (Table III). Similarly, there is a considerable increase in iron content in the callus tissue. The carotene values decreased in the newly formed tissue despite the increase in lipid content. Carotenes or its products (vitamin A), or both, have been implicated in the growth and development (morphogenesis) of tissues for a long time. In view

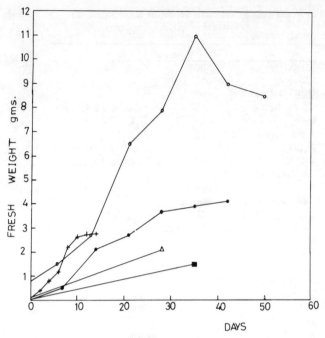

Fig. 1. Comparison of growth rates of different plant Calli on various growth media. (o) Tobacco callus in standard basal medium (Murashige and Skoog, 1962). (+) Rice callus in R-2 medium (Ohira et al., 1973). (■) Growth of *Xanthium* callus in defined medium (Frattarelli et al., 1972). (△) Tomato callus (Padmanabhan et al., 1974). (●) Our studies on *Amaranthus viridis.*

Table II. Chromosomal Analysis of Callus Tissues of *Amaranthus viridis*

Euploids			
Diploids	34 (39)[a]	Tetraploids	68 (5)
Hexaploids	102 (2)	Octoploids	136 (1)

Aneuploids
28(1),[a] 31(1), 33(3)
35(2), 36(1), 37(1), 38(1), 39(2), 44(1), 47(1), 49(2)
52(2), 53(1), 57(2), 58(1), 59(1), 60(1), 65(1)
69(2), 70(1), 72(2), 79(1), 81(2), 83(1)
93(1), 98(2), 99(3)
103(1), 104(1), 108(2), 111(1), 112(1), 113(1), 118(1)
123(1), 127(1)
143(1), 149(1)
163(1)

[a]Chromosome number of cells with the number of metaphase cells counted in parentheses.

Table III. Biochemical Studies on the
Explants and Callus of *Amaranthus Viridis*

Constituent	Explant[a]	Callus[a]
DNA	6	4.5
RNA	41	50
Soluble proteins	1025	1275
Soluble carbohydrates	247	388
Triglycerides	63	93
Carotenes	0.32	0.27
Iron (μg/g tissue)	0.52	0.83
Moisture (%)	75%	86%

[a]Expressed in μg/100 mg wet wt. tissue.

of these findings, the alteration of carotene content in this newly formed tissue is very interesting.

ACKNOWLEDGMENT

This work was supported by research grant No. SU-CH-46 from the Pakistan Science Foundation, Islamabad. We are very grateful to this foundation for providing all the funds to undertake this work, including the salary of one of us (A.N.). Miss Rafat and Mr. Parvez performed the biochemical analysis of the tissue.

REFERENCES

Bothwell, T. H. and Finch, C. A. (1962). *Iron Metabolism,* pp. 18–19. Little, Brown, Boston.

Dische, Z. (1955). *Color Reactions of Nucleic Acid Components in the Nucleic Acids,* Vol. I (Chargaff, E. and Davidson, J. N., eds.), pp. 286–301. Academic Press, New York.

Fales, F. W. (1951). The assimilation and degradation of carbohydrate by yeast cells. *J. Biol. Chem. 193*:113–124.

Frattarelli, F. J., Rier, J. P., and Reid, H. B. (1972). Growth of *Xanthium* stem callus on a defined culture medium. *Physiol. Plant 27*:439–440.

Gamborg, O. L., Miller, R. A., and Ojima, K. (1968). Nutrient requirement of suspension cultures of Soybean root cells. *Exp. Cell Res. 50*:151–158.

Hawk, B., Oser, B. L., and Summerson, W. H. (1954). *Practical Physiological Chemistry,* 13th ed. 1329 pp. McGraw Hill, New York.

Kidwai, I. M., Zain, B. K., and Zain-ul-Abedin, M. (1969). Nutritive value of some common plants. *Pak. J. Biochem. 11*:28–32.

Methods of Vitamin Assay,(1951). Prepared and edited by the Assoc. of Vitamin Chemists., 2nd ed., pp. 63–66, Interscience Publications, New York.

Murashige, T. (1974). Plant propagation through tissue cultures. *Annu. Rev. Plant Physiol.* 25:135–166.

Murashige, T. and Skoog, F. (1962). A revised medium for rapid growth and bioassays with tobacco tissue cultures. *Physiol. Plant. 15*:473–497.

Neuhoff, V. (1973). Micro determination of phospholipids in micromethods in Molecular biology. *Mol. Biol. Biochem. Biophys. 14*:162–174.

Nitsch, J. P. and Nitsch, C. (1969). Haploid plants from pollen grains. *Science 163*:85–87.

Ohira, K., Ojima, K., and Fujiwara, A. (1973). Studies on the nutrition of rice cell culture. I. A simple defined medium for rapid growth in suspension culture. *Plant and Cell Physiol. 14*:1113–1121.

Padmanabham, V., Paddock, E. F., and Sharp, W. R. (1974). Plantlet formation from *Lycopersicon esculentum* leaf callus. *Can. J. Bot. 52*:1429–1432.

Scrimshaw, N. S. (1963a). World-wide importance of protein malnutrition and progress towards its prevention. *Am. J. Pub. Health 53*:1781–1786.

Scrimshaw, N. S. (1963b). Malnutrition and the health of children. *J. Am. Diet. Assoc. 42*:203–208.

Shimada, T. and Tabata, M. (1967). Chromosome numbers in cultured pith tissue of tobacco. *Jap. J. Genet. 42*:195–201.

Stern, I. and Shapiro, B. (1953). Rapid simple method for determination of esterified fatty acids and total fatty acids in the blood. *J. Chem. Pathol. 6*:158–160.

Stringam, G. R. (1970). A simple mordant technique for plants with small chromosomes. *Can. J. Bot. 48*:1134–1135.

Welander, T. (1974). Callus and root formation in explants of *Beta vulgaris*. *Physiol. Plant. 32*:305–307.

40

Molecular Mechanisms in Genetic Transformation

Jane K. Setlow

Brookhaven National Laboratory
Upton, New York

ABSTRACT

Molecular mechanisms of recombination of genetic material are most readily studied in microorganisms; a great deal is known about recombination of transforming DNA, introduced into the cell from the medium, with DNA inside bacteria. At present, it is doubtful that this type of transformation will be of use in improving crop plants. However, a new technique of making recombinant DNA molecules from two or more highly divergent organisms may turn out to have great practical importance for agriculture.

INTRODUCTION

In order to attempt to understand genetic recombination in higher organisms, such as plants, it is useful to consider what is known about recombination in lower organisms, such as bacteria, as some of the fundamental mechanisms of rearrangement of DNA molecules are expected to be the same for both types of organisms.

Figure 1 shows what is meant by bacterial transformation. A bacterium has a certain characteristic designated A^+ (e.g., resistance to an antibiotic, such as streptomycin). DNA is extracted from the bacterium and may be purified. Another closely related strain of bacteria lacks the particular character A^+ and is

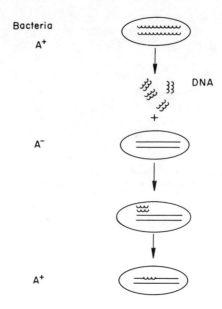

Fig. 1. Schematic diagram of bacterial transformation.

thus called A⁻. By manipulating the physiological condition of the A⁻ bacteria, they can be induced to take up the DNA from the medium. Some of the A⁺ DNA within the A⁻ cell becomes linearly inserted as a single-strand piece in the genome of the cell, thereby replacing a homologous section of the recipient DNA. If this piece happens to contain the A⁺ character, then the cell containing the A⁺ piece in its DNA becomes A⁺. When the cell DNA replicates in the usual semiconservative fashion, there results one A⁺ daughter cell, and from the opposite strand an A⁻ daughter cell.

The final step in the recombination process shown in Fig. 1 has been studied in the bacterium *Hemophilus influenzae.* The transforming DNA does not go into the recipient DNA at random, but instead always goes to a matching part of the recipient cell's DNA. The problem is how, starting with two double-stranded DNA molecules, it is possible for a piece of the incoming DNA to find its correct place in the cell DNA. Two discoveries were recently made in our laboratory that help in the understanding of this process. The first is that DNA newly synthesized in cells able to take up DNA from the medium (called competent cells) and also able to recombine incoming DNA and recipient DNA has a very different structure than is normally found in the cell (LeClerc and Setlow, 1974, 1975). To show this we have used two different radioactive labels for the cell's DNA. One of the labels (^{14}C) is left in for a number of generations before the competence regime. The other (^{3}H) is applied for a short time to cells that have become highly competent. The DNA is centrifuged in an alkaline sucrose gradient, which gives a measure of the size of single strands of DNA (Fig. 2). In the wild-type competent cell, the newly synthesized (pulse-labeled) DNA sediments less rapidly than the prelabeled DNA, and is therefore much smaller. However, there is no such large peak of single-stranded material in the exponentially growing wild-type cells. Figure 2 also shows the results of similar experiments with two recombination-defective mutants: *rec2* does not have the big peak of small single-stranded material, but *rec1* does. The mutant *rec1* undergoes the first part of the recombination process, but in *rec2* the transforming DNA taken up by the competent cell does not become associated with the cell's DNA (LeClerc and Setlow, 1974), evidence that the production of single-strand nicks or gaps in competent cell DNA is essential for an early step in recombination.

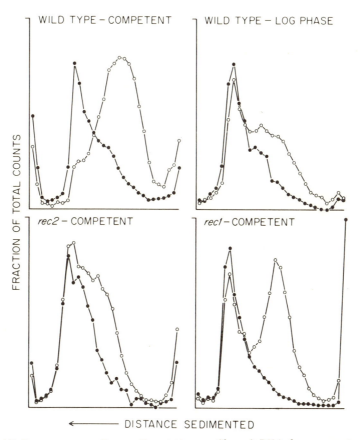

Fig. 2. Alkaline sucrose gradient sedimentation profiles of DNA from competent and exponentially growing wild type and competent recl and rec2 cells. Cells were prelabeled with [¹⁴C] dThd (●) and pulse labeled with [³H] dThd (o) 10 min before sedimentation.

Another way to observe the peculiar structure of DNA in competent cells is to make use of benzoylated, naphthoylated diethylaminoethyl (BND)–cellulose column chromatography, which makes it possible to separate double-stranded DNA with partly single-stranded regions from completely double-stranded DNA. Figure 3 shows that in the newly synthesized DNA of the competent wild-type cell labeled with ^{3}H there is a large peak of material in the region where partly single-stranded DNA elutes (in the right-hand portion of the profile). Such a peak is not present either in competent *rec2* or growing, noncompetent, wild-type cells.

Experiments with single-strand-specific nuclease have demonstrated that the newly synthesized DNA contains single-stranded tails (LeClerc and Setlow, 1975). The partially single-stranded material probably arises in competent cells by a mechanism known as strand displacement (Masamune and Richardson, 1971), shown schematically in Fig. 4. A DNA polymerase molecule (p) binds to a nick in the DNA (a) and begins to replicate the DNA while simultaneously

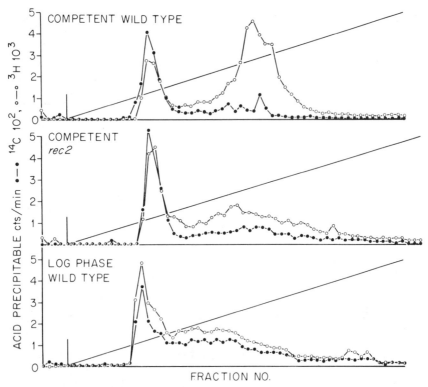

Fig. 3. BND-cellulose column chromatography of DNA from competent and exponentially growing wild type and competent rec2 cells. Labeling was as in Fig. 2. The gradient buffer was 0.3–1.0 *M* NaCl–Tris-EDTA and 0–2% caffeine.

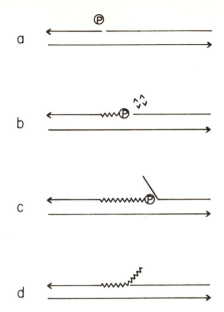

Fig. 4. Schematic diagram of DNA strand displacement.

degrading the other strand (b), finally pushing it back (c). This structure can readily turn into the structure of Fig. 4d, with a dangling, single-stranded end all ready to pair with an homologous, single-stranded end on a piece of transforming DNA.

We have recently found that transforming DNA after it enters the wild-type cell has single-stranded ends (Sedgwick and Setlow, 1976). These single-stranded ends are formed as a result of preliminary reaction between the transforming DNA and the cell DNA, after which pairing between the correct single-stranded regions in the two DNAs can occur, followed by single-strand insertion, which represents completed recombination.

The studies of recombination in bacteria show that cells go to great lengths to ensure that inserted genetic material goes to the correct place on the recipient DNA molecule. Furthermore, a great deal of homology between DNA molecules is required in order for pairing to occur. An example of the types of results obtained in transforming various drug-resistance markers into *H. influenzae from* resistant *H. influenzae* and from a closely related species, *H. parainfluenzae* (Beattie and Setlow, 1970), is shown in Table I. These two species contain DNA that is about 50% homologous (Boling, 1972), but the transformation between the species is much lower than within one species, and in the case of one of the genetic markers, novobiocin resistance, is four orders of magnitude lower.

Because of the problems of incompatibility of DNA molecules, the prospects for use of transformation between distantly related species for improvement of

**Table I. Transformation of *H. influenzae* by DNA from
H. influenzae and by DNA from *H. parainfluenzae*
Bearing Various Antibiotic Resistance Markers**

	Number of transformants/mliter		
DNA	Streptomycin	Novobiocin	Erythromycin
H. influenzae	3×10^7	3×10^7	4×10^7
H. parainfluenzae	4×10^5	3×10^3	4×10^6

agricultural products are not very bright. However, a new technique that resulted from studies of *H. influenzae* by Hamilton Smith and his collaborators (Kelly and Smith, 1970; Smith and Wilcox, 1970) provides a novel method of making recombinant DNA molecules. This technique may be the most important advance in biology since the discovery of the structure and function of DNA. It is likely that application of the new technique will eventually be of tremendous importance in agriculture.

Figure 5 shows an example of what can be done with the new technique. There is a special enzyme found in *H. influenzae* that cuts DNA in the particular way shown. This enzyme, called a restriction enzyme, recognizes only the particular sequence in DNA. The sequence is also remarkable for the fact that it reads the same forward and backward (the top sequence being AAGCTT, left to right, is identical to the bottom sequence, right to left). When the DNA is cut in the manner shown, what are produced are single-stranded ends that are homolo-

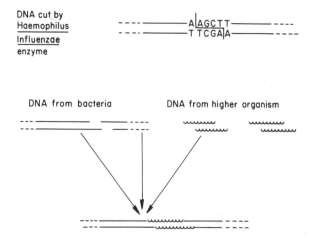

Fig. 5. Schematic diagram of method of making recombinant DNA molecules.

gous. This property of the enzyme, i.e., the production of single-stranded ends that can pair with each other, makes it possible to combine DNA from entirely different organisms. What the cell cannot do when the incoming DNA has too little homology with the cell DNA, the biochemist can accomplish with restriction enzymes of this type.

No miracles have been wrought as yet with this new technique. It has been shown to be possible to replicate such recombinant molecules in bacteria (Morrow et al., 1974), and much progress has been made with the aid of this technique in the problem of organizing the genome of some higher organisms (Glover et al., 1975; Kedes et al., 1975). A real possibility exists that in the future the new technique will make it possible to do "molecular farming," in which the most desirable genes are inserted at will into plants.

ACKNOWLEDGMENT

Work at the Brookhaven National Laboratory was performed under the auspices of the U.S. Energy Research and Development Administration.

REFERENCES

Beattie, K. L. and Setlow, J. K. (1970). Transformation between *Haemophilus influenzae* and *Haemophilus parainfluenzae*. *J. Bacteriol. 104*:390–400.

Boling, M. E. (1972). Homology between the deoxyribonucleic acids of *Haemophilus influenzae* and *Haemophilus parainfluenzae*. *J. Bacteriol. 112*:745–750.

Glover, D. M., White, R. L., Finnegan, D. J. and Hogness, D. S. (1975). Characterization of six cloned DNAs from *Drosophila melanogaster,* including one that contains the genes for rRNA. *Cell 5*:149–157.

Kedes, L. H., Cohn, R. H., Lowry, J. C., Chang, A. C. Y., and Cohen, S. N. (1975). The organization of sea urchin histone genes. *Cell 6*:359–369.

Kelly, T. J., Jr. and Smith, H. O. (1970). A restriction enzyme from *Haemophilus influenzae*. II. Base sequence of the recognition site. *J. Mol. Biol. 51*:393–409.

LeClerc, J. E. and Setlow, J. K. (1974). Transformation in *Haemophilus influenzae*. In *Mechanisms in Recombination* (Grell, R. F., ed.), pp. 187–207. Plenum Press, New York.

LeClerc, J. E. and Setlow, J. K. (1975). Single-strand regions in the deoxyribonucleic acid of competent *Haemophilus influenzae*. *J. Bacteriol. 122*:1091–1102.

Masamune, Y. and Richardson, C. C. (1971). Strand displacement during deoxyribonucleic acid synthesis at single strand breaks. *J. Biol. Chem. 246*:2692–2701.

Morrow, J. F., Cohen, S. N., Chang, A. C. Y., Boyer, H. W., Goodman, H. M., and Helling, R. B. (1974). Replication and transcription of eukaryotic DNA in *Escherichia coli*. *Proc. Natl. Acad. Sci. USA 71*:1743–1747.

Sedgwick, B. and Setlow, J. K. (1976). Single-stranded regions in transforming deoxyribonucleic acid after uptake by competent *Haemophilus influenzae*. *J. Bacteriol. 125*: 588–594.

Smith, H. O. and Wilcox, K. W. (1970). A restriction enzyme from *Haemophilus influenzae*. I. Purification and general properties. *J. Mol. Biol. 51*:379–391.

41

Unconventional Methods in Plant Breeding*

Georg Melchers

Max-Planck-Institut für Biologie
Tübingen, Federal Republic of Germany

ABSTRACT

There are three ways whereby unconventional methods of plant genetics can be used for applied plant breeding.

1. The time necessary for breeding by recombination can be shortened, making use of the discovery that plants can be obtained directly from the products of meiosis, the "Gonen." Two new cultivars bred in tobacco by this method already exist.

2. Microbiological methods may be applied to mutation and selection in haploid or dihaploid cell cultures. New cultivars bred by this method have not yet been published, but it should be possible to make use of this technique in plant breeding.

3. Somatic hybridization of plants by fusion of protoplasts or by uptake of nuclei and other organelles (plastids, mitochondria) or pure nucleic acids is another useful method. There exist up to now somatic hybrid plants (a) between mutants of the liverwort *Sphaerocarpos donnellii,* (b) some varieties of tobacco, and (c) two species of *Nicotiana.* All these hybrids can also be produced by conventional sexual hybridization. It is impossible to predict how often incompatibility for cross-fertilization can be surmounted by somatic hybridization, as incompatibility between two genomes must not be restricted to the fertilization process, but it can work on any stage of the development of the hybrid.

---

*Closing Remarks of the Chairperson. More detail is given in an evening lecture "Recent methods in plant genetics" in the Goethe-Institute, Lahore, March 4 (unpublished).

SHORTENING OF TIME FOR RECOMBINATION BREEDING

This method, which makes use of the discovery that plants can be obtained directly from the products of meiosis, has not been mentioned in this volume, despite the fact that the discovery that embryos could be regenerated from microspores during anther culture was made on this subcontinent by Guha and Maheswari (1964, 1966). New cultivars of tobacco have already been obtained by this method in Japan and China (Nakamura et al., 1974; Cooperative Group, 1974). Furthermore, on a visit to the Genetic Institute of the Academia Sinica, China in 1975, the author observed a new cultivar of rice, produced through anther culture, which was growing in the experimental field of the Red Star people's commune near Peking.

In the immediate future there are two approaches that can and should be used for plant-breeding purposes.

1. The search for new and interesting gene combinations in plants which have already yielded to anther culture (tobacco, *Hyoscyamus, Datura, Atropa,* and so on; see Kasha, 1974).
2. The improvement of anther or isolated microspore culture techniques for important cultivated food plants (cereals, corn, rape, potatoes, and others—Cooperative Group, Academia Sinica (1974); Lab. of Genetics, Kwantung Institute (1975); Lab. of Plant Cell Culture (1975); Ouyang et al. 1973); Thomas and Wenzel (1975); Thomas et al. (1975, 1976); C. C. Wang et al. (1973, 1974); Y. S. Wang et al. (1973); Wenzel and Thomas (1974); Wenzel et al. (1975).

MICROBIOLOGICAL METHODS

We can now apply microbiological methods for mutagenesis and mutant selection in haploid or dihaploid cell cultures. This volume has discussed the interesting plans as well as some promising results of Brock and Scowcroft, but so far no mention has been made of the new cultivars obtained by these methods. Indeed, the fundamental ideas and first experiments in this field are not particularly new (cf. Melchers and Bergmann, 1958–1959; Melchers, 1960; Binding et al., 1970; Maliga et al., 1973; Kasha, 1974). Yet again, new cultivars of agriculturally important plants superior to the existing cultivars (in disease resistance, yield, amount, and quality of particular products, etc.) have not yet been produced by these methods. For 15 years, although it has been known that under certain conditions haploid plants may also be used as the experimental material without the necessity of using cell cultures (Melchers, 1960; Melchers and Labib, 1970), the technique has not been applied.

The first two methods mentioned above can both be used to serve the purposes of practical plant breeding. Unfortunately, the efforts made so far in this direction have seldom been adequate for this great task. Therefore, it is not certain whether we can achieve, in the immediate future, striking success comparable to that already obtained with conventional plant-breeding methods. In this volume, Johnson has given a good example of the success of conventional methods for the improvement of protein quality and quantity in wheat.

SOMATIC HYBRIDIZATION

It is now possible to obtain somatic hybridization of plants by protoplast fusion or by the uptake of nuclei and other organelles (plastids, mitochondria) or pure nucleic acids. These methods have been the subject of much discussion for some time. Some authors like to draw attention to their work by the use of pretentious titles, such as "manipulation of genes," or "genetic engineering." However, there are only a few experimental facts existing in this field. The chances of achieving practical results using these methods are too low to justify the optimism raised by some authors through their publications. We are simply crossing the borders of an unknown country with hardly any good experimental results. At the moment, no one can predict whether we will discover a fertile, cultivated land or a desert.

Those plant physiologists and biochemists who make such claims naively presume that barriers of incompatibility between two genomes exist only during pollination and not at other plant developmental stages. Admittedly, the isolation of detached populations from a large mother population is an important determinative factor in evolution, and for this purpose incompatibility at any one stage of fertilization is sufficient (pollen germination, pollen tube growth, gametic fusion). However, isolation can also be produced by disturbance in embryo or the endosperm development, or both, or through abortive vegetative or generative growth during hybrid development (e.g., Hollingshead, 1930a,b; Melchers, 1939; Stebbins, 1950). Therefore, although pollen incompatibility generally may be considered a major factor in evolution, it cannot be certain that some somatic hybrids do not present other incompatibility barriers. At this moment, indeed, we cannot predict whether or not other incompatibilities exist that partially or completely affect other developmental stages (cell division, regeneration to embryos or plants, failure in meiosis, and so on; cf. Binding, 1976).

When we consider the "parasexual hybrid" between *N. glauca* and *N. langsdorffii* (Carlson et al., 1972; Kung et al., 1975; and critically discussed by Melchers, 1977), that of *Sphaerocarpos donnellii* (Schieder, 1975), and the hybrid specimens produced between tobacco varieties (Melchers and Labib,

1973; Gleba et al., 1975; Melchers and Sacristán, 1977), it will be realized that at the present time there are only three cases of somatic hybrid production by fusion of the protoplasts of green plants. Furthermore, all three of these hybrids can be sexually produced. Extensive experiments in the author's laboratory on fusions between *Nicotiana tabacum* and *Petunia hybrida,* which do not normally produce viable seeds after fertilization (Zenkteler and Melchers, in preparation), have not yet been successful. It is therefore particularly interesting that while working as a guest at the author's laboratory in the summer of 1975 Zenkteler obtained fertilization and a few succeeding cell divisions after sexually crossing *N. tabacum* and *P. hybrida in vitro,* but he never observed the development of real embryos (see Zenkteler and Melchers, 1977). Sexual hybrids between *N. tabacum* and *P. parodii* are not known to be very vigorous, but are at least normal (Pogliaga, 1952), which indicates that the suggested embryonic barrier is genus specific in this case. Hence, although hybrid cells and their initial divisions are known following the fusion of soybean and pea as well as soybean and barley (Kao et al., 1974), this does not necessarily mean that regeneration of plants from these hybrid cells is possible. Many callus cultures (e.g., *N. tabacum*) lose the ability to regenerate plants when subjected to continuous subculture, primarily because of abnormal chromosome sets, or they lose the ability to produce chlorophyll (cf. Melchers, 1965; Sacristán and Melchers, 1969).

Some critical remarks have been levied by the author against our sometimes too-optimistic colleagues, whose results in somatic hybridization experiments are

---

Fig. 1. Scheme summarizing conventional sexual (×) and somatic (+) hybridization. Selection of somatic hybrid cells, calluses, and plants complemented to normal chlorophyll color and light resistance from two light-sensitive nonallelic recessive tobacco mutants *ss* and *vv,* indicating the diploid and *s* and *v* the haploid condition. Two pairs of chromosomes symbolize the situation in the genome. The situation in the plastom is also indicated (●○)—no difference in the case of (*s* × *v*) and (*v* × *s*) (Melchers and Labib, 1974), but with differences in the peptide pattern of the large subunit of Fraction I protein (cf. Sakano et al., 1974) in the sexual hybrids of (*N. glauca* ♀ × *N. langsdorffii* ♂) and (*N. langsdorffi* ♀ × *N. glauca* ♂), respectively. The identity of the so-called parasexual hybrid of Carlson et al. (1972) with respect to plastid genetics with the sexual hybrid (*N. glauca* ♀ × *N. langsdorffii* ♂) (cf. Kung et al., 1975) is not easily understandable. This scheme presents as well (1) the production of "haploids" according to Guha and Maheswari (1966); (2) the culture of plants of the "haploid embryos" in faint light (800 lux) to more or less normal green plants; (3) the preparation of protoplasts out of these plants; and (4) the fusion of protoplasts from *s* and *v* and the selection in high light intensity of the hybrid callus and plants from it, or slow growth and pale color of plants out of the nonhybridized protoplasts in 10,000 lux. *Abbreviations:* (PMC) pollen mother cells; (PO) pollen with tube (microgametophyte); (ES) embryo sac; (PL) plastids or proplastids only transmitted by the egg cell, not by the pollen tube and mixed after fusion (after Melchers and Labib, 1974).

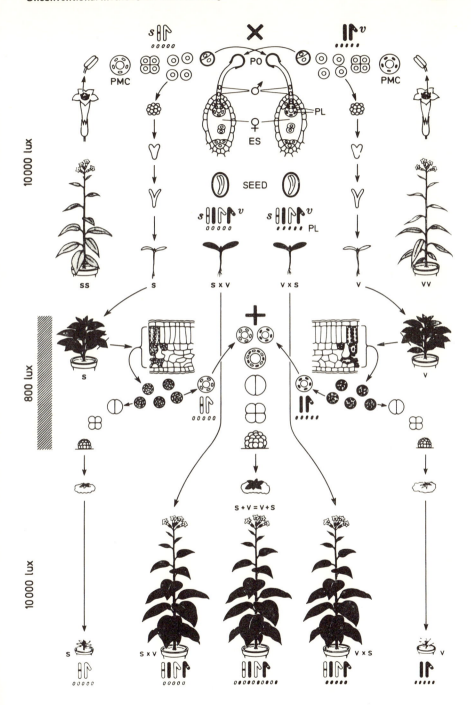

even poorer than the results mentioned earlier. Nevertheless, such remarks should not deter efforts to extend our knowledge and abilities so that we may change the genetic information of our most important cultivated plants in an unconventional way. At the moment, however, it seems irresponsible to lead plant breeders and their sponsors to expect revolutionary results in practical plant breeding for the immediate future. The transformation experiments with pure nucleic acid, using an especially well-adapted test material for an impressive demonstration, as reported earlier in this volume by Ledoux, as well as similar results of other authors, are not yet very promising for plant breeding.

Besides its possible utilization in plant breeding, somatic hybridization by protoplast fusion can be interesting in other respects. Figure 1 compares nuclear heredity to plastid heredity. In the case of two sexually compatible species in the genus *Nicotiana,* each may possess genetically different plastids. Because the plastids are not transferred by the pollen tube, maternal heredity takes place in the sexual hybrid, e.g., in *N. glauca* X *N. langsdorffii* (Sakano et al., 1974). In contrast, in a somatic hybrid, the plastid genetic elements (the plastome, Renner, 1934) of both parents should be present. Kung et al. (1975) found that the large subunit of the Fraction I protein of the "parasexual hybrid", genetically informed by plastic genes, resembles that of *N. glauca* and is unlike that of *N. langsdorffii.* These workers are therefore of the opinion that the genetic information of plastids of *N. langsdorffii* is "not expressed" in the hybrid. The author subscribes to the simple hypothesis that the parasexual hybrid is indeed sexual, in the sense that it does not contain any *N. langsdorffii* plastids arisen by an experimental mistake. This hypothesis can easily be disproved when the offspring of several additional parasexual hybrid plants become available. Parenthetically, the single plant reported was obtained with the use of $NaNO_3$ as fusion medium, a method that has not been used successfully by any other investigator, despite several attempts. For two years it has been possible to produce hybrids repeatedly using two well-established fusion media (high pH and calcium and polyethyleneglycol (Keller and Melchers, 1973; Kao and Michayluk, 1974). Using these methods, it is a relatively simple matter to produce many hybrids. One could then determine if the large subunit of the Fraction I protein always resembles that of *N. glauca,* or if it sometimes resembles that of *N. langsdorffii,* or, again, whether it is sometimes a mixture of both. At the moment it is uncertain as to which is the case.

In order to be successful in somatic hybridization, it is necessary to have not only a well-functioning fusion medium, but also a selection system that favors the growth or identification of hybrid cells, calluses, or regenerated plantlets. Especially suitable are pairs of recessive mutations that retard growth or development of the parents, but show complementation in the hybrid to give normal development. We chose two chlorophyll-deficient, light-sensitive tobacco varieties, the F_1 hybrid of which is not obviously different in its plastome and which exhibits complementation for both normal chlorophyll color and light resistance. In this manner, as a result of four independent protoplast fusion experiments, we found 20–40 somatic hybrid plants (Figs. 2–5). Figure 6 shows that among these plants arose many normal somatic hybrids identical in their chromosome characteristics and offspring with the sexually produced hybrids. However, we also found hybrids with aneuploid, triploid, and tetraploid chromosome numbers. In the latter two cases the plants may have resulted from fusion involving more than two protoplasts, although because similar deviations in chromosome numbers also occur during callus culture, it is possible that these deviations occurred following a normal fusion of two protoplasts. The surprising factor is that the deviations appeared after only a short period of callus culture (large deviations in the chromosome number are often observed after prolonged culture of calluses; Melchers and Sacristán, 1977).

Some additional remarks about the fusion technique are appropriate at this point. During the preparation of protoplasts from a particular species, "spontaneous fusion," caused by the contact of adjacent cells via their plasmodesmata, takes place. The always existing "fusion" of cells in a normal plant tissue by plasmodesmata rarely remains in the preparation procedure. T. Nagata, while a fellow of the Humboldt Foundation and a guest scientist at the author's laboratory, measured the negative surface charge of tobacco protoplasts by electrophoresis experiments (unpublished). He found a negative ζ-potential of approximately 30 mV. In such an electrostatic condition, spontaneous fusion cannot occur. However, in a solution containing Ca^{2+} ions, the surface charge is reduced almost to zero, and under these conditions contact and fusion become

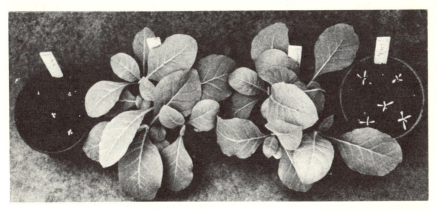

Fig. 2. *Seedlings after 1.5 months of growing after germination in a normal greenhouse in winter. Left–right:* (1) sublethal, *ss;* (2) $(s \times v)F_1$; (3) $(v \times s)F_1$; and (4) virescent, *vv* demonstrating the light sensitivity of *s* and *v*, the complementation in the hybrids, and the identity of $(s \times v)$ and $(v \times s)$. (No differences in the plastom!)

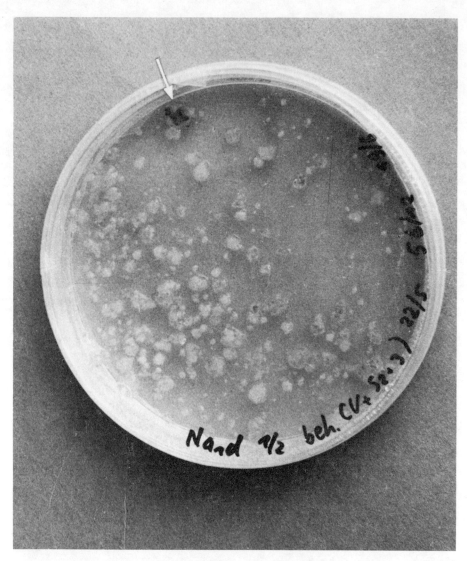

Fig. 3. A Petri dish with calluses after one of the first successful fusion experiments (5/2/74) cultivated in Nagata-Takebe-medium without auxin with reduced concentration (0.2) of organic compounds and in high light intensity. One callus with a dark green regenerate, shown afterward to have 48 chromosomes, normal hybrid characters, and an offspring with *s*- and *v*-like plants.

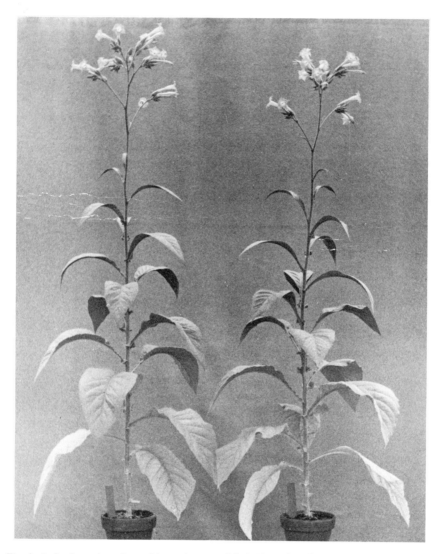

Fig. 4. Left: flowering plant of (v × s) = sexual hybrid. Right: flowering plant of (v + s) = somatic hybrid.

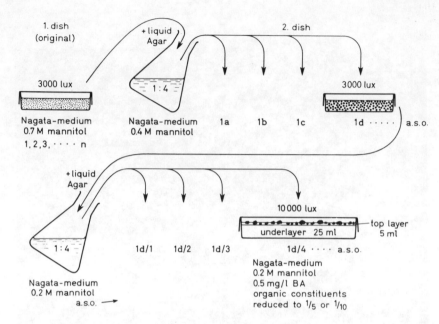

Fig. 5. Schematic representation of the culture of protoplasts and the calluses originating out of them after a fusion experiment. Mornings: preparation of protoplasts. Early afternoon: Fusion, immediate plating in the first dishes (φ 60 mm). Numbering of the dishes (1, 2, 3, etc.). Culture temperature always 28°C. 72 h at 300 lux followed by 3000 lux for approximately 2 weeks. Then diluted approximately 1 : 4 with liquid agar, with reduced mannitol concentrations of 0.4 M. Second set of dishes numbers 1a, 1b, 1c, etc. As soon as necessary (usually after about 2 more weeks) another dilution with liquid agar, decreased mannitol concentration of 0.2 M, no auxin, 0.5 mg/liter BA, organic constituents reduced to 0.2 or 0.1. Plating into top layer of Petri dishes (Ø 90 mm). Culture under approx. 10,000 lux. Labeling of plates 1d/1, 1d/2, 1d/3, etc. (after Melchers and Sacristán, 1977.)

possible. Nagata tried not only to reduce the surface charge, but also to change the value from a negative to a positive one. He accomplished this by removing the negative phosphate groups enzymatically, but the protoplasts did not survive the treatment. However, using a phospholipid synthesized by H. Eibl (MP Institute of Biophysical Chemistry, Göttingen) a change to a low positive value could be induced without affecting vitality. The positive charge (+ 5 mV ζ-potential) was rather weak, so that, although the protoplasts do not adhere very strongly to negatively charged surfaces, such as glass or plastic, they adhere slightly to each other. We are still trying to induce artificial sexuality in somatic cells by increasing the positive charge of one protoplast while maintaining the negative charge of another protoplast type. Such a method would increase the ratio of hybrid fusions to nonhybrid fusions with obvious advantages, especially in cases in which no efficient system of hybrid selection exists.

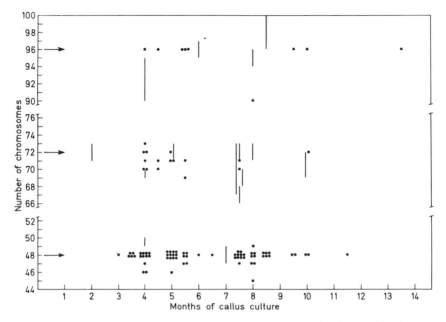

Fig. 6. The chromosome numbers of somatic hybrids originated by fusion of haploid (24) chromosomic protoplasts of two tobacco varieties in relation to the time of callus culture. For further details see text and Melchers and Sacristán (1977).

ACKNOWLEDGMENT

The author is very grateful to Dr. Emrys Thomas, Max-Planck Institut für Pflanzengenetik, Project group "Haploids in Plant Breeding," 6802 Ladenburg/Rosenhof, for translating the closing remarks expressed in this chapter.

REFERENCES

Binding, H. (1976). Somatic hybridization experiments in solanaceous species. *Mol. Gen. Genet. 144*:171–175.

Binding, H., Binding, K., and Straub, J. (1970). Selektion in Gewebekulturen mit haploiden Zellen. *Naturwissenschaften 57*:136–139.

Carlson, P. S., Smith, H. H., and Dearing, R. (1972). Parasexual interspecific plant hybridization. *Proc. Natl. Acad. Sci. USA 69*:2292–2294.

Cooperative Group of Haploid Breeding of Tobacco of Shangtung Institute of Tobacco and Peking Institute of Botany, Academia Sinica (1974). Success of breeding the new tobacco cultivar "Tan-Yuk Nr.1." (Chinese with English summary.) *Acta Bot. Sin. 16*:300–303.

Gleba, Y. Y., Butenko, R. G., and Sytnik, K. M. (1975). Protoplast fusion and parasexual hybridization in *Nicotiana tabacum*. *XII International Botanical Congress, Leningrad*, p. 290 (Abst.).

Guha, S. and Maheswari, S. C. (1964). In vitro production of embryos from anthers of *Datura*. *Nature (London) 204*:497.

Guha, S. and Maheswari, S. C. (1966). Cell division and differentiation of embryos in the pollen grains of *Datura* in vitro. *Nature (London) 212*:97 -98.

Hollingshead, L. (1930*a*). A lethal factor in *Crepis* effective only in an interspecific hybrid. *Genetics 15*:114–140.

Hollingshead, L. (1930*b*). Cytological investigations of hybrids and hybrid derivatives of *Crepis capillaris* and *Crepis tectorum. Univ. Calif. Publ. Agri. Sci. 6*:55–94.

Kao, K. N. and Michayluk, M. R. (1974). A method for high frequency intergeneric fusion of plant protoplasts. *Planta (Berlin) 115*:355–367.

Kao, K. N., Constabel, F., Michayluk, M. R. and Gamborg, O. L. (1974). Plant protoplast fusion and growth of intergeneric hybrid cells. *Planta 120*:215–227.

Kasha, K. J., ed. (1974). *Proceedings 1st International Symposium Haploids in Higher Plants—Advances and Potential, June, 1974*, Univ. of Guelph, Canada.

Keller, W. A. and Melchers, G. (1973). The effect of high pH and calcium on tobacco leaf protoplast fusion. *Z. Naturforsch. 28c*:737–741.

Kung, S. D., Gray, J. C., Wildman, S. G. and Carlson, P. S. (1975). Polypeptide composition of fraction I protein from parasexual hybrid plants in the genus *Nicotiana*. *Science 187*:353–355.

Laboratory of Plant Cell and Tissue Culture, 401 Research Group, Institute of Genetics, Academia Sinica (1975). Primary study on induction of pollen plants of *Zea mays*. (Chinese with English summary.) *Acta Genet. Sinica 2*:138–143.

Laboratory of Genetics, Kwantung Institute of Botany (1975). Studies on anther culture in vitro in *Oryza sativa* subsp. Shien I. The role of basic medium and supplemental constituents in callus induced from anther and in differentiation of root and shoot. *Acta Genet. Sin. 2*:81–89.

Maliga, P., Breznovits, A., and Marton, L. (1973). Streptomycin resistant plants from callus culture of haploid tobacco. *Nature New Biol. 244*:29–30.

Melchers, G. (1939). Genetik und Evolution. Bericht eines Botanikers. *Z. Vererbungslehre 76*:229–259.

Melchers, G. (1960). Haploide Blütenpflanzen als Material der Mutations-Züchtung. Beispiele: Blattfarbmutanten und Mutatio *wettsteini* von *Antirrhinum majus. Züchter 30*:129–134.

Melchers, G. (1965). Einige genetische Gesichtspunkte zu sogenannten Gewebekulturen. *Ber. Deut. Bot. Ges. 78*:21–29.

Melchers, G. (1973). Summation: Haploid research in higher plants. In *Proc. Haploids in Higher Plants—Advances and Potential, Int. Symp., Guelph, Canada* (Kasha, K. J., ed.), pp. 391–401. Univ. of Guelph, Canada.

Melchers, G. (1977). Protoplast fusion and plants from fusion. *(12th Int. Bot. Congress, Leningrad, 1975)* In *Physiology and Biochemistry of Cultural Plants*.

Melchers, G. and Bergmann, L. (1958–1959). Untersuchungen an Kulturen von haploiden Geweben von *Antirrhinum majus. Ber. Deut. Bot. Ges. 71*:459–473.

Melchers, G. and Labib, G. (1970). Die Bedeutung haploider höherer Pflanzen für Pflanzenphysiologie und -züchtung. Die durch Antherenkultur erzeugten Haploiden, ein neuer Durchbruch für die Pflanzenzüchtung. *Ber. Deut. Bot. Ges. 83*:129–150.

Melchers, G. and Labib, G. (1973). Plants from protoplasts, significance for genetics and breeding. *Collogn. Int. CNRS No. 212, Protoplastes et fusion de cellules somatiques végétales*, pp. 367–372.

Melchers, G. and Labib, G. (1974). Somatic hybridization of plants by fusion of protoplasts. I. Selection of light resistant hybrids of "haploid" light sensitive varieties of tobacco. *Mol. Gen. Genet. 135*:277–294.

Melchers, G. and Sacristán, M. D. (1977). Somatic hybridization of plants by fusion of protoplasts. II. The chromosome numbers of somatic hybrid plants of 4 different fusion experiments. *Recueil de Travaux Dédiés à "la mémoire de G. Morel"* (Gautheret, G. J., ed.). Masson et Cie, Paris.

Nakamura, A., Yamada, I., Kadotani, N., and Itagaki, R. (1974). Improvement of flue-cured tobacco variety MC 1610 by means of haploid breeding method and investigations on some problems of this method. *Proc. Haploids in Higher Plants–Advances and Potential,* (Kasha, K. J. ed.), pp. 277–278. University of Guelph, Canada.

Ouyang, T. W., Hu, H., Chuang, C. C., and Tseng, C. C. (1973). Induction of pollen plants from anthers of *Triticum aestivum* L. cultured in vitro. *Sci. Sin. 16*:79–95.

Pogliaga, H. H. (1952). Hibrido intergenerico *"Nicotiana* X *Petunia"*. *Rev. Argent. Agron. 19*:171–178.

Renner, O. (1934). Die pflanzlichen Plastiden als selbständige Elemente der genetischen Konstitution. *Ber. Math. Phys. Klasse Sächsischen Akad. Wiss. 86*:241–266.

Sacristán, M. D. and Melchers, G. (1969). The caryological analysis of plants regenerated from tumorous and other callus cultures of tobacco. *Mol. Gen. Genet. 105*:317–333.

Sakano, K., Kung, S. D., and Wildman, S. G. (1974). Identification of several chloroplast DNA genes which code for the large subunit of *Nicotiana* Fraction I proteins. *Mol. Gen. Genet. 130*:91–97.

Schieder, O. (1975). Selektion einer somatischen Hybriden nach Fusion vom Protoplasten auxotropher Mutanten von *Sphaerocarpos donnellii. Aust. Z. Pflanz. 74*:357–364.

Stebbins, L. (1950). *Variation and Evolution in Plants.* Columbia Univ. Press, New York.

Thomas, E. and Wenzel, G. (1975). Embryogenesis from microspores of *Brassica napus. Z. Pflanz. 74*:77–81.

Thomas, E., Hoffmann, F., and Wenzel, G. (1975). Haploid plantlets from microspore of rye. *Z. Pflanz. 75*:106–113.

Thomas, E., Hoffman, F., Potrykus, I., and Wenzel, G. (1976). Protoplast regeneration and stem embryogenesis of haploid androgenetic rape. *Mol. Gen. Genet. 145*:245–247.

Wang, C. C., Chu, C. C. Sun, C. S., Wu, S. H., Yin, K. C., and Hsu, C. (1973). The androgenesis in wheat (*Triticum aestivum*) anthers cultured in vitro. *Sci. Sin. 16*:218–222.

Wang, C. C., Sun, C. S., and Chu, Z. C. (1974). On the conditions for the induction of rice pollen plantlets and certain factors affecting the frequency of induction., (Chinese with English summary.) *Acta Bot. Sin. 16*:45–54.

Wang, Y. S., Sun, C. S., Wang, C. C., and Chien, N. F. (1973). The induction of the pollen plantlets of *Triticale* and *Capsicum annuum* from anther culture. *Sci. Sin. 16*:147–151.

Wenzel, G. and Thomas, E. (1974). Observations on the growth in culture of anthers of *Secale cereale. Z. Pflanz. 72*:89–94.

Wenzel, G., Hoffmann, F., Potrykus, I., and Thomas, E. (1975). The separation of viable rye microspores from mixed populations and their development in culture. *Mol. Gen. Genet. 138*:293–297.

Zenkteler, M. and Melchers, G. (1977). Self and cross-pollination of ovules of several species in the test tubes. (In preparation.)

Participants

Abedin, M. Zain-ul–Dean, Faculty of Science, Karachi University, Karachi, Pakistan.

Ahmad, M.–Department of Plant Breeding and Genetics, University of Agriculture, Lyall-pur, Pakistan.

Ahmad, W.–Department of Plant Breeding and Genetics, University of Agriculture, Lyall-pur, Pakistan.

Ahmad, Z.–Department of Plant Breeding and Genetics, University of Agriculture, Lyall-pur, Pakistan.

Ahmed, Jamil–Department of Botany, Karachi University, Karachi, Pakistan.

Ahmed, Munir–Scientific Officer, Nuclear Institute for Agriculture and Biology, Lyallpur, Pakistan.

Ahmed, Shaukat–Director, Atomic Energy Agricultural Research Center, Tandojam, Pakistan.

Akbar, Muhammad–Senior Scientific Officer, Nuclear Institute for Agriculture and Biology, Lyallpur, Pakistan.

Akhtar, Muhammad–Plant Pathologist, Punjab Agricultural Research Institute, Lyallpur, Pakistan.

Akram, M.–Department of Plant Breeding and Genetics, University of Agriculture, Lyall-pur, Pakistan.

Aksel, Rustem–Department of Genetics, University of Alberta, Edmonton, Alberta, T6G 2E9, Canada.

Alam, Khurshid–Associate Professor, Department of Plant Breeding and Genetics, University of Agriculture, Lyallpur, Pakistan.

Ali, Mahboob–Director, Cotton Research Institute, Multan, Pakistan.

Allard, R.W.–Department of Agronomy and Range Science, University of California, Davis 95616, California, U.S.A.

Andrabi, S. Sharifuddin–Director, Agriculture Department, Azad Kashmir, Muzzaffarabad, Azad Kashmir.

Ansari, Nabi N.–Principal, Agricultural College, Tandojam, Pakistan.

Arain, A. Ghafoor–Senior Scientific Officer, Atomic Energy Agricultural Research Center, Tandojam, Pakistan.

Arshad, M.–Department of Agronomy, University of Agriculture, Lyallpur, Pakistan.

Aslam, Muhammad–Plant Pathologist, Agricultural Research Institute, Tarnab, Peshawar, Pakistan.

Aslam, Muhammad—Dean, Faculty of Agriculture, University of Agriculture, Lyallpur, Pakistan.

Aslam, Muhammad—Scientific Officer, Nuclear Institute for Agriculture and Biology, Lyallpur, Pakistan.

Aslamkhan, M.—Geneticist, Pakistan Medical Research Center, Lahore, Pakistan.

Auckland, A. K.—Plant Breeder, International Crops Research Institute for the Semi-arid tropics, Experimental Station Patancheru, Bombay Road, Hyderabad, India.

Awan, M. Afsar—Scientific Officer, Nuclear Institute for Agriculture and Biology, Lyallpur, Pakistan.

Azmi, A. Razzaq—Head of Bio-sciences, Pakistan Atomic Energy Commission, Islamabad, Pakistan.

Bandesha, Akbar A.—Assistant Scientific Officer, Nuclear Institute for Agriculture and Biology, Lyallpur, Pakistan.

Bano, H.—Lecturer, Department of Genetics, University of Karachi, Karachi, Pakistan.

Bari, Ghulam—Senior Scientific Officer, Atomic Energy Agricultural Research Center, Tandojam, Pakistan.

Bell, E. A.—School of Biological Sciences, University of London, King's College, 68 Half Moon Lane, London SE24 9JF, U.K.

Bernstein, L.—Volunteer Executive, International Executive Service Corps, 622 Third Avenue, New York, N.Y. 10017, U.S.A.

Bhatti, Hayat M.—Agriculture Chemist (Soils), Punjab Agricultural Research Institute, Lyallpur, Pakistan.

Bhatti, I. M.—Director, Rice Research Institute, Dokri, Pakistan.

Bhutta, Manzoor A.—Lecturer, Department of Plant Breeding and Genetics, University of Agriculture, Lyallpur, Pakistan.

Boulter, D. A.—Department of Botany, Faculty of Science, University of Durham, Old Shire Hall, Durham, U.K.

Brock, R. D.—CSIRO, Division of Plant Industry, P.O. Box 1600, Canberra City, A.C.T. 2601, Australia.

Cheema, Akbar A.—Assistant Scientific Officer, Nuclear Institute for Agriculture and Biology, Lyallpur, Pakistan.

Choudhry, M. Asif—Lecturer, Department of Plant Breeding and Genetics, University of Agriculture, Lyallpur, Pakistan.

Choudhry, M. Boota—Scientific Officer, Nuclear Institute for Agriculture and Biology, Lyallpur, Pakistan.

Choudhry, M. Hussain—Economic Botanist, Bahawalpur, Pakistan.

Choudhry, M. Karim—Principal, Agriculture Training School, Muzaffarabad, Azad Kashmir.

Döbereiner, J.—Universidade Federal Rural, Rio de Janeiro, Brazil.

Doll, H.—Danish Atomic Energy Commission, Research Establishment Riso, DK-4000, Roskilde, Denmark.

Eggum, B. O.—Institute of Animal Science, Rolighedevej, Denmark 25 Copenhagen, Denmark.

Farzana, N.—Department of Genetics, University of Karachi, Karachi, Pakistan.

Foard, D. E.—Biology Division, Oak Ridge National Laboratory, P.O. Box 'Y', Oak Ridge, Tennessee 37830, U.S.A.

Frankel, O. H.—CSIRO, Division of Plant Industry, P.O. Box 1600, Canberra City, A.C.T. 2601, Australia.

Gale, M. D.—Plant Breeding Institute, Maris Lane, Trumpington, U. K.

Ghoddousi, H.—Atomic Energy Center, Tehran, Iran.

Groth, J.—Assistant Professor, University of Minnesota, U.S.A.

Hafeez, A.—Project Manager, Regional Project Field Food Crops, F.A.O., P.O. Box 2223, Cairo, Egypt.

Haq, M. Ahsanul—Scientific Officer, Nuclear Institute for Agriculture and Biology, Lyallpur, Pakistan.

Hashmi, Naeem I.—Scientific Officer, Nuclear Institute for Agriculture and Biology, Lyallpur, Pakistan.

Hashmi, Z. A.—Chairman, Pakistan Science Foundation, Islamabad, Pakistan.

Hassan, M.—Assistant Scientific Officer, Nuclear Institute for Agriculture and Biology, Lyallpur, Pakistan.

Hussain, Altaf—Vegetable Botanist, Punjab Agricultural Research Institute, Lyallpur, Pakistan.

Hussain, M. Kamil—Assistant Professor, Department of Plant Breeding and Genetics, University of Agriculture, Lyallpur, Pakistan.

Johnson, V. A.—Plant Science Research Division, USDA, Lincoln, Nebraska 68503, U.S.A.

Kausar, A. G.—Director, Advanced Studies and Research, University of Agriculture, Lyallpur, Pakistan.

Khairunnissa—Department of Genetics, University of Karachi, Karachi, Pakistan.

Khaliq, A.—Lecturer, Department of Plant Breeding and Genetics, University of Agriculture, Lyallpur, Pakistan.

Khan, Alauddin—Cereal Botanist, Agricultural Research Institute, Tarnab, Peshawar, Pakistan.

Khan, Iftikhar A.—Lecturer, Department of Plant Breeding and Genetics, University of Agriculture, Lyallpur, Pakistan.

Khan, M. Amin—Senior Research Officer, Cotton Research Institute, Multan, Pakistan.

Khan, Manzoor A.—Professor, Department of Plant Breeding and Genetics, University of Agriculture, Lyallpur, Pakistan.

Khan, M. Iqbal—Senior Scientific Officer, Atomic Energy Agricultural Research Center, Tandojam, Pakistan.

Khan, M. Ishaq—Associate Professor, Department of Botany, Karachi University, Karachi, Pakistan.

Khan, Riaz A.—Associate Professor, Department of Agronomy, University of Agriculture, Lyallpur, Pakistan.

Khan, Saeed I.—Scientific Officer, Nuclear Institute for Agriculture and Biology, Lyallpur, Pakistan.

Khan, Shamshad A.—Oilseed Botanist, Punjab Agricultural Research Institute, Lyallpur, Pakistan.

Khan, Waheed S.—Cotton Botanist, Punjab Agricultural Research Institute, Lyallpur, Pakistan.

Khullas, B.—Department of Plant Breeding and Genetics, University of Agriculture, Lyallpur, Pakistan.

Kimber, G.—Department of Agronomy, University of Missouri, Columbia, Missouri 65201, U.S.A.

Knowles, P.—USDA/ARC Advisor (Oilseed), Agriculture Research Council, P.O. Box 1251, Islamabad, Pakistan.

Ledoux, L.—Radiobiology, Centre d'Etude de l'Energie Nucleaire, S.C.K.-C.E.N., B-2400 Mol, Belgium.

Leghari, M.Z.A.—Department of Plant Breeding and Genetics, University of Agriculture, Lyallpur, Pakistan.

Majeed, A.—Director, Rice Research Institute, Kala Shah Kaku, Pakistan.

Malik, Feroze K.—Scientific Officer, Nuclear Institute for Agriculture and Biology, Lyallpur, Pakistan.

Malik, Kausar A.—Senior Scientific Officer, Nuclear Institute for Agriculture and Biology, Lyallpur, Pakistan.

Maqsood, Farooq—Karachi Nuclear Power Plant, Karachi, Pakistan.

Maryam, B.—Department of Plant Breeding and Genetics, University of Agriculture, Lyallpur, Pakistan.

Mehdi, S. S.—Department of Plant Breeding and Genetics, University of Agriculture, Lyallpur, Pakistan.

Melchers, G.—Director, Max Planck Institut für Biologie, 74 Tubingen, West Germany.

Mian, M. Asghar—Lecturer, Department of Plant Breeding and Genetics, University of Agriculture, Lyallpur, Pakistan.

Muhammad, Nek—Wheat Botanist, Agricultural Research Institute, Quetta, Pakistan.

Muhammed, Amir—Vice-Chancellor, University of Agriculture, Lyallpur, Pakistan.

Mujahid, M. Y.—Department of Plant Breeding and Genetics, University of Agriculture, Lyallpur, Pakistan.

Nafees, Amtul—Research Officer, Biological Research Center, University of Karachi, Karachi, Pakistan.

Naqvi, S. H. Mujtaba—Director, Nuclear Institute for Agriculture and Biology, Lyallpur, Pakistan.

Nawaz, H.—Department of Plant Breeding and Genetics, University of Agriculture, Lyallpur, Pakistan.

Osman, A. A. M.—Department of Plant Breeding and Genetics, University of Agriculture, Lyallpur, Pakistan.

Qureshi, M. Jamil—Senior Scientific Officer, Nuclear Institute for Agriculture and Biology, Lyallpur, Pakistan.

Qureshi, S. A.—Cereal Botanist, Punjab Agricultural Research Institute, Lyallpur, Pakistan.

Rafiq, M.—Professor of Botany, University of Karachi, Karachi, Pakistan.

Rajput, Mushtaq A.—Senior Scientific Officer, Atomic Energy Agricultural Research Center, Tandojam, Pakistan.

Rao, A. R.—Assistant Professor, Department of Botany, University of Agriculture, Lyallpur, Pakistan.

Razzaki, Tashmeem—Lecturer, Department of Botany, University of Karachi, Karachi, Pakistan.

Rehman, A.—Professor, Department of Plant Breeding and Genetics, University of Agriculture, Lyallpur, Pakistan.

Rehman, A.—Department of Agronomy, University of Agriculture, Lyallpur, Pakistan.

Rehman, H.—Assistant Professor, Department of Botany, Peshawar University, Peshawar, Pakistan.

Rehman, S.—Department of Plant Breeding and Genetics, University of Agriculture, Lyallpur, Pakistan.

Sadia, M.—Department of Botany, University of Karachi, Karachi, Pakistan.

Sadiq, M. Siddique—Scientific Officer, Nuclear Institute for Agriculture and Biology, Lyallpur, Pakistan.

Sadiq, M.—Assistant Scientific Officer, Nuclear Institute for Agriculture and Biology, Lyallpur, Pakistan.

Sajjad, M. S.—Assistant Scientific Officer, Nuclear Institute for Agriculture and Biology, Lyallpur, Pakistan.

Salah-ud-Din, Muhammad—Senior Scientific Officer, Atomic Energy Agricultural Research Center, Tandojam, Pakistan.

Sandhu, G. R. – Principal Scientific Officer, Nuclear Institute for Agriculture and Biology, Lyallpur, Pakistan.

Scowcroft, W. R. – CSIRO, Division of Plant Industry, P.O. Box 1600, Canberra City, A.C.T. 2601, Australia.

Sethi, J. M. – Department of Plant Breeding and Genetics, University of Agriculture, Lyallpur, Pakistan.

Setlow, J. K. – Brookhaven National Laboratory, Associated Universities Inc., Upton, N.Y. 11973, U.S.A.

Shah, S. A. – Associate Professor, Department of Botany, University of Agriculture, Lyallpur, Pakistan.

Shah, S. Meer Muhammad – Associate Professor, Engineering College, Sind University, Jamshoro, Pakistan.

Shakoor, A. – Senior Scientific Officer, Nuclear Institute for Agriculture and Biology, Lyallpur, Pakistan.

Shehla, A. – Department of Genetics, University of Karachi, Karachi, Pakistan.

Shuaib, M. – Senior Scientific Officer, Atomic Energy Agricultural Research Center, Tandojam, Pakistan.

Siddiqui, Khushnood A. – Principal Scientific Officer, Atomic Energy Agricultural Research Center, Tandojam, Pakistan.

Siddiqui, K. M. – Forest Geneticist, Pakistan Forest Research Institute, Peshawar, Pakistan.

Siddiqui, Shamim H. – Senior Scientific Officer, Atomic Energy Agricultural Research Center, Tandojam, Pakistan.

Sigurbjornsson, B. – Director, Agricultural Research Institute, Government of Iceland, Roykjavik.

Soomro, B. A. – Associate Professor, Department of Botany, Agricultural College, Tandojam, Pakistan.

Tahir, Muhammad – Wheat Co-ordinator, Agriculture Research Council, Islamabad, Pakistan.

Tariq, A. – Assistant Botanist, Pakistan Central Cotton Committee, Multan, Pakistan.

Tufail, Muhammad – Millet Botanist, Punjab Agricultural Research Institute, Lyallpur, Pakistan.

Vasti, S. M. – Senior Scientific Officer, Atomic Energy Agricultural Research Center, Tandojam, Pakistan.

von Borstel, R. C. – Department of Genetics, University of Alberta, Edmonton, Alberta, T6G 2E9, Canada.

Yildirim, M. B. – Department of Agronomy and Genetics, Faculty of Agriculture, Ege University, Bornova, Izmir, Turkey.

Yousaf, Muhammad – Professor, Department of Plant Breeding and Genetics, University of Agriculture, Lyallpur, Pakistan.

Zahoor, M. S. – Department of Botany, Punjab University, Lahore, Pakistan.

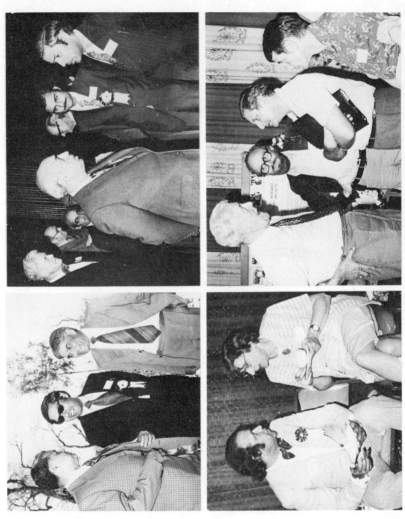

Plate 1. Top: Sahib Dad Khan, Amir, Sadiq/Melchers, Eggum, Bernstein, Governor Abbasi, Brock, Naqvi, Amir. Bottom: Jamil, Setlow/Melchers, Doll, Boulter, Foard.

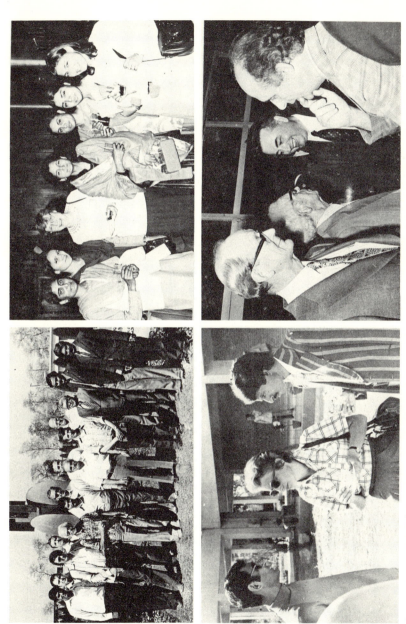

Plate 2. Top: Akbar, Yildirim, Gale, Boulter, Frankel, Sadiq, Johnson, Bernstein, Ledoux, Foard, Eggum, Ghoddousi, Naqvi, Rao/ Farhat, Amtul Nafeez, Setlow, Fazilat, Bushra, Shamshad, Shagufta. Bottom: Soomro, Döbereiner, Iftikhar/Brock, Frankel, Ledoux, Kimber.

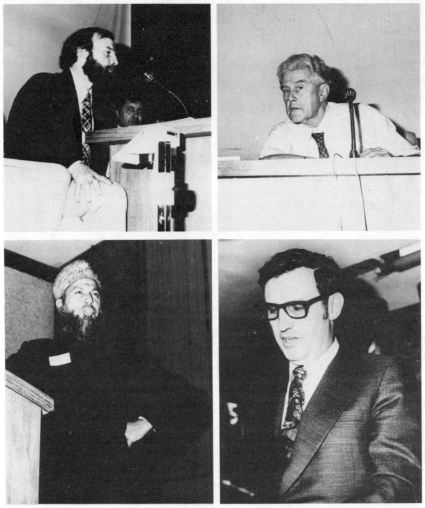

Plate 3. Top: Groth, von Borstel/Melchers. Bottom: Akhtar/Wheeler.

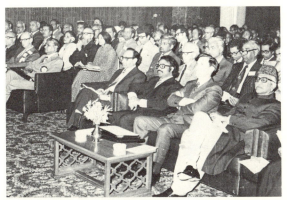

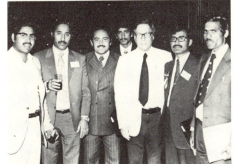

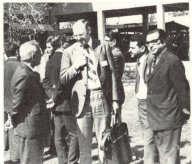

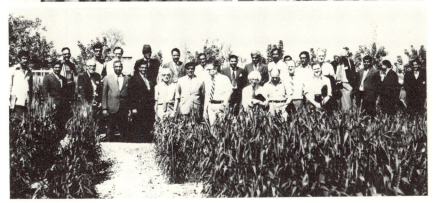

Plate 4. Top: Naeem, Brock, Shaukat, Tashmeem Razzaki, Yusuf, Aslam Khan, Wheeler, Bucha. Middle: Feroz, Ghafoor, Saif, Zulfikar, Allard, Ahsan, Akram/Jamil Qureshi, Eggum, Akmal, Rashid. Bottom: Falak Sher, Rao, Qureshi, Doll, Soomro, Manzoor, Allard, Rahman, Naz, Frankel, Tufail, Amir, Siraj Din Shah, Johnson, Akmal, Aksel, Yusuf, Kimber, Noor, Eggum, Saleem, Bell, Sigurbjornsson, Melchers, Khurshid, Kausar, Niaz.

Author Index

Subject Index